Feature Articles on Obesity and Weight Loss Treatments

Feature Articles on Obesity and Weight Loss Treatments

Guest Editor

Jose M. Soriano del Castillo

MDPI

Basel • Beijing • Wuhan • Barcelona • Belgrade • Novi Sad • Cluj • Manchester

Guest Editor
Jose M. Soriano del Castillo
Food & Health Laboratory
University of Valencia
Paterna
Spain

Editorial Office
MDPI AG
Grosspeteranlage 5
4052 Basel, Switzerland

This is a reprint of the Special Issue, published open access by the journal *Nutrients* (ISSN 2072-6643), freely accessible at: https://www.mdpi.com/journal/nutrients/special_issues/5774778QZZ.

For citation purposes, cite each article independently as indicated on the article page online and as indicated below:

Lastname, A.A.; Lastname, B.B. Article Title. *Journal Name* **Year**, *Volume Number*, Page Range.

ISBN 978-3-7258-8429-2 (Hbk)
ISBN 978-3-7258-8430-8 (PDF)
https://doi.org/10.3390/books978-3-7258-8430-8

Contents

About the Editor

Jose M. Soriano del Castillo

Jose M. Soriano del Castillo is affiliated with the Food & Health Laboratory, Institute of Materials Science, University of Valencia, Spain. His research interests include nutrition, medicinal plants, natural products, human health and bioactive compounds, with a particular focus on public health nutrition and the relationship between diet, health and disease prevention. He has developed academic and research activity in nutrition and food science and has participated in national and international collaborations. His work combines clinical, epidemiological and translational approaches to improve understanding of nutritional status, dietary interventions and health promotion.

Preface

Obesity and weight loss treatments remain central challenges for nutrition science, clinical practice and public health. This Reprint was prepared to gather contributions that examine obesity beyond a single-discipline perspective, integrating dietary approaches, anthropometry, biomarkers, body composition, molecular nutrition, cultural factors and new technologies. Its purpose is to provide readers with a concise and updated collection of studies and reviews that may support safer, more personalized and evidence-based strategies for weight management. The Reprint is addressed to researchers, clinicians, dietitians, public health professionals and students interested in the prevention and treatment of obesity.

Jose M. Soriano del Castillo
Guest Editor

nutrients

MDPI

Article

Periconceptional Maternal Protein Intake from Animal and Plant Sources and the Impact on Early and Late Prenatal Growth and Birthweight: The Rotterdam Periconceptional Cohort

Sofie van Zundert [1,2], Simone van der Padt [1], Sten Willemsen [1,3], Melek Rousian [1], Mina Mirzaian [2], Ron van Schaik [2], Régine Steegers-Theunissen [1,*] and Lenie van Rossem [1]

1 Department of Obstetrics and Gynecology, Erasmus MC, University Medical Center, P.O. Box 2040, 3000 CA Rotterdam, The Netherlands
2 Department of Clinical Chemistry, Erasmus MC, University Medical Center, P.O. Box 2040, 3000 CA Rotterdam, The Netherlands
3 Department of Biostatistics, Erasmus MC, University Medical Center, P.O. Box 2040, 3000 CA Rotterdam, The Netherlands
* Correspondence: r.steegers@erasmusmc.nl

Abstract: Plant-based diets continue to rise in popularity, including among women of reproductive age, while consequences for pregnancy outcomes have hardly been studied. During pregnancy, maternal diet is the only source of proteins for the developing fetus. Hence, we investigated the effects of periconceptional maternal animal and plant protein intake on prenatal growth and birthweight. 501 pregnancies were included from the prospective Rotterdam Periconceptional Cohort. Embryonic growth was depicted by crown-rump length (CRL) and embryonic volume (EV) at 7, 9 and 11 weeks using 3D ultrasound scans. Estimated fetal weight (EFW) at 20 weeks and birthweight were retrieved from medical records and standardized. Multivariable mixed models were used for CRL and EV trajectories, and linear regression for EFW and birthweight. A 10 g/day higher maternal animal protein intake was positively associated with increased embryonic growth (CRL: $\beta = 0.023$ $\sqrt{\text{mm}}$, $p = 0.052$; EV: $\beta = 0.015$ $\sqrt[3]{\text{cm}}$, $p = 0.012$). A positive association, albeit non-significant, was found between maternal animal protein intake and EFW, and birthweight. No clear associations emerged between maternal plant protein intake and prenatal growth and birthweight, with effect estimates close to zero. In conclusion, maternal animal protein intake during the periconception period was positively associated with early and late prenatal growth and birthweight, while no associations were found between maternal plant protein intake and prenatal growth and birthweight.

Keywords: periconception period; pregnancy; nutrition; crown-rump length; embryonic volume; estimated fetal weight; birthweight

1. Introduction

In recent years, there has been a shift towards diets consisting of fewer animal products and more plant-based foods due to their lower impact on environment and climate change [1]. It is widely known that the protein quality, which is determined by its ability to meet the requirements for essential amino acids and its digestibility, of plant proteins is generally lower than that of animal proteins [2]. However, adherence to plant-based diets reduces the incidence of non-communicable diseases in the general population. So far, less attention has been devoted to the potential risks of adherence to plant-based diets during pregnancy [3–5]. Maternal dietary quality is especially important during the periconception period, which is defined as the 14 weeks before conception until the 10 weeks thereafter. During this critical time window, epigenetic programming can affect the development of the gametes, embryo and placenta, and can induce long-term health effects on the offspring [6].

Our earlier studies have shown that periconceptional maternal dietary patterns have an impact on reproduction and prenatal growth and development [7]. Existing research on maternal protein intake has mainly focused on birthweight and most studies revealed a positive association [8–11]. In contrast, Morisaki, et al. [12] found a non-linear (inverse U-curve) association between maternal protein intake and fetal growth and birthweight. A few studies have distinguished between animal and plant proteins [8,10,11]. A higher birthweight and a lower risk of fetal growth restriction was found in women who consumed more animal proteins during pregnancy. The associations between plant proteins and fetal growth and birthweight were, however, less evident and inconsistent [8,10,11]. Despite the importance of embryonic growth as a determinant for fetal growth, birthweight and health later in life, the relationship between periconceptional maternal protein intake and embryonic growth is unknown [13–15].

Since maternal diet is the primary source of proteins required for embryonic and fetal growth, we hypothesize that periconceptional maternal protein intake is positively associated with prenatal growth and birthweight. Considering the higher protein quality of animal proteins compared to plant proteins, we hypothesize that the associations are stronger for animal proteins than for plant proteins when distinguishing between protein source. The objectives of this study are to determine the associations between periconceptional maternal protein intake, including animal and plant protein intake, and embryonic growth. A secondary objective is to investigate the relationship with fetal growth and birthweight.

2. Materials and Methods

2.1. Study Design and Participants

The data used for this study were collected prospectively within the Rotterdam Periconceptional Cohort (Predict Study), an ongoing periconceptional prospective tertiary hospital-based cohort study conducted at the Department of Obstetrics and Gynecology of the Erasmus MC, University Medical Center, Rotterdam, The Netherlands (Erasmus MC) from 2010 onwards. Approval for the Predict Study was granted by the Central Committee on Research in The Hague and the local Medical Ethics Committee of the Erasmus MC (15 October 2004, MEC-2004-277). All participants gave written informed consent before inclusion [7,16]. Data on periconceptional maternal protein intake from animal and plant sources have been obtained from the Food Frequency Questionnaire (FFQ) since November 2014 [17]. Therefore, only women who entered the Predict Study from November 2014 onwards were included in this study. Additionally, women had to be 18 years or older, familiar with the Dutch language and less than 8 weeks pregnant.

In total, 1365 pregnancies were included between November 2014 and December 2020. Pregnancies conceived after oocyte donation (n = 15) were excluded, because no information on maternal diet of the donors was collected. Furthermore, multiple pregnancies (n = 13) and pregnancies with an a-priori increased risk of impaired embryonic growth were excluded: miscarriages (n = 78), live-born with congenital anomalies (n = 96), terminated pregnancies because of congenital anomalies (n = 15), and fetal and neonatal deaths (n = 26) [18,19]. Pregnancies were also excluded when missing first-trimester ultrasound data (n = 115), missing FFQ data (n = 158) or unreliable FFQ data (n = 209) according to the Goldberg cut-off method explained further in Section 2.2.3. We additionally excluded naturally conceived pregnancies with an unreliable gestational age (GA) (n = 121), as GA is an important determinant of embryonic and fetal growth. Our definition of an unreliable GA can be found in Section 2.2.1. When women participated twice within the Predict study, only the first pregnancy (n = 18) was included in the current study to avoid clustering. This resulted in a total study population of 501 pregnancies (Figure 1).

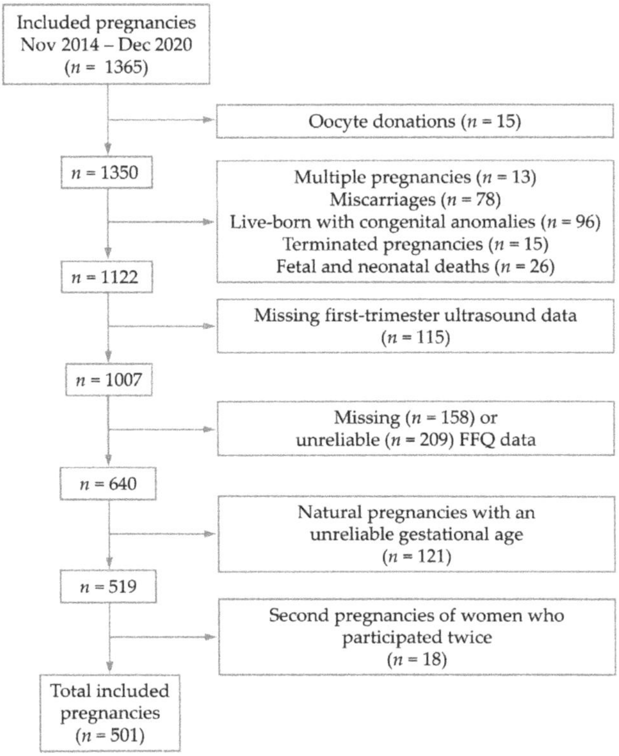

Figure 1. Selection of the study population from the Rotterdam Periconceptional cohort (Predict Study). FFQ = Food Frequency Questionnaire.

2.2. Data Collection

2.2.1. Embryonic Growth and Gestational Age

Embryonic growth was depicted by longitudinal CRL and EV measurements using three dimensional (3D) ultrasound scans and virtual reality (VR) techniques performed in the 7th, 9th and 11th week of gestation by trained medical doctors. A comprehensive description of the 3D ultrasound scans and measurements of CRL and EV using VR techniques has been described extensively in previous publications [7,16,20]. The acquired 3D ultrasound scans were transferred and visualized using VR systems by trained researchers following a standard protocol. An interactive 3D hologram is created by these VR systems, allowing real depth perception and precise measurements of the embryo [20]. The CRL measurement is performed manually, while the EV measurement is performed using a semi-automated method. Both CRL and EV are reliable and reproducible measurements, proven by inter-observer and intra-observer variability analyses (intra-class correlation coefficients (ICC) > 0.99) [7,20].

As CRL was a primary outcome measure, it was not used to estimate the GA of the embryo. Naturally conceived pregnancies also included pregnancies after ovulation induction (OI) and intrauterine insemination (IUI). For naturally conceived pregnancies, the GA was calculated from the first day of the last menstrual period (LMP) of a regular menstrual cycle. If the menstrual cycle was <25 days or >31 days, the GA was adjusted for the length of the menstrual cycle. The GA of a naturally conceived pregnancy was considered unreliable when the menstrual cycle was irregular, the LMP was missing or when the calculated GA differed more than 7 days from the estimated GA based on the CRL. For pregnancies conceived after in vitro fertilization (IVF) or intracytoplasmic sperm injection (ICSI), the GA was calculated from the conception date, which was the oocyte retrieval day minus 14 days for fresh embryo transfers, and the embryo transfer day minus 19 days for cryopreserved embryo transfers.

2.2.2. Fetal Growth and Birthweight

Data on fetal growth parameters were retrieved from the routine transabdominal mid-pregnancy anomaly scans at around 20 weeks of pregnancy (n = 422). Estimated fetal weight (EFW) was calculated using the Hadlock formula based on the head circumference (HC), abdominal circumference (AC) and femur length (FL) in centimeters [21]:

$$\mathrm{EFW} = 10^{1.3596 - 0.00386 \times \mathrm{AC} \times \mathrm{FL} + 0.0064 \times \mathrm{HC} + 0.00061 \times \mathrm{BPD} \times \mathrm{AC} + 0.0424 \times \mathrm{AC} + 0.174 \times \mathrm{FL}} \quad (1)$$

Birthweights were retrieved from medical records. For EFW and birthweight standard scores (z-scores) were calculated based on Dutch reference growth curves adjusted for GA, and additionally for fetal sex, respectively [22,23].

2.2.3. Food Frequency Questionnaire

To assess information on periconceptional maternal protein intake, participants received a standardized semi-quantitative FFQ at enrollment. The FFQ was developed at the Division of Human Nutrition and Health, Wageningen University, The Netherlands, and covered the dietary intake of participants during the previous four weeks [24]. The FFQ included questions regarding preparation methods, portion sizes and additions, and was validated for the intake of macronutrients and energy in women of reproductive age [25]. The amount of energy and the nutritional values of the food items were determined using the Dutch food composition table and were presented in commonly used units using Dutch household measures [26]. FFQ data were considered unreliable when the reported energy intake was below the calculated individual's energy intake based on basal metabolic rate and physical activity (Goldberg cut-off) as proposed by Black [27]. The 95% lower confidence limit of the calculated Goldberg cut-off provided the cut-off energy intake for each individual. A more detailed description of the rationale and calculation of the Goldberg cut-off can be found in the recently published study of Smit et al. [28].

2.2.4. Maternal Characteristics

Data on maternal characteristics such as date of birth, geographical background, educational level, parity, conception mode and periconceptional lifestyle factors (smoking, alcohol consumption, drug use and folic acid supplement use) were obtained from general questionnaires filled out by participants before their intake appointment in the first trimester of pregnancy. Height and weight were measured by a research nurse at the intake appointment in the first trimester of pregnancy, and body mass index (BMI) was calculated by dividing weight (kg) by the square of height (m). Age at conception was calculated by the difference between the date of birth and the conception date as described in Section 2.2.1. Geographical background was categorized into western and non-western and educational level as high, intermediate or low according to the Dutch central bureau of statistics (CBS) [29,30]. Parity was divided into nulliparous and multiparous. Conception mode was verified by medical records and divided into naturally conceived pregnancies and IVF/ICSI pregnancies. Folic acid supplement use was considered adequate when started before conception.

2.3. Statistical Analysis

The baseline characteristics were presented as means with standard deviation (SD) or as numbers of individuals with percentages. To study differences in baseline characteristics between those with a low and those with a high protein intake relative to their energy intake, participants were divided into tertiles based on protein intake as percentage of energy intake.

To illustrate whether the protein intake of our study population met the recommended daily intake (RDI), the RDI was calculated for each individual per trimester of pregnancy according to the EFSA Panel on Dietetic Products [31]:

$$\begin{aligned} &\text{RDI (g/day)} = 0.83 \times \text{weight (kg)}\ {}^{*} \\ &{}^{*} +1\ \text{g/day in the first trimester, } +9\ \text{g/day in the second trimester, and} \\ &+28\ \text{g/day in the third trimester of pregnancy} \end{aligned} \quad (2)$$

Model 1 included GA and energy intake, and animal and plant protein intake were mutually adjusted for each other. Model 2 (the adjusted model) was additionally adjusted for the following covariates based on previous research and a Directed Acyclic Graph: age, BMI, geographical background, educational level, parity, conception mode, fetal sex, smoking, and folic acid supplement use [32–39]. The percentage of missing values of the covariates did not exceed 5%. Since GA is the strongest determinant of prenatal growth, it was further evaluated by adding a cubic spline function for GA and interaction terms between GA and all the other above mentioned covariates. Only the non-linear GA improved our model fit and was included in all models.

Mixed models were used to determine the associations between periconceptional maternal protein intake and longitudinal CRL and EV measurements, taking into account subject-specific trajectories. CRL and EV were transformed ($\sqrt{\text{CRL}}$ and $\sqrt[3]{\text{EV}}$) to obtain a constant variance and a normal distribution of the residuals given the covariates. Three different types of sensitivity analyses were performed to assess the robustness of the main findings. First, the nutrient density method was used to correct for differences in protein intake due to differences in energy intake [40]. Model 1 and 2 were again used for analyses, but included protein intake as percentage of energy intake instead of grams per day. Next, as animal protein sources contain generally more iron than plant protein sources, which is an important micronutrient for prenatal growth, iron intake could potentially explain the effect of animal protein intake [5]. Therefore, as a second sensitivity analysis iron intake was additionally added to Model 2 (Model 3). Finally, in the last sensitivity analysis, analyses using Model 1 and Model 2 were repeated only in women with a BMI within the normal range (18.5–24.9 kg/m^2), who are least likely to under- or over-report their dietary intake [41,42].

Linear regression models were used to determine the associations between periconceptional maternal protein intake with EFW and birthweight. For EFW and birthweight, standard scores (z-scores) were calculated based on Dutch reference growth curves [22,23]. The reference curve of EFW was adjusted for GA and that of birthweight for GA and fetal sex. Except for the covariates GA and fetal sex, the models were built up in the same way as Model 1 and Model 2 with embryonic growth as outcome. In short, Model 1 included energy intake, and either maternal animal or plant protein intake (mutually adjusted for each other). Model 2 also included the covariates age, BMI, geographical background, educational level, parity, conception mode, fetal sex (only in models with standardized EFW as outcome), smoking, and folic acid supplement use.

All analyses were performed using R version 4.2.1. of R Core Team [43]. Results were reported as effect estimates with 95% confidence intervals (95% CI). A p-value ≤ 0.05 was considered statistically significant.

3. Results

3.1. Baseline Characteristics

Table 1 shows the baseline characteristics of the total study population and stratified by tertiles of energy intake derived from total protein intake. Women who consumed more total protein as percentage of energy intake were slightly older (T3 vs. T1: 33.3 (3.9) vs. 32.1 (4.5) years) and less frequently low-educated (T3 vs. T1: 2.5% vs. 12.3%). Furthermore, women with a higher energy intake from total protein had a lower total energy intake (T3 vs. T1: 1740 (383) vs. 2100 (699) kcal/day), were more likely to start folic acid supplement use preconceptionally (T3 vs. T1: 91.8% vs. 85.2%), and were less likely to smoke (T3 vs.

T1: 8.8% vs. 17.9%) or use drugs (T3 vs. T1: 0.6% vs. 3.7%). Women in the highest tertile of energy intake from total protein were more often western (T3 vs. T1: 90.6% vs. 87.0%) and nulliparous (T3 vs. T1: 45.0% vs. 39.5%), and conceived after IVF/ICSI (T3 vs. T1: 57.5% vs. 52.7%) compared with those in the lowest tertile. No dose-response relationship was found between total protein intake as percentage of energy intake and BMI (T3 vs. T1: 24.6 (3.5) vs. 24.7 (4.2) kg/m^2), and alcohol consumption (T3 vs. T1: 25.0% vs. 24.1%).

Table 1. Baseline characteristics of the study population and stratified by tertiles of total protein intake as percentage of energy intake.

Maternal Characteristics	**Total Study Population (*n* = 501)**	**Tertile 1 (*n* = 167) 8.3–14.1%**	**Tertile 2 (*n* = 167) 14.2–16.0%**	**Tertile 3 (*n* = 167) 16.1–23.4%**
Age at conception (years)				
Mean (SD)	32.7 (4.3)	32.1 (4.5)	32.8 (4.4)	33.3 (3.9)
Missing	0	0	0	0
Geographical background				
Non-western	50 (10.4%)	21 (13.0%)	14 (8.8%)	15 (9.4%)
Western	431 (89.6%)	141 (87.0%)	145 (91.2%)	145 (90.6%)
Missing	20	5	8	7
Educational level				
Low	33 (6.9%)	20 (12.3%)	9 (5.6%)	4 (2.5%)
Medium	159 (33.0%)	64 (39.5%)	45 (28.1%)	50 (31.3%)
High	290 (60.2%)	78 (48.1%)	106 (66.3%)	106 (66.3%)
Missing	19	5	7	7
Parity				
Nulliparous	205 (42.4%)	64 (39.5%)	69 (42.9%)	72 (45.0%)
Multiparous	278 (57.6%)	98 (60.5%)	92 (57.1%)	88 (55.0%)
Missing	18	5	6	7
Conception mode				
IVF/ICSI	271 (54.1%)	87 (52.1%)	87 (52.1%)	96 (57.5%)
Natural	230 (45.9%)	80 (47.9%)	80 (47.9%)	71 (42.5%)
Missing	0	0	0	0
Body Mass Index (kg/m^2)				
Mean (SD)	24.7 (4.1)	24.7 (4.2)	24.6 (4.5)	24.6 (3.5)
Missing	0	0	0	0
Folic acid supplement use				
Inadequate	62 (12.9%)	24 (14.8%)	25 (15.5%)	13 (8.2%)
Adequate	420 (87.1%)	138 (85.2%)	136 (84.5%)	146 (91.8%)
Missing	19	5	6	8
Smoking				
Yes	66 (13.7%)	29 (17.9%)	23 (14.3%)	14 (8.8%)
No	417 (86.3%)	133 (82.1%)	138 (85.7%)	146 (91.3%)
Missing	18	5	6	7
Alcohol				
Yes	139 (28.8%)	39 (24.1%)	60 (37.3%)	40 (25.0%)
No	344 (71.2%)	123 (75.9%)	101 (62.7%)	120 (75.0%)
Missing	18	5	6	7
Drugs				
Yes	10 (2.1%)	6 (3.7%)	3 (1.9%)	1 (0.6%)
No	473 (97.9%)	156 (96.3%)	158 (98.1%)	159 (99.4%)
Missing	18	5	6	7

Table 1. *Cont.*

Maternal Characteristics	Total Study Population (n = 501)	Tertile 1 (n = 167) 8.3–14.1%	Tertile 2 (n = 167) 14.2–16.0%	Tertile 3 (n = 167) 16.1–23.4%
Energy intake (kcal/day)				
Mean (SD)	1940 (562)	2100 (699)	1990 (498)	1740 (383)
Missing	0	0	0	0

Tertile 1 includes the lowest total protein intake (8.3% of energy) and Tertile 3 includes the highest total protein intake (23.4% of energy). Continuous data are presented as means with standard deviation (SD) and categorical data as numbers of individuals with percentages.

The baseline characteristics of the included (n = 501) and excluded population (n = 864) are shown in Table S1 (Supplementary Material). In contrast to the included pregnancies, the majority of the excluded pregnancies were naturally conceived (64.3% vs. 45.9%). Furthermore, excluded women more often had a non-western geographical background (16.6% vs. 10.4%), had a higher BMI (27.1 (5.5) vs. 24.7 (4.1) kg/m^2) despite a lower reported total energy intake (1590 (678) vs. 1940 (562) kcal/day), and started folic acid supplement use less often in the preconception period (75.3% vs. 87.1%) than the included women.

3.2. Protein Intake

The intake of protein in our study population is summarized in Table 2. For protein intake, we refer to maternal protein intake during the periconception period. The mean protein intake was 72.8 g/day, which was 13.5 g/day more than the first trimester RDI, 5.5 g/day more than the second trimester RDI, but 13.5 g/day less than the third trimester RDI [31]. Slightly more than half of the total protein intake was derived from animal sources (56.0%). The contribution of protein intake to energy intake was 15.2%, of which animal protein intake accounted for 8.6% and plant protein intake for 6.5%.

Table 2. Periconceptional maternal protein intake.

Maternal Nutrient Intake	g/Day	% of Energy	% of Protein
Total protein	72.8 (20.5)	15.2 (2.4)	
Animal protein	41.4 (15.8)	8.6 (2.6)	56.0 (10.6)
Plant protein	31.4 (10.1)	6.5 (1.3)	44.0 (10.6)
RDI first trimester	59.3 (10.5)		
RDI second trimester	67.3 (10.5)		
RDI third trimester	86.3 (10.5)		

Data are presented as means with standard deviation (SD). RDI = Recommended Daily Intake.

3.3. Embryonic Growth

Model 1 shows a positive association between total protein intake and embryonic growth (Table 3). After adjustment for covariates (Model 2), this positive association persisted with comparable effect estimates. These effect estimates indicate that a 10 g/day higher total protein intake increases the $\sqrt{CRL}$ by 0.022 mm (p = 0.061) and $\sqrt[3]{EV}$ by 0.014 cm^2 (p = 0.17), respectively. Furthermore, animal protein intake was positively associated with embryonic growth in both the unadjusted (Model 1) and adjusted (Model 2) analysis. In the adjusted analysis (Model 2), a 10 g/day higher animal protein intake was associated with an increase of $\sqrt{CRL}$ and $\sqrt[3]{EV}$ by 0.023 mm (p = 0.052) and 0.015 cm^2 (p = 0.012), respectively. In essence, this means that in the total study population, at 11 weeks of pregnancy, the difference in CRL between −2SD and +2SD protein intake is 2.493 mm, which is an increase of 6.0% in CRL, and corresponds with 0.2 days according to Verburg, et al. [44]. Figure 2 illustrates the positive associations of animal protein intake with CRL and EV trajectories. No statistically significant associations were found between plant protein intake and embryonic growth.

Table 3. Associations between periconceptional maternal protein intake for each additional 10 g/day and embryonic growth measurements.

Total Study Population	**Model 1**		**Model 2**	
(n = 501)	**β (95% CI)**	**p-Value**	**β (95% CI)**	**p-Value**
$\sqrt{\text{CRL}}$ (mm)				
For each additional 10 g/day				
Total protein intake	0.024 (0.002, 0.046)	0.031	0.022 (−0.001, 0.045)	0.061
Animal protein intake	0.025 (0.003, 0.047)	0.027	0.023 (−0.0002, 0.046)	0.052
Plant protein intake	0.011 (−0.031, 0.054)	0.597	0.0001 (−0.045, 0.046)	0.998
$\sqrt[3]{\text{EV}}$ (cm^3)				
For each additional 10 g/day				
Total protein intake	0.011 (0.001, 0.022)	0.033	0.014 (0.003, 0.025)	0.017
Animal protein intake	0.012 (0.002, 0.023)	0.024	0.015 (0.003, 0.026)	0.012
Plant protein intake	−0.004 (−0.024, 0.016)	0.698	−0.01 (−0.028, 0.016)	0.617

Model 1 is adjusted for GA and energy intake. Model 2 is as Model 1, but additionally adjusted for age, BMI, geographical background, educational level, parity, conception mode, fetal sex, smoking, and folic acid supplement use. In both models animal and plant protein intake were mutually adjusted for each other. BMI = Body Mass Index; CRL = Crown-Rump Length; EV = Embryonic Volume.

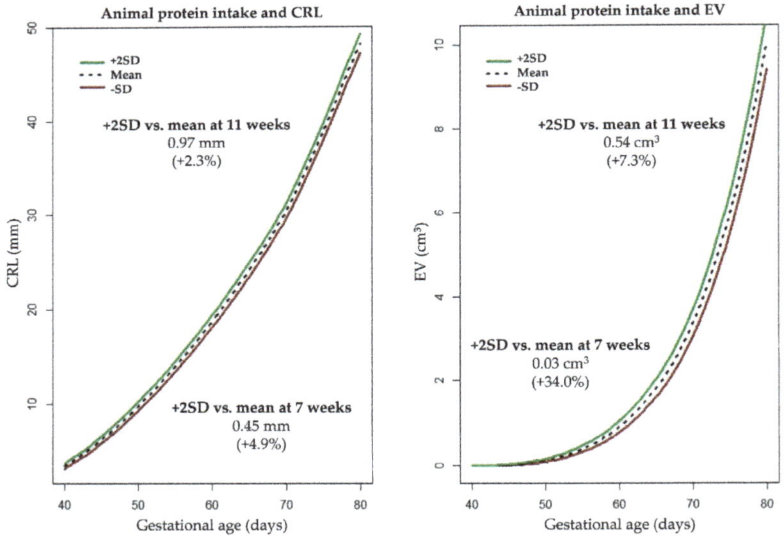

Figure 2. Embryonic growth according to periconceptional maternal animal protein intake. CRL = Crown-Rump Length, EV = Embryonic Volume.

A series of sensitivity analyses were performed. First, the nutrient density method was used to correct for differences in protein intake due to differences in energy intake. Analyses with protein intake as percentage of energy intake increased the effect estimates and decreased the width of the confidence intervals, suggesting more precise estimates (Table 4). Adjustment for covariates did not influence the associations much. The adjusted analysis (Model 2) showed that a 10% higher total protein intake increased $\sqrt{\text{CRL}}$ by 0.119 mm (p = 0.035) and $\sqrt[3]{\text{EV}}$ by 0.061 cm^2 (p = 0.024). Similarly, a 10% higher animal protein intake increased $\sqrt{\text{CRL}}$ and $\sqrt[3]{\text{EV}}$ by 0.110 mm (p = 0.049) and 0.062 cm^2 (p = 0.021), respectively. In the adjusted model including iron intake (Model 3), the effect estimates were quite similar to those of Model 2, suggesting that iron intake did not affect the relationship (Table 5). Lastly, the effect estimates were slightly stronger in women with a normal BMI (18.5–24.9 kg/m^2), but were not substantially different from the associations in the total study population, indicating limited bias by under- or over-reporting of dietary intake (Table 6).

Table 4. Associations between periconceptional maternal protein intake for each 10% increase as percentage of energy intake and embryonic growth measurements.

Total Study Population	**Model 1**		**Model 2**	
(n = 501)	**β (95% CI)**	***p*-Value**	**β (95% CI)**	***p*-Value**
$\sqrt{CRL}$ (mm)				
For each 10% increase				
Total protein intake	0.118 (0.015, 0.222)	0.025	0.119 (0.009, 0.229)	0.035
Animal protein intake	0.113 (0.009, 0.216)	0.034	0.011 (0.004, 0.220)	0.049
Plant protein intake	0.083 (−0.127, 0.294)	0.437	0.043 (−0.187, 0.273)	0.716
$\sqrt[3]{EV}$ (cm^3)				
For each 10% increase				
Total protein intake	0.048 (−0.0004, 0.097)	0.052	0.061 (0.008, 0.114)	0.024
Animal protein intake	0.050 (0.002, 0.099)	0.043	0.062 (0.009, 0.115)	0.021
Plant protein intake	−0.020 (−0.120, 0.081)	0.701	−0.028 (−0.138, 0.083)	0.623

Model 1 is adjusted for GA and energy intake. Model 2 is as Model 1, but additionally adjusted for age, BMI, geographical background, educational level, parity, conception mode, fetal sex, smoking, and folic acid supplement use. In both models animal and plant protein intake were mutually adjusted for each other. BMI = Body Mass Index; CRL = Crown-Rump Length; EV = Embryonic Volume.

Table 5. Associations between periconceptional maternal protein intake for each additional 10 g/day and embryonic growth measurements adjusted for iron intake.

Total Study Population	**Model 2**		**Model 3**	
(n = 501)	**β (95% CI)**	***p*-Value**	**β (95% CI)**	***p*-Value**
$\sqrt{CRL}$ (mm)				
For each additional 10 g/day				
Total protein intake	0.022 (−0.001, 0.045)	0.061	0.028 (0.003, 0.054)	0.027
Animal protein intake	0.023 (−0.0002, 0.046)	0.052	0.027 (0.001, 0.053)	0.040
Plant protein intake	0.0001 (−0.045, 0.046)	0.998	0.0001 (−0.046, 0.046)	0.998
$\sqrt[3]{EV}$ (cm^3)				
For each additional 10 g/day				
Total protein intake	0.014 (0.003, 0.025)	0.017	0.018 (0.006, 0.031)	0.004
Animal protein intake	0.015 (0.003, 0.026)	0.012	0.015 (0.032, 0.026)	0.012
Plant protein intake	−0.01 (−0.028, 0.016)	0.617	−0.006 (−0.028, 0.016)	0.617

Model 2 is adjusted for GA, energy intake, age, BMI, geographical background, educational level, parity, conception mode, fetal sex, smoking, and folic acid supplement use. Model 3 is as Model 2, but additionally adjusted for iron intake. In both models animal and plant protein intake were mutually adjusted for each other. BMI = Body Mass Index; CRL = Crown-Rump Length; EV = Embryonic Volume.

Table 6. Associations between periconceptional maternal protein intake for each additional 10 g/day and embryonic growth measurements in women with a normal BMI.

Women with a BMI: 18.5–25 kg/m^2	Model 2		Model 3	
(n = 286)	β (95% CI)	p-Value	β (95% CI)	p-Value
$\sqrt{CRL}$ (mm) For each additional 10 g/day				
Total protein intake	0.046 (0.017, 0.076)	0.002	0.044 (0.012, 0.076)	0.007
Animal protein intake	0.047 (0.017, 0.077)	0.002	0.044 (0.012, 0.075)	0.007
Plant protein intake	0.036 (−0.021, 0.094)	0.212	0.020 (−0.042, 0.082)	0.519
$\sqrt[3]{EV}$ (cm^3) For each additional 10 g/day				
Total protein intake	0.016 (0.002, 0.031)	0.021	0.017 (0.002, 0.033)	0.024
Animal protein intake	0.016 (0.003, 0.030)	0.021	0.018 (0.003, 0.033)	0.023
Plant protein intake	0.001 (−0.027, 0.029)	0.939	0.001 (−0.030, 0.031)	0.973

Model 2 is adjusted for GA and energy intake. Model 3 is as Model 2, but additionally adjusted for age, BMI, geographical background, educational level, parity, conception mode, fetal sex, smoking, and folic acid supplement use. In both models animal and plant protein intake were mutually adjusted for each other. BMI = Body Mass Index; CRL = Crown-Rump Length; EV = Embryonic Volume.

3.4. Fetal Growth and Birthweight

In both the unadjusted and adjusted analyses, no statistically significant associations were found between protein intake and fetal growth and birthweight (Table 7). Though not statistically significant, protein intake was positively associated with fetal growth (Model 1). Adjustment for covariates did not considerably change the estimated associations (Model 2). In the unadjusted analyses (Model 1), protein intake was also positively associated with birthweight. However, after adjustment for covariates the effect estimates decreased and the width of the confidence intervals increased (Model 2).

Table 7. Associations between periconceptional maternal protein intake for each additional 10 g/day and standardized EFW and birthweight (z-scores).

Total Study Population	Model 1		Model 2	
	β (95% CI)	p-Value	β (95% CI)	p-Value
Standardized EFW (n = 422) For each additional 10 g/day				
Total protein intake	0.062 (−0.025, 0.150)	0.161	0.060 (−0.029, 0.150)	0.186
Animal protein intake	0.064 (−0.024, 0.151)	0.155	0.062 (−0.028, 0.151)	0.178
Plant protein intake	0.032 (−0.131, 0.194)	0.702	0.021 (−0.151, 0.193)	0.810
Birthweight (n = 501) For each additional 10 g/day				
Total protein intake	0.049 (−0.036, 0.134)	0.259	0.019 (−0.069, 0.107)	0.667
Animal protein intake	0.049 (−0.036, 0.134)	0.256	0.019 (−0.069, 0.107)	0.675
Plant protein intake	0.038 (−0.123, 0.198)	0.647	−0.001 (−0.174, 0.173)	0.993

Model 1 is adjusted for energy intake. Model 2 is as Model 1, but additionally adjusted for age, BMI, geographical background, educational level, parity, conception mode, fetal sex, smoking, and folic acid supplement use. Fetal sex was not included in the models for standardized birthweight. BMI = Body Mass Index; EFW = Estimated Fetal Weight.

4. Discussion

4.1. Main Findings

The primary aim of this study was to investigate the associations between periconceptional maternal protein intake from animal and plant sources and embryonic growth. Furthermore, associations with fetal growth and birthweight were examined. This study showed that, even in women with a protein intake that generally met the nutritional requirements, periconceptional protein intake, and in particular from animal sources, was positively associated with embryonic growth. In addition, periconceptional maternal total and animal protein intake were associated with higher EFW and birthweight, though not statistically significantly. In this study, no associations between periconceptional maternal plant protein intake and prenatal growth and birthweight were found (Figure 3).

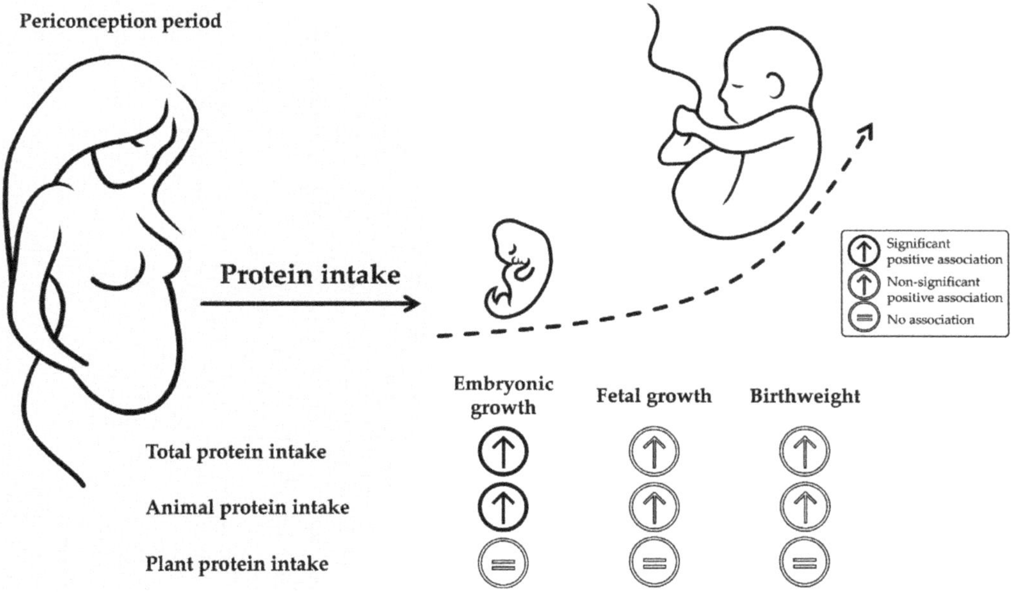

Figure 3. Graphical summary of the findings.

4.2. Interpretation of Findings and Comparison with Previous Studies

4.2.1. Maternal Protein Intake

The positive associations between periconceptional maternal protein intake and embryonic growth, fetal growth and birthweight are in line with previous research, which showed that maternal protein intake was associated with a reduced risk of fetal growth restriction and a higher birthweight [8,9,11,45]. In contrast, one cohort study found a non-linear (inverse U-curve) association between maternal protein intake and birthweight [12]. This inconsistency can be at least partly explained by the study population as it included Japanese women with other dietary habits, and thus protein and energy intake, amino acid composition and micronutrient content were different from our study population, consisting of mainly Dutch women. In the current study, no non-linear function of maternal protein intake was included, since none of the participants had a protein intake below the RDI. It could be that, in a larger more diverse population regarding protein intake, we would have found a non-linear association with prenatal growth and birthweight. The findings of the current study support our hypothesis that periconceptional maternal protein intake plays an important role in prenatal growth. Maternal protein intake is the primary source of amino acids for the developing fetus during pregnancy, which are involved in multiple metabolic pathways. Disruption of these metabolic pathways can cause epigenetic alterations, which may affect the expression of genes involved in growth of the fetus [6,46,47].

Although we did find a positive association between periconceptional maternal protein intake with EFW and birthweight, this association was not statistically significant. The consistency of the direction of the associations with EFW and birthweight suggests a positive trend overall. A possible explanation for attenuation of the effect later in pregnancy might be the transition from histio-trophic nutrition in the first trimester of pregnancy to hemo-trophic nutrition in the second and third trimester of pregnancy [48]. There is increasing evidence that during early pregnancy nutrients for the developing embryo are provided by uterine glands which discharge secretions into the intervillous space, and by accumulation of maternal proteins within coelomic cavity fluid from which these are taken up by the (secondary) yolk sac. Once the placenta is developed, hemo-trophic nutrition with exchange between the maternal and fetal circulation becomes predominant [48]. Even though we have previously shown that maternal diet also affects development and function of the placenta, the specific effect of periconceptional maternal protein intake on placental health fell beyond the scope of our study [49]. Another explanation may be that the relative effect of maternal protein intake is smaller later in pregnancy, because of an increasing role of other (non-nutritional) factors. Finally, less standardized methods of measurement may explain the attenuation. Fetal growth parameters and birthweight were retrieved from medical records and therefore measurement errors cannot be ruled out.

4.2.2. Maternal Animal Protein Intake

The findings of the current study suggest that the positive association of maternal protein intake during the periconception period with prenatal growth and birthweight can be predominantly ascribed to protein intake from animal sources. Periconceptional maternal animal protein intake was statistically significantly associated with increased embryonic growth, and also with higher EFW and birthweight, though not statistically significantly. In line with these results, an additional analysis including an 'animal/plant protein intake' ratio (data available on request) showed that consuming more animal proteins relative to plant proteins was associated with increased prenatal growth and birthweight. These findings correspond with other studies that showed a positive association between maternal animal protein intake and fetal growth and birthweight [8,10,11,45]. To our knowledge, the current study is the first study that investigated the effect of protein sources on embryonic growth. In our study population, the CRL and EV of embryos of women with +2SD animal protein intake (absolute increase of 30 g/day) were 0.45 mm (+4.9%) and 0.03 cm^3 (+34.0%) larger at 7 weeks of pregnancy and 0.97 mm (2.3%) and 0.54 cm^3 (7.3%) larger at 11 weeks of pregnancy compared to those of women with the mean animal protein intake. As an illustration, the CRL and EV of embryos of women who did not use folic acid supplements or started folic acid supplement use post-conception were 0.75 mm (−7.8%) and 0.01 cm^3 (−19.5%) smaller at 7 weeks of pregnancy and 1.63 mm (−3.7%) and 0.86 cm^3 (−12.2%) than those of women who started folic acid supplement use preconceptionally [7,35].

4.2.3. Maternal Plant Protein Intake

Surprisingly, no associations were found between periconceptional plant protein intake and prenatal growth. Previous research on maternal plant protein intake and prenatal growth and birthweight is limited and yielded inconsistent results [8,10,11]. One study found a positive association with birthweight, while other studies found a non-linear (inverse U-curve) association [8,10,11]. Our findings may be partly explained by low digestibility of plant proteins due to anti-nutritional factors and fibers in plant protein sources [2,50]. Moreover, in general, animal proteins are complete protein sources providing all essential amino acids, while plant proteins are deficient in one or more essential amino acids, such as lysine and threonine [2,5]. Therefore, without careful assortment of plant protein sources, the amino acid requirements for fetal growth may not be met [2]. The results may also be related to the differences in micronutrient content. For example, compared to animal protein sources, plant protein sources contain less iron, which is important for fetal growth [5]. However, the effect estimates of the model adjusted for iron intake were comparable to those of the other models, which suggests that iron intake did not affect the relationship between animal protein intake and embryonic growth. Lastly, dietary exposure to pesticides used in agriculture may have affected the associations between periconceptional maternal plant protein intake and prenatal growth. However, further research should be undertaken to investigate this.

4.3. Strengths and Limitations

The most important strength of this study is the extensive longitudinal data collection providing information on many patient characteristics and fetal growth. Potential confounding bias is limited as the analyses were adjusted for a comprehensive set of covariates [32–39]. Nevertheless, considering the complexity of the effect of maternal nutrition on prenatal growth, residual confounding from unobserved and unknown factors may still be present. However, as adjusting for covariates had little effect on the effect estimates, we do not think that residual confounding can explain our findings.

Furthermore, the serial 3D ultrasound scans performed in the first trimester of pregnancy by trained medical doctors are unique. Using VR systems and V-Scope software developed at the Erasmus MC accurate CRL and EV measurements were performed, which have been proven reliable (ICC > 0.99) [7,20]. Moreover, in order to assess maternal protein intake, a validated FFQ was used, as it provides semi-quantitative information on macronutrient and energy intake during four weeks within the periconception period [25]. Even though the FFQ is a validated questionnaire, response bias, in particular social-desirability bias, cannot be ruled out. To reduce the number of patients underreporting their dietary intake, we applied the Goldberg cut-off, which was based on the personalized basal metabolic rate and physical activity [27,28]. Additionally, the study population was restricted to patients with a normal BMI, which revealed stronger effect estimates, but no substantial changes of the associations. This indicates limited bias by overreporting or underreporting dietary intake, though underestimation of our results is more likely than overestimation [41,42].

The recruitment of patients in a tertiary hospital may have affected the generalizability of our results. However, the protein intake as percentage of energy intake was 15.2% in our study population, which is between 10% and 20%, as recommended for adults in the general population by the EFSA Panel on Dietetic Products [31]. Even though the patients included in our study are at higher risk of developing pregnancy complications, we think that the direction of the associations is the same as in the general population.

4.4. Implications for Future Research

The results of our study suggest that maternal protein intake during the periconception period, and in particular protein intake from animal sources, has a significant effect on embryonic growth and potentially on fetal growth and birthweight. The impact is substantial, since prenatal growth can affect health later in life, and even health of future offspring [6]. Even though knowledge regarding optimal growth of an embryo is still largely unknown, smaller embryos have been associated with fetal growth restriction, reduced birthweight and an increased risk of cardiovascular risk factors later in life [13–15,19]. As previous research has demonstrated that maternal diet hardly changes during pregnancy, early health interventions should target women already in the preconception period [51]. These interventions should aim for a well-balanced diet from a variety of sources containing an appropriate intake of macro- and micronutrients. Future research on amino acid composition, nutrient metabolism, digestibility and the interaction with microbiota are warranted to further investigate the association between protein sources and prenatal growth and birthweight. Future studies should also take into account the residues of pesticides and veterinary medicine in plant and animal products, since they have been associated with endocrine disruption and teratogenic effects [52–54].

5. Conclusions

This study has shown that even in women with a protein intake that met the nutritional recommendations, periconceptional total protein intake and animal protein intake was associated with increased embryonic growth. In addition a positive association was found between periconceptional maternal total and animal protein intake with fetal growth and birthweight, though not statistically significant. This study was, however, unable to demonstrate an association between periconceptional maternal plant protein intake and prenatal growth and birthweight. Our findings highlight the importance of a well-balanced diet during the periconception period and its impact on prenatal growth.

Supplementary Materials: The following supporting information can be downloaded at: https://www.mdpi.com/article/10.3390/nu14245309/s1, Table S1: Baseline characteristics of the included and excluded pregnancies.

Author Contributions: Conceptualization, S.v.Z., S.v.d.P., S.W., M.R., M.M., R.v.S., R.S.-T. and L.v.R.; methodology, S.W., M.R., R.S.-T. and L.v.R.; formal analysis, S.v.Z., S.v.d.P., S.W. and L.v.R.; data curation, S.v.Z. and S.v.d.P.; resources, R.v.S. and R.S.-T.; writing—original draft preparation, S.v.Z., S.v.d.P. and L.v.R.; writing—review and editing, S.W., M.R., M.M., R.v.S., R.S.-T. and L.v.R.; supervision, M.M., R.v.S., R.S.-T. and L.v.R.; project administration, R.S.-T. All authors have read and agreed to the published version of the manuscript.

Funding: This research was funded by the Department of Obstetrics and Gynecology and the Department of Clinical Chemistry of the Erasmus MC, University Medical Center, Rotterdam, The Netherlands. The APC was funded by the Department of Obstetrics and Gynecology and the Department of Clinical Chemistry of the Erasmus MC, University Medical Center, Rotterdam, The Netherlands.

Institutional Review Board Statement: The study was conducted in accordance with the Declaration of Helsinki and approved by the Central Committee on Research in The Hague and the local Medical Ethics Committee of the Erasmus MC (15 October 2004, MEC-2004-277).

Informed Consent Statement: Informed consent was obtained from all subjects involved in the study.

Data Availability Statement: The data presented in this study are available on request from the corresponding author.

Acknowledgments: We wish to thank all women of the Rotterdam Periconceptional cohort (Predict Study) for their participation. In addition, we appreciate the help provided by the researchers for recruiting participants, collecting data and carrying out 3D ultrasound scans. Finally, we gratefully acknowledge the financial support of the Department of Obstetrics and Gynecology for the Predict Study, and the department of Clinical Chemistry for financially supporting the current study.

Conflicts of Interest: The authors declare no conflict of interest.

References

1. World Health Organization. *Plant-Based Diets and Their Impact on Health, Sustainability and the Environment: A Review of the Evidence: WHO European Office for the Prevention and Control of Noncommunicable Diseases*; Regional Office for Europe: Copenhagen, Denmark, 2021.
2. Hertzler, S.R.; Lieblein-Boff, J.C.; Weiler, M.; Allgeier, C. Plant Proteins: Assessing Their Nutritional Quality and Effects on Health and Physical Function. *Nutrients* **2020**, *12*, 3704. [CrossRef] [PubMed]
3. Khan, N.; Afaq, F.; Mukhtar, H. Cancer chemoprevention through dietary antioxidants: Progress and promise. *Antioxid. Redox Signal.* **2008**, *10*, 475–510. [CrossRef] [PubMed]
4. Jenkins, D.J.; Kendall, C.W.; Marchie, A.; Jenkins, A.L.; Augustin, L.S.; Ludwig, D.S.; Barnard, N.D.; Anderson, J.W. Type 2 diabetes and the vegetarian diet. *Am. J. Clin. Nutr.* **2003**, *78*, 610S–616S. [CrossRef] [PubMed]
5. Sebastiani, G.; Herranz Barbero, A.; Borrás-Novell, C.; Alsina Casanova, M.; Aldecoa-Bilbao, V.; Andreu-Fernández, V.; Pascual Tutusaus, M.; Ferrero Martínez, S.; Gómez Roig, M.D.; García-Algar, O. The Effects of Vegetarian and Vegan Diet during Pregnancy on the Health of Mothers and Offspring. *Nutrients* **2019**, *11*, 557. [CrossRef]
6. Steegers-Theunissen, R.P.; Twigt, J.; Pestinger, V.; Sinclair, K.D. The periconceptional period, reproduction and long-term health of offspring: The importance of one-carbon metabolism. *Hum. Reprod. Update* **2013**, *19*, 640–655. [CrossRef]

7. Rousian, M.; Schoenmakers, S.; Eggink, A.J.; Gootjes, D.V.; Koning, A.H.; Koster, M.P.; Mulders, A.G.; Baart, E.B.; Reiss, I.K.; Laven, J.S.; et al. Cohort profile update: The Rotterdam periconceptional cohort and embryonic and fetal measurements using 3D ultrasound and virtual reality techniques. *Int. J. Epidemiol.* **2021**, *50*, 1426–1427. [CrossRef]
8. Cucó, G.; Arija, V.; Iranzo, R.; Vilà, J.; Prieto, M.T.; Fernández-Ballart, J. Association of maternal protein intake before conception and throughout pregnancy with birth weight. *Acta Obstet. Gynecol. Scand.* **2006**, *85*, 413–421. [CrossRef]
9. Moore, V.M.; Davies, M.J.; Willson, K.J.; Worsley, A.; Robinson, J.S. Dietary composition of pregnant women is related to size of the baby at birth. *J. Nutr.* **2004**, *134*, 1820–1826. [CrossRef]
10. Salavati, N.; Bakker, M.K.; Lewis, F.; Vinke, P.C.; Mubarik, F.; Erwich, J.H.M.; van der Beek, E.M. Associations between preconception macronutrient intake and birth weight across strata of maternal BMI. *PLoS ONE* **2020**, *15*, e0243200. [CrossRef]
1. Yang, J.; Chang, Q.; Tian, X.; Zhang, B.; Zeng, L.; Yan, H.; Dang, S.; Li, Y.H. Dietary protein intake during pregnancy and birth weight among Chinese pregnant women with low intake of protein. *Nutr. Metab.* **2022**, *19*, 43. [CrossRef]
2. Morisaki, N.; Nagata, C.; Yasuo, S.; Morokuma, S.; Kato, K.; Sanefuji, M.; Shibata, E.; Tsuji, M.; Senju, A.; Kawamoto, T.; et al. Optimal protein intake during pregnancy for reducing the risk of fetal growth restriction: The Japan Environment and Children's Study. *Br. J. Nutr.* **2018**, *120*, 1432–1440. [CrossRef]
3. Van Uitert, E.M.; Exalto, N.; Burton, G.J.; Willemsen, S.P.; Koning, A.H.; Eilers, P.H.; Laven, J.S.; Steegers, E.A.; Steegers-Theunissen, R.P. Human embryonic growth trajectories and associations with fetal growth and birthweight. *Hum. Reprod.* **2013**, *28*, 1753–1761. [CrossRef]
4. Jaddoe, V.W.; de Jonge, L.L.; Hofman, A.; Franco, O.H.; Steegers, E.A.; Gaillard, R. First trimester fetal growth restriction and cardiovascular risk factors in school age children: Population based cohort study. *BMJ* **2014**, *348*, g14. [CrossRef]
5. Mook-Kanamori, D.O.; Steegers, E.A.; Eilers, P.H.; Raat, H.; Hofman, A.; Jaddoe, V.W. Risk factors and outcomes associated with first-trimester fetal growth restriction. *JAMA* **2010**, *303*, 527–534. [CrossRef]
6. Steegers-Theunissen, R.P.; Verheijden-Paulissen, J.J.; van Uitert, E.M.; Wildhagen, M.F.; Exalto, N.; Koning, A.H.; Eggink, A.J.; Duvekot, J.J.; Laven, J.S.; Tibboel, D.; et al. Cohort profile: The Rotterdam periconceptional cohort (Predict study). *Int. J. Epidemiol.* **2016**, *45*, 374–381. [CrossRef]
7. Feunekes, G.I.; Van Staveren, W.A.; De Vries, J.H.; Burema, J.; Hautvast, J.G. Relative and biomarker-based validity of a food-frequency questionnaire estimating intake of fats and cholesterol. *Am. J. Clin. Nutr.* **1993**, *58*, 489–496. [CrossRef]
8. DeVilbiss, E.A.; Mumford, S.L.; Sjaarda, L.A.; Connell, M.T.; Plowden, T.C.; Andriessen, V.C.; Perkins, N.J.; Hill, M.J.; Silver, R.M.; Schisterman, E.F. Prediction of pregnancy loss by early first trimester ultrasound characteristics. *Am. J. Obstet. Gynecol.* **2020**, *223*, 242.e1–242.e22. [CrossRef]
9. Baken, L.; van Heesch, P.N.; Wildschut, H.I.; Koning, A.H.; van der Spek, P.J.; Steegers, E.A.; Exalto, N. First-trimester crown-rump length and embryonic volume of aneuploid fetuses measured in virtual reality. *Ultrasound Obstet. Gynecol.* **2013**, *41*, 521–525. [CrossRef]
0. Rousian, M.; Koning, A.H.; van Oppenraaij, R.H.; Hop, W.C.; Verwoerd-Dikkeboom, C.M.; van der Spek, P.J.; Exalto, N.; Steegers, E.A. An innovative virtual reality technique for automated human embryonic volume measurements. *Hum. Reprod.* **2010**, *25*, 2210–2216. [CrossRef]
1. Hadlock, F.P.; Harrist, R.B.; Sharman, R.S.; Deter, R.L.; Park, S.K. Estimation of fetal weight with the use of head, body, and femur measurements—A prospective study. *Am. J. Obstet. Gynecol.* **1985**, *151*, 333–337. [CrossRef]
2. Gaillard, R.; de Ridder, M.A.; Verburg, B.O.; Witteman, J.C.; Mackenbach, J.P.; Moll, H.A.; Hofman, A.; Steegers, E.A.; Jaddoe, V.W. Individually customised fetal weight charts derived from ultrasound measurements: The Generation R Study. *Eur. J. Epidemiol.* **2011**, *26*, 919–926. [CrossRef] [PubMed]
3. Hoftiezer, L.; Hukkelhoven, C.W.; Hogeveen, M.; Straatman, H.M.; van Lingen, R.A. Defining small-for-gestational-age: Prescriptive versus descriptive birthweight standards. *Eur. J. Pediatr.* **2016**, *175*, 1047–1057. [CrossRef] [PubMed]
4. Fayet, F.; Flood, V.; Petocz, P.; Samman, S. Relative and biomarker-based validity of a food frequency questionnaire that measures the intakes of vitamin B(12), folate, iron, and zinc in young women. *Nutr. Res.* **2011**, *31*, 14–20. [CrossRef] [PubMed]
5. Verkleij-Hagoort, A.C.; de Vries, J.H.; Stegers, M.P.; Lindemans, J.; Ursem, N.T.; Steegers-Theunissen, R.P. Validation of the assessment of folate and vitamin B12 intake in women of reproductive age: The method of triads. *Eur. J. Clin. Nutr.* **2007**, *61*, 610–615. [CrossRef]
6. NEVO-Online Versie 2021/7.0. Available online: https://www.rivm.nl/nederlands-voedingsstoffenbestand (accessed on 3 January 2022).
7. Black, A.E. Critical evaluation of energy intake using the Goldberg cut-off for energy intake:basal metabolic rate. A practical guide to its calculation, use and limitations. *Int. J. Obes. Relat. Metab. Disord.* **2000**, *24*, 1119–1130. [CrossRef]
8. Smit, A.J.P.; Hojeij, B.; Rousian, M.; Schoenmakers, S.; Willemsen, S.P.; Steegers-Theunissen, R.P.M.; van Rossem, L. A high periconceptional maternal ultra-processed food consumption impairs embryonic growth: The Rotterdam periconceptional cohort. *Clin. Nutr.* **2022**, *41*, 1667–1675. [CrossRef]
9. Schneider, S.L. The international standard classification of education 2011. In *Class and Stratification Analysis*; Emerald Group Publishing Limited: Bingley, UK, 2013.
0. Alders, M. Classification of the population with a foreign background in The Netherlands. In Proceedings of the Measure and Mismeasure of Populations. The Statistical Use of Ethnic and Racial Categories in Multicultural Societies, Paris, France, 17–18 December 2001; p. 18.

31. EFSA Panel on Dietetic Products, N.a.A.N. Scientific Opinion on Dietary Reference Values for protein. *EFSA J.* **2012**, *10*, 2557. [CrossRef]
32. Bukowski, R.; Smith, G.C.; Malone, F.D.; Ball, R.H.; Nyberg, D.A.; Comstock, C.H.; Hankins, G.D.; Berkowitz, R.L.; Gross, S.J.; Dugoff, L.; et al. Human sexual size dimorphism in early pregnancy. *Am. J. Epidemiol.* **2007**, *165*, 1216–1218. [CrossRef]
33. Shah, P.S. Parity and low birth weight and preterm birth: A systematic review and meta-analyses. *Acta Obstet. Gynecol. Scand.* **2010**, *89*, 862–875. [CrossRef]
34. Van Uitert, E.M.; van der Elst-Otte, N.; Wilbers, J.J.; Exalto, N.; Willemsen, S.P.; Eilers, P.H.; Koning, A.H.; Steegers, E.A.; Steegers-Theunissen, R.P. Periconception maternal characteristics and embryonic growth trajectories: The Rotterdam Predict study. *Hum. Reprod.* **2013**, *28*, 3188–3196. [CrossRef]
35. Van Dijk, M.R.; Borggreven, N.V.; Willemsen, S.P.; Koning, A.H.J.; Steegers-Theunissen, R.P.M.; Koster, M.P.H. Maternal Lifestyle Impairs Embryonic Growth: The Rotterdam Periconception Cohort. *Reprod. Sci.* **2018**, *25*, 916–922. [CrossRef]
36. Van Duijn, L.; Rousian, M.; Laven, J.S.E.; Steegers-Theunissen, R.P.M. Periconceptional maternal body mass index and the impact on post-implantation (sex-specific) embryonic growth and morphological development. *Int. J. Obes.* **2021**, *45*, 2369–2376. [CrossRef]
37. Bottomley, C.; Daemen, A.; Mukri, F.; Papageorghiou, A.T.; Kirk, E.; Pexsters, A.; De Moor, B.; Timmerman, D.; Bourne, T. Assessing first trimester growth: The influence of ethnic background and maternal age. *Hum. Reprod.* **2009**, *24*, 284–290. [CrossRef]
38. Eindhoven, S.C.; van Uitert, E.M.; Laven, J.S.; Willemsen, S.P.; Koning, A.H.; Eilers, P.H.; Exalto, N.; Steegers, E.A.; Steegers-Theunissen, R.P. The influence of IVF/ICSI treatment on human embryonic growth trajectories. *Hum. Reprod.* **2014**, *29*, 2628–2636. [CrossRef]
39. Jackson, R.A.; Gibson, K.A.; Wu, Y.W.; Croughan, M.S. Perinatal outcomes in singletons following in vitro fertilization: A meta-analysis. *Obstet. Gynecol.* **2004**, *103*, 551–563. [CrossRef]
40. Mackerras, D. Energy adjustment: The concepts underlying the debate. *J. Clin. Epidemiol.* **1996**, *49*, 957–962. [CrossRef]
41. Mendez, M.A.; Popkin, B.M.; Buckland, G.; Schroder, H.; Amiano, P.; Barricarte, A.; Huerta, J.-M.; Quirós, J.R.; Sánchez, M.-J.; González, C.A. Alternative methods of accounting for underreporting and overreporting when measuring dietary intake-obesity relations. *Am. J. Epidemiol.* **2011**, *173*, 448–458. [CrossRef]
42. Willett, W. *Nutritional Epidemiology;* Oxford University Press: Oxford, UK, 2012.
43. R Core Team. *R: A Language and Environment for Statistical Computing;* R Foundation for Statistical Computing: Vienna, Austria, 2022.
44. Verburg, B.O.; Steegers, E.A.; De Ridder, M.; Snijders, R.J.; Smith, E.; Hofman, A.; Moll, H.A.; Jaddoe, V.W.; Witteman, J.C. New charts for ultrasound dating of pregnancy and assessment of fetal growth: Longitudinal data from a population-based cohort study. *Ultrasound Obstet. Gynecol.* **2008**, *31*, 388–396. [CrossRef]
45. Godfrey, K.; Robinson, S.; Barker, D.J.; Osmond, C.; Cox, V. Maternal nutrition in early and late pregnancy in relation to placental and fetal growth. *BMJ* **1996**, *312*, 410–414. [CrossRef]
46. Wu, G.; Bazer, F.W.; Cudd, T.A.; Meininger, C.J.; Spencer, T.E. Maternal nutrition and fetal development. *J. Nutr.* **2004**, *134*, 2169–2172. [CrossRef]
47. Peral-Sanchez, I.; Hojeij, B.; Ojeda, D.A.; Steegers-Theunissen, R.P.M.; Willaime-Morawek, S. Epigenetics in the Uterine Environment: How Maternal Diet and ART May Influence the Epigenome in the Offspring with Long-Term Health Consequences. *Genes* **2021**, *13*, 31. [CrossRef] [PubMed]
48. Burton, G.J.; Hempstock, J.; Jauniaux, E. Nutrition of the human fetus during the first trimester—A review. *Placenta* **2001**, *22* (Suppl. A), S70–S77. [CrossRef] [PubMed]
49. Reijnders, I.F.; Mulders, A.; van der Windt, M.; Steegers, E.A.P.; Steegers-Theunissen, R.P.M. The impact of periconceptional maternal lifestyle on clinical features and biomarkers of placental development and function: A systematic review. *Hum. Reprod. Update* **2019**, *25*, 72–94. [CrossRef] [PubMed]
50. Day, L.; Cakebread, J.A.; Loveday, S.M. Food proteins from animals and plants: Differences in the nutritional and functional properties. *Trends Food Sci. Technol.* **2021**, *119*, 428–442. [CrossRef]
51. Crozier, S.R.; Robinson, S.M.; Godfrey, K.M.; Cooper, C.; Inskip, H.M. Women's dietary patterns change little from before to during pregnancy. *J. Nutr.* **2009**, *139*, 1956–1963. [CrossRef]
52. Widyawati, S.A.; Suhartono, S.; Mexitalia, M.; Soejoenoes, A. The Relationship between Pesticide Exposure and Umbilical Serum IGF-1 Levels and Low-birth Weight: A Case-control Study in Brebes, Indonesia. *Int. J. Occup. Environ. Med.* **2020**, *11*, 15–23. [CrossRef]
53. Petit, C.; Chevrier, C.; Durand, G.; Monfort, C.; Rouget, F.; Garlantezec, R.; Cordier, S. Impact on fetal growth of prenatal exposure to pesticides due to agricultural activities: A prospective cohort study in Brittany, France. *Environ. Health* **2010**, *9*, 71. [CrossRef]
54. Beyene, T. Veterinary drug residues in food-animal products: Its risk factors and potential effects on public health. *J. Vet. Sci. Technol.* **2016**, *7*, 285. [CrossRef]

nutrients

MDPI

Article

Plasma FGF21 Levels Are Not Associated with Weight Loss or Improvements in Metabolic Health Markers upon 12 Weeks of Energy Restriction: Secondary Analysis of an RCT

Anouk Gijbels , Sophie Schutte, Diederik Esser, Charlotte C. J. R. Michielsen, Els Siebelink, Monica Mars , Marco Mensink and Lydia A. Afman *

Division of Human Nutrition and Health, Department of Agrotechnology and Food Sciences, Wageningen University & Research, Stippeneng 4, 6708 WE Wageningen, The Netherlands
* Correspondence: lydia.afman@wur.nl

Abstract: Recent studies suggest that circulating fibroblast growth factor 21 (FGF21) may be a marker of metabolic health status. We performed a secondary analysis of a 12-week randomized controlled trial to investigate the effects of two energy restriction (ER) diets on fasting and postprandial plasma FGF21 levels, as well as to explore correlations of plasma FGF21 with metabolic health markers, (macro)nutrient intake and sweet-taste preference. Abdominally obese subjects aged 40–70 years (n = 110) were randomized to one of two 25% ER diets (high-nutrient-quality diet or low-nutrient-quality diet) or a control group. Plasma FGF21 was measured in the fasting state and 120 min after a mixed meal. Both ER diets did not affect fasting or postprandial plasma FGF21 levels despite weight loss and accompanying health improvements. At baseline, the postprandial FGF21 response was inversely correlated to fasting plasma glucose ($\rho = -0.24$, $p = 0.020$) and insulin ($\rho = -0.32$, $p = 0.001$), HOMA-IR ($\rho = -0.34$, $p = 0.001$), visceral adipose tissue ($\rho = -0.24$, $p = 0.046$), and the liver enzyme aspartate aminotransferase ($\rho = -0.23$, $p = 0.021$). Diet-induced changes in these markers did not correlate to changes in plasma FGF21 levels upon intervention. Baseline higher habitual polysaccharide intake, but not mono- and disaccharide intake or sweet-taste preference, was related to lower fasting plasma FGF21 ($p = 0.022$). In conclusion, we found no clear evidence that fasting plasma FGF21 is a marker for metabolic health status. Circulating FGF21 dynamics in response to an acute nutritional challenge may reflect metabolic health status better than fasting levels.

Keywords: FGF21; fibroblast growth factor 21; overweight; obesity; caloric restriction; energy restriction; weight loss; dietary intervention; liver fat; metabolic health

1. Introduction

Fibroblast growth factor 21 (FGF21) is a peptide hormone that regulates metabolic homeostasis [1,2]. The exact biological functions and regulation of FGF21 vary widely between tissues and are not completely understood [1,2]. Circulating FGF21 levels are typically elevated in conditions of impaired metabolic health, such as obesity, non-alcoholic fatty liver disease (NAFLD) and type 2 diabetes (T2DM) [3,4]. Accordingly, circulating FGF21 levels have been reported to positively associate with BMI, body fat, liver fat content, blood pressure, insulin resistance (IR) and atherogenic lipid profiles [5,6], as well as predict incident metabolic syndrome and T2DM [7,8]. It is unclear whether and how weight loss and accompanying health improvements affect FGF21 levels, with some trials reporting reduced levels of circulating FGF21 upon diet-induced weight loss [9–13], and others reporting no effects on FGF21 [14–20].

Recently, FGF21 has been implicated in the metabolic adaptations to both under- and overfeeding. In the DIETFITS trial, fasting FGF21 level was associated with diet-induced weight loss, with higher FGF21 levels at baseline being associated with larger weight loss in response to a 12-month low-fat or low-carbohydrate diet [20,21]. Furthermore, in a 6-week trial, the change in circulating FGF21 upon energy restriction was associated with weight loss, with individuals with larger increases in fasting FGF21 achieving greater weight loss [22]. In addition, in a short-term trial, greater increases in fasting plasma FGF21 in response to a 1-day hypercaloric low-protein, high-fat diet were associated with larger weight loss in free-living conditions after 6 months [23]. Plasma FGF21 (response) thus seems to be related to the ability to lose weight.

Next to its metabolic effects, FGF21 also appears to play a role in the regulation of nutrient intake via central nervous system (CNS) signaling. Multiple large human genome-wide association studies (GWAS) have reported associations between *FGF21* gene variants and carbohydrate, sugar, and alcohol consumption and sweet-taste preference [24–27]. Furthermore, higher fasting FGF21 levels have been associated with lower sweet-taste preference [26] and lower soda consumption [28]. Animal studies suggest that in response to carbohydrate and in particular sugar intake, FGF21 is induced in the liver, enters the circulation and subsequently acts as negative feedback signal via the liver-brain-axis to suppress further sweet-taste preference and carbohydrate intake [29–31]. As of yet, evidence from human studies on the link between plasma FGF21 and nutrient intake and taste preference is sparse.

We previously reported the effects of two 12-week energy restriction (ER) diets differing in nutrient quality in overweight and obese adults [32]. Both ER diets resulted in substantial weight loss and concomitant improvements in various health parameters, including reduced liver fat, and decreased fasting glucose and insulin levels. In the present study, we investigated whether these diet-induced changes in body weight and related health outcomes were accompanied by changes in fasting and postprandial FGF21 levels. Additionally, we explored correlations of plasma FGF21 with markers of metabolic health, weight loss, habitual (macro)nutrient intake and sweet-taste preference.

2. Materials and Methods

The present study is a secondary analysis of a 12-week parallel randomized controlled trial (RCT) that was performed at Wageningen University, the Netherlands, in 2014. The aim of this trial was to investigate the effects of two different ER diets on weight loss and cardiometabolic health outcomes. Details have been described previously [32].

2.1. Participants and Study Design

The study population consisted of 110 women and men aged 40–70 years with abdominal obesity (BMI > 27 kg/m^2 or waist circumference > 88 cm for women or >102 cm for men). Exclusion criteria were diagnosis of diabetes, heavy alcohol consumption, smoking, unstable body weight, diagnosis of long-term medical condition, and use of medication that is known to interfere with glucose or lipid metabolism.

Eligible subjects were randomly assigned to one of three intervention groups: a 25% ER high-nutrient-quality diet (n = 40), a 25% ER low-nutrient-quality diet (n = 40), or a control group (n = 30). At baseline and after 12 weeks of intervention, participants visited hospital Gelderse Vallei (Ede, the Netherlands) for an MRI scan and—on a separate day—visited Wageningen University after an overnight fast for measurements of general health and blood metabolites in the fasting state, as well as in response to a mixed meal.

2.2. Dietary Intervention

The dietary intervention strategy has been described in detail previously [32]. Briefly, both the ER diets were energy restricted by 25% of the estimated energy requirement of each participant. The high-nutrient-quality diet (HQ) was designed to improve metabolic health and contained an increased amount of soy protein, fiber, monounsaturated fat (MUFA), and omega-3 fatty acids. The low-nutrient-quality diet (LQ) contained an increased amount of saturated fat (SFA), animal protein, and fructose. The control group did not receive an intervention and was instructed to maintain their usual dietary habits. Participants in the ER groups received dietary advice and key food products. Adherence to the ER diets was assessed based on participants' food diaries, taking reported deviations from the dietary advice and leftover key food products into account [32].

2.3. General Health Measures

Systolic and diastolic blood pressure were measured automatically for 10 min with a 3-min interval using a DINAMAP PRO100. After an overnight fast, blood samples were collected from an intravenous cannula before and 30, 60, 120, 180, 240, and 360 min after consumption of a liquid mixed meal (3833 kJ; 76.3 g carbohydrates, 17.6 g protein, 60 g fat). To estimate IR, we used the homeostatic model assessment of insulin resistance (HOMA-IR), which is calculated as (fasting glucose [mmol/L] × fasting insulin [mU/L])/22.5 [33]. IR was defined as HOMA-IR > 2.5 [34]. Incremental area under the curves (iAUC) for glucose and insulin were calculated using the trapezoid method.

2.4. Plasma FGF21

Plasma FGF21 levels were measured in plasma samples from the fasting state and 120 min after consumption of the mixed meal using ELISA, according to manufacturer's instructions (FGF-21 Human ELISA Kit, ab125966, Abcam, Cambridge, UK). The inter- and intra-assay coefficients of variation were 12.4% and 5.9%, respectively. All samples from two subjects and one sample from another subject fell outside of the range of the standard curve and were therefore excluded from analyses.

2.5. Intra-Hepatic Lipid Content and Abdominal Fat Distribution

Intra-hepatic lipid content (IHL) was quantified using proton magnetic spectroscopy (^{1}H-MRS) on a 3T whole-body scanner (Siemens, Munich, Germany). Details have been described previously [32]. MRS spectra were analyzed using jMRUI software v5.2. NAFLD was defined as IHL > 5.56% [35]. Abdominal fat distribution was evaluated as subcutaneous (SAT) and visceral adipose tissue (VAT) areas in the abdomen and assessed using magnetic resonance imaging (MRI). SAT and VAT were quantified in a single-slice transverse image at the inter-vertebral space L3-L4 using the semi-automatic software program HippoFatTM [36].

2.6. Clinical Chemistry

Plasma glucose, insulin, and triglycerides, as well as serum total cholesterol, HDL cholesterol and safety parameters of liver function (aminotransferase [ALAT], aspartate aminotransferase [ASAT], and gamma-glutamyl transferase [γGT]) were analyzed photometrically (Cobas 8000, Roche Diagnostic Limited, Switzerland) by a center for medical diagnostics (Stichting Huisartsenlaboratorium Oost, Velp, the Netherlands). Plasma free fatty acids (FFA) were determined with an enzymatic assay (INstruchemie, Delfzijl, The Netherlands). HbA1c was determined in whole blood by hospital Gelderse Vallei (Ede, The Netherlands).

2.7. Habitual Dietary Intake and Sweet-Taste Preference

Habitual dietary intake including alcohol consumption was assessed by a validated 131-item semi-quantitative food frequency questionnaire (FFQ) [37,38]. Preference for sweet foods was assessed by a digital food preference ranking task [39]. Sweet-taste preference scores range from 1.5 to 3.5, with higher scores indicating greater preference for sweet foods compared to savory foods.

2.8. Statistical Analyses

Normality of variables was visually inspected using residual Q-Q plots. Skewed variables (plasma FGF21, VAT/SAT ratio, IHL, iAUC plasma glucose, fasting plasma insulin, iAUC plasma insulin, fasting plasma triglycerides, fasting plasma FFA, HOMA-IR, ASAT, and γGT) were log transformed (log2) to improve normality. Treatment effects on fasting FGF21 levels were analyzed using a general linear model for univariate analysis

(ANCOVA), with baseline FGF21 level as covariate. Treatment effects on the postprandial FGF21 response were analyzed using ANOVA with the change in postprandial response as dependent variable. Correlations between variables were tested using Spearman's correlation coefficient. Differences in plasma FGF21 levels between tertiles of nutrient intake were analyzed using ANCOVA with adjustment for gender, and LSD post-hoc testing was used if overall differences were statistically significant. To evaluate the robustness of the results, we performed sensitivity analyses excluding outliers. Outliers were defined as plasma FGF21 levels that deviated more than two standard deviations (SD) from the mean. Data analysis was performed using IBM SPSS Statistics version 25.0 (IBM Corp., Armonk, NY, US). Two-tailed $p < 0.05$ was considered statistically significant.

3. Results

A total of 100 subjects completed the study ($n = 6$ drop-outs in HQ, $n = 1$ drop-out in LQ, and $n = 3$ drop-outs in the control group [32]). Plasma FGF21 data were available from 98 subjects. Approximately half of the study population were women, median age was 62 years and median BMI was 30.8 kg/m^2. Baseline demographics and clinical characteristics were similar across intervention groups (Table 1).

Table 1. Baseline characteristics of study participants with available FGF21 data.

	High-Nutrient-Quality Diet (n = 34)	Low-Nutrient-Quality Diet (n = 38)	Control Group (n = 26)
Women, n (%)	18 (52.9%)	21 (55.3%)	13 (50.0%)
Age, years	62 (53,65)	64 (54, 65)	61 (56, 66)
BMI, kg/m^2	31.1 (28.7, 33.8)	30.8 (28.9, 33.4)	30.3 (28.1, 32.6)
Intra-hepatic lipid content, %	3.1 (1.4, 10.2)	4.9 (2.6, 9.7)	3.7 (2.1, 8.4)
NAFLD, n (%)	9 (26.5%)	14 (36.8%)	7 (26.9%)
HbA1c, mmol/mol	37 ± 3	36 ± 2	35 ± 3
HOMA-IR	2.7 (2.0, 4.9)	2.8 (1.6, 5.0)	2.6 (1.9, 4.4)
HOMA-IR > 2.5, n (%)	19 (55.9%)	21 (55.3%)	14 (53.8%)
Plasma glucose, mmol/L	5.7 ± 0.5	5.6 ± 0.7	5.7 ± 0.4
Plasma insulin, mU/L	10.9 (8.2, 17.5)	11.6 (7.0, 18.6)	10.9 (7.9, 17.0)
Plasma triglycerides, mmol/L	1.5 (1.1, 1.9)	1.7 (1.3, 2.3)	1.7 (1.4, 2.1)
Serum total cholesterol, mmol/L	5.5 ± 0.8	5.8 ± 1.0	5.5 ± 1.0
Serum HDL cholesterol, mmol/L	1.4 ± 0.4	1.3 ± 0.4	1.3 ± 0.4
Plasma free fatty acids, mmol/L	0.5 (0.4, 0.6)	0.4 (0.3, 0.5)	0.4 (0.3, 0.5)
Systolic blood pressure, mmHg	131 ± 15	126 ± 19	126 ± 14
Diastolic blood pressure, mmHg	76 ± 9	72 ± 8	75 ± 9
Alanine aminotransferase, U/L	24 (19, 33)	24 (20, 33)	25 (20, 33)
Aspartate aminotransferase, U/L	22 (19, 26)	22 (19, 25)	24 (20, 32)
Gamma-glutamyl transferase, U/L	23 (18, 33)	26 (18, 36)	23 (17, 32)

Data are presented as mean ± SD or median (25th percentile, 75th percentile). Abbreviations: BMI, body mass index; NAFLD, non-alcoholic fatty liver disease; HbA1c, glycated hemoglobin A1c; HOMA-IR, homeostatic model assessment of insulin resistance; HDL, high-density lipoprotein.

In five participants ($n = 2$ in HQ, $n = 1$ in LQ, and $n = 2$ in the control group), plasma FGF21 levels deviated more than 2 SD from the mean both in the fasting and postprandial state, and both at baseline and after 12 weeks of intervention. Another two participants ($n = 1$ in HQ and $n = 1$ in LQ) had deviating plasma FGF21 levels in the postprandial state at baseline or in the fasting state after 12 weeks of intervention, respectively.

The reported dietary intakes of participants on the ER diets were in agreement with the advised (macro)nutrient composition, with higher intakes of MUFA, polyunsaturated fat, plant-based protein, and fiber, and lower intakes of SFA and fructose in the high-nutrient-quality diet compared to the low-nutrient-quality diet [32].

3.1. Effects of Dietary Interventions on Plasma FGF21

As has been previously reported, 12 weeks of 25% ER resulted in substantial weight loss (mean ± SD: −8.4 ± 3.2 kg in HQ and −6.3 ± 3.9 kg in LQ) and concomitant improvements in markers of metabolic health, including more favorable abdominal fat distribution, and reductions in IHL, fasting glucose, and fasting insulin levels [32]. On average, plasma FGF21 levels were not affected by the interventions, nor did the interventions affect the postprandial FGF21 response (Table 2; Figure 1). Pooling of the ER groups together yielded similar results (ER: Δ fasting FGF21 −0.11 ng/ml, 95% CI −0.20 to −0.01, p ER vs. control group = 0.29; Δ postprandial FGF21 response −0.02 ng/ml, 95% CI −0.10 to 0.06, p ER vs. control group = 0.62). Exclusion of outliers did not affect the results (all $p > 0.19$).

Table 2. Change in fasting plasma FGF21 and the postprandial FGF21 response upon a 12-week energy restriction diet (low or high nutrient quality) compared to a control group.

	Baseline [a]	Change after 12 Wks [b]	p-Value [c]
Fasting FGF21 (ng/mL)			
Control group (n = 26)	0.95 ± 1.86	−0.01 (−0.17, 0.16)	
Low-Nutrient-Quality Diet (n = 38)	0.77 ± 1.89	−0.08 (−0.21, 0.05)	0.48
High-Nutrient-Quality Diet (n = 34)	0.71 ± 1.92	−0.14 (−0.28, 0.004)	
Postprandial FGF21 (ng/mL)			
Control group (n = 26)	0.82 ± 2.00	0.00 (−0.15, 0.15)	
Low-Nutrient-Quality Diet (n = 37)	0.71 ± 1.93	−0.09 (−0.21, 0.04)	0.57
High-Nutrient-Quality Diet (n = 32)	0.64 ± 1.88	−0.10 (−0.24, 0.04)	
Postprandial FGF21 response (ng/mL)			
Control group (n = 26)	−0.12 ± 0.22	−0.02 (−0.15, 0.11)	
Low-Nutrient-Quality Diet (n = 37)	−0.02 ± 0.27	0.01 (−0.10, 0.12)	0.86
High-Nutrient-Quality Diet (n = 32)	−0.05 ± 0.34	0.03 (−0.09, 0.15)	

[a] Values are geometric means ± SD (fasting and postprandial FGF21) or means ± SD (postprandial FGF21 response). [b] Values are (adjusted) means with 95% confidence intervals. [c] Differences between the groups were analyzed using ANCOVA with baseline FGF21 levels as covariate (fasting and postprandial FGF21) or using univariate ANOVA (postprandial FGF21 response).

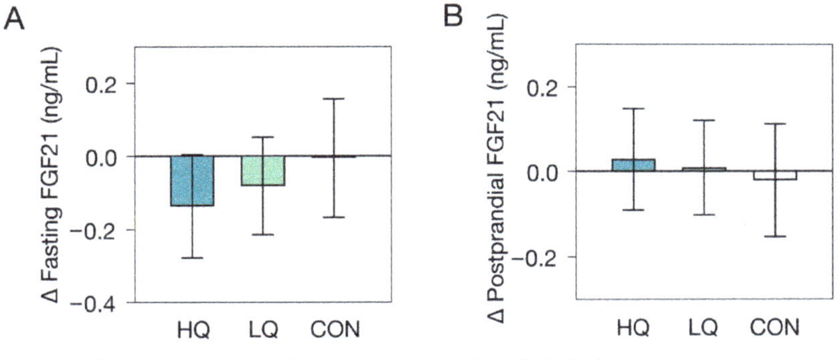

Figure 1. Effects of two 12-week energy restriction diets (HQ, high-nutrient-quality diet; LQ, low-nutrient-quality diet) or control group (CON) on fasting and postprandial plasma FGF21 levels. (**A**) Geometric mean (95% CI) change in fasting plasma FGF21 upon a 12-week diet, as tested by ANCOVA with adjustment for baseline fasting FGF21 levels. (**B**) Geometric mean (95% CI) change in postprandial FGF21 response (Δ120–0 min) to a mixed meal upon a 12-week diet, as tested by univariate ANOVA.

3.2. Postprandial Plasma FGF21 Response at Baseline

On average, plasma FGF21 tended to decrease 120 min after consumption of the mixed meal (Δ −0.06 ng/ml, 95% CI −0.11 to 0.001, p = 0.055), although inter-individual variation in response was high (Figure 2A). Exclusion of outliers strengthened this effect (Δ −0.12 ng/ml, 95% CI −0.23 to −0.02, p = 0.026).

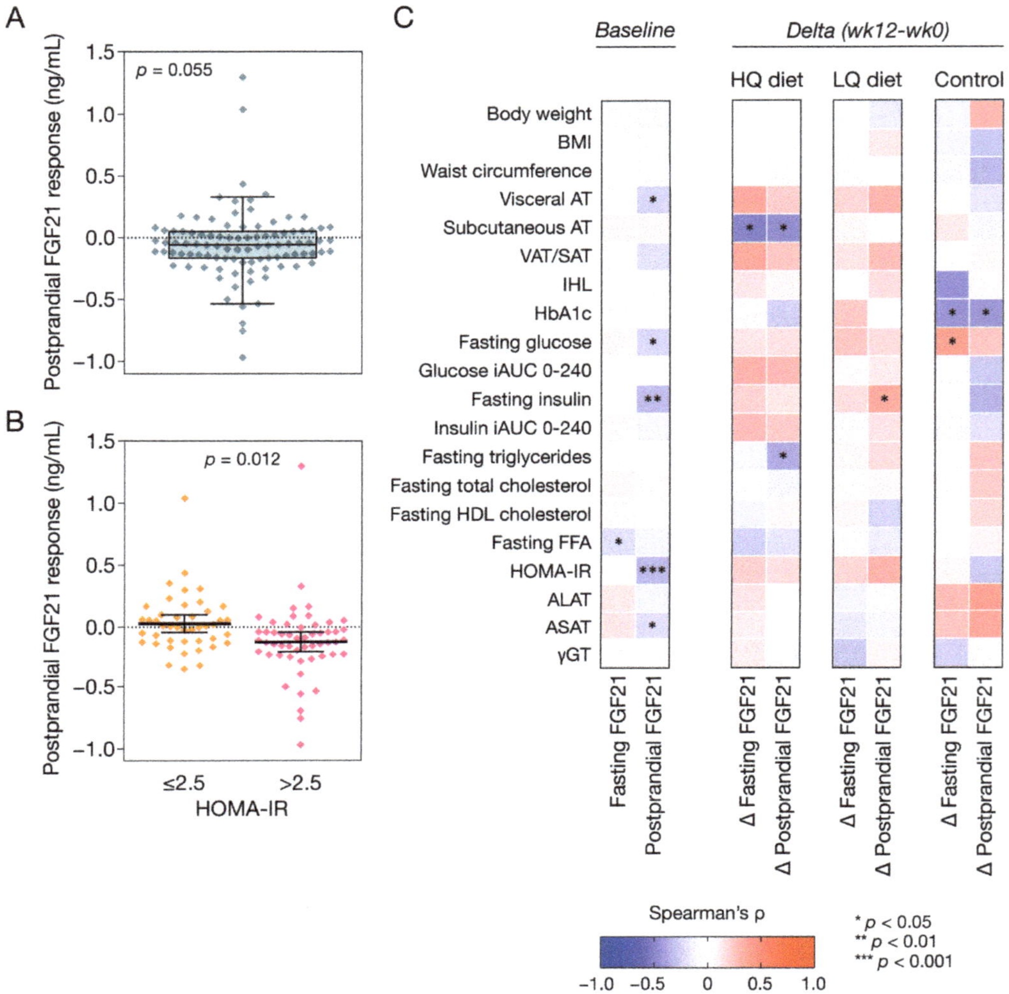

Figure 2. Postprandial FGF21 response at baseline and correlations between plasma FGF21 and markers of metabolic health. (**A**) Box plot with individual data points of the change in plasma FGF21 levels from the fasting state to 120 min after the consumption of the mixed meal in the complete population at baseline ($p = 0.055$, as tested using a paired-samples T-test). The box plot represents the 5th percentile, first quartile, median, third quartile, and 95th percentile. (**B**) Individual postprandial FGF21 responses according to baseline HOMA-IR: ≤ 2.5 or >2.5 ($p = 0.012$ for the difference between groups, as tested with ANCOVA, adjusted for fasting FGF21, age, gender, and BMI. (**C**) Spearman correlations between fasting FGF21 and the postprandial FGF21 response with cardiometabolic parameters at baseline (left) and in response to a 12-week intervention (right). Abbreviations: BMI, body mass index; AT, adipose tissue; IHL, intra-hepatic lipid content; HbA1c, glycated hemoglobin A1c; iAUC, incremental area under the curve; HDL, high-density lipoprotein; HOMA-IR, homeostatic model assessment of insulin resistance; ALAT, aminotransferase; ASAT, aspartate aminotransferase; γGT, gamma-glutamyl transferase.

3.3. Plasma FGF21 and Correlations with Markers of Metabolic Health

At baseline, fasting plasma FGF21 concentrations were inversely correlated to plasma FFA ($\rho = -0.22$, $p = 0.03$), and not correlated to BMI, IHL, HOMA-IR or any of the other assessed cardiometabolic parameters (Figure 2C and Figure S1; Table S1). The change in plasma FGF21 from the fasting state to 120 min postprandially was inversely correlated to fasting plasma glucose, fasting insulin, HOMA-IR, VAT and ASAT ($\rho = -0.34$ to -0.23, all $p < 0.05$), but did not correlate with IHL or the postprandial response of plasma glucose or insulin (Figure 2C and Figure S1; Table S1). Exclusion of outliers attenuated the inverse correlations of the postprandial FGF21 response with plasma glucose ($\rho = -0.19$, $p = 0.069$) and ASAT ($\rho = -0.20$, $p = 0.051$), annulled the correlation with VAT ($\rho = -0.18$, $p = 0.14$), and did not affect the other correlations.

To further explore the relationship between the postprandial FGF21 response and HOMA-IR, we stratified the total study population into insulin-sensitive ($n = 44$) and insulin-resistant ($n = 53$) subjects based on HOMA-IR ≤ 2.5 and >2.5 [38]. In insulin sensitive subjects, FGF21 did not change from fasting to 120 min postprandially, while in insulin resistant subjects, FGF21 declined 120 min after consumption of the mixed meal, also after adjustment for fasting FGF21, age, gender, and BMI ($\Delta -0.03$ ng/ml, 95% CI -0.06 to 0.11 vs. $\Delta -0.13$ ng/ml, 95% CI -0.20 to -0.05; $p = 0.012$) (Figure 2B). Exclusion of outliers ($p = 0.007$) or additional adjustment for NAFLD status (IHL $\leq 5.56\%$ or $> 5.56\%$ [39]) or IHL did not affect this result ($p = 0.013$ and $p = 0.018$, respectively).

Next to testing correlations at baseline, we also explored correlations between the change in fasting and postprandial FGF21 response and change in markers of metabolic health. In the high-nutrient-quality diet group, change in both fasting FGF21 and the postprandial FGF21 response upon the 12 weeks of intervention was inversely correlated to the reduction in abdominal SAT ($\rho = -0.49$, $p = 0.012$; $\rho = -0.45$, $p = 0.023$, respectively) (Figure 2C; Tables S2 and S3). Furthermore, in the high-nutrient-quality diet group, the change in postprandial FGF21 response was inversely correlated to the reduction in fasting plasma triglycerides ($\rho = -0.36$, $p = 0.041$) (Figure 2C; Table S3). In the low-nutrient-quality diet, the change in postprandial FGF21 response was positively correlated to the reduction in fasting insulin levels ($\rho = 0.35$, $p = 0.034$) (Figure 2C; Table S3). In the control group, changes in both fasting and postprandial FGF21 response were inversely correlated to change in HbA1c, and change in fasting FGF21 levels was positively correlated to change in fasting glucose levels (Figure 2C; Table S3). These latter three correlations, however, were driven by data points from two participants, and exclusion of these data points resulted in a loss of significant correlations ($\rho = -0.30$ to 0.25, $p > 0.13$).

Exclusion of outliers resulted in positive correlations between the change in fasting FGF21 and the change in fasting insulin, iAUC insulin, and HOMA-IR in the high-nutrient-quality diet group ($\rho = 0.36$ to 0.51, all $p < 0.05$). In addition, exclusion of outliers attenuated the inverse correlation between the change in postprandial FGF21 response and change in fasting plasma triglycerides in the high-nutrient-quality diet group ($\rho = -0.31$, $p = 0.097$), annulled the positive correlation between change in postprandial FGF21 response and change in fasting insulin in the low-nutrient-quality diet group ($\rho = 0.27$, $p = 0.11$), and did not affect the other correlations.

3.4. Plasma FGF21 and Habitual (Macro)Nutrient Intake and Sweet-Taste Preference

Since FGF21 has been linked to (macro)nutrient intake and preference, we compared fasting plasma FGF21 levels between tertiles of habitual nutrient intake, alcohol consumption, and sweet-taste preference. Fasting FGF21 levels were lower in individuals in the highest tertile of habitual polysaccharide intake compared to individuals in lower tertiles of polysaccharide intake (overall $p = 0.022$; tertile 3 vs. tertile 1, $p = 0.035$; tertile 3 vs. tertile 2, $p = 0.009$; Figure 3C). FGF21 levels did not differ between individuals in tertiles of habitual intake of carbohydrates, protein, fat, mono- and disaccharides (sugars), or alcohol consumption (Figure 3). In addition, plasma FGF21 levels did not differ according to sweet-taste preference (Figure 3G). The ranges and means of the tertiles of habitual nutrient intake, alcohol consumption, and sweet-taste preference are reported in Table S4. Exclusion of outliers attenuated the differences in fasting FGF21, according to habitual polysaccharide intake (overall $p = 0.098$; tertile 3 vs. tertile 1, $p = 0.066$; tertile 3 vs. tertile 2, $p = 0.063$).

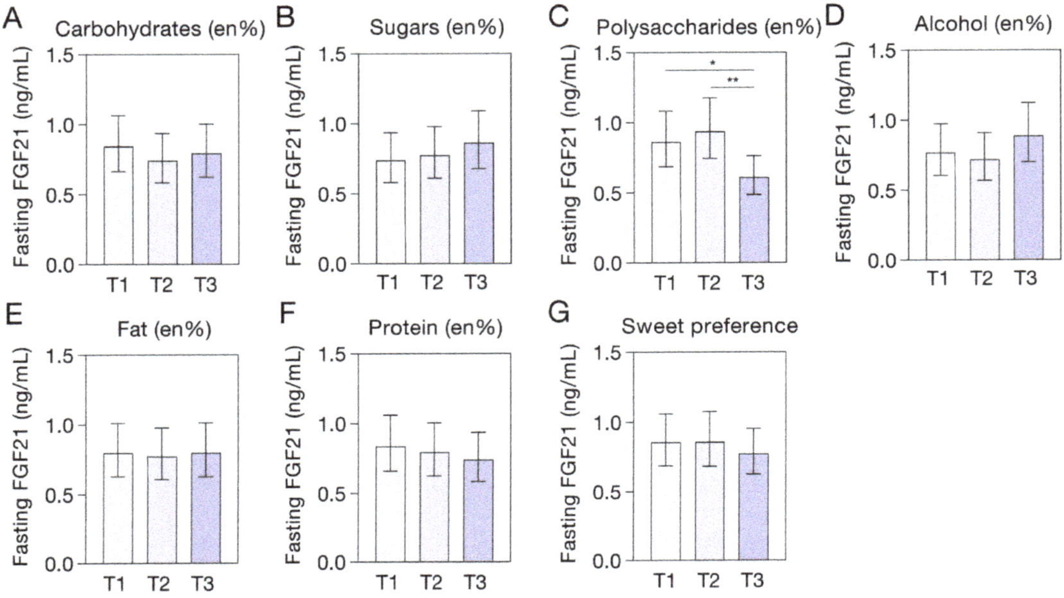

Figure 3. Fasting plasma FGF21 levels (adjusted geometric means with 95% CI) according to tertiles (T1: lowest tertile, T3: highest tertile) of habitual (macro)nutrient intake as % of daily energy intake (en%) (**A–C**,**E**,**F**), habitual alcohol consumption (**D**), and sweet-taste preference (**G**). FGF21 levels were lower in the highest tertile of polysaccharide intake compared to the lower tertiles (overall $p = 0.022$; tested by ANCOVA with adjustment for gender and LSD post-hoc testing; * $p = 0.035$; ** $p = 0.009$) and did not differ between tertiles of other nutrient intakes.

3.5. Baseline Plasma FGF21 and Weight Loss

In an explorative analysis, we examined whether fasting plasma FGF21 and the FGF21 postprandial response at baseline were associated with weight loss after 12 weeks of ER intervention. Fasting plasma FGF21 levels at baseline were not correlated to weight loss in either of the ER groups (HQ: $\rho = -0.01$, $p = 0.96$; LQ: $\rho = -0.27$, $p = 0.10$; HQ and LQ combined: $\rho = -0.08$, $p = 0.50$ Figure 4A). The postprandial change in FGF21 at baseline was borderline positively associated with weight change in the low-nutrient-quality diet group ($\rho = 0.30$, $p = 0.065$) but not in the high-nutrient-quality diet group or in the two groups combined (HQ: $\rho = -0.23$, $p = 0.19$; HQ and LQ combined: $\rho = 0.06$, $p = 0.63$ Figure 4B). Exclusion of outliers resulted in an inverse correlation between fasting FGF21 at baseline and weight loss ($\rho = -0.33$, $p = 0.048$) and attenuated the correlation with the postprandial FGF21 response in the low-nutrient-quality diet group ($\rho = 0.27$, $p = 0.10$).

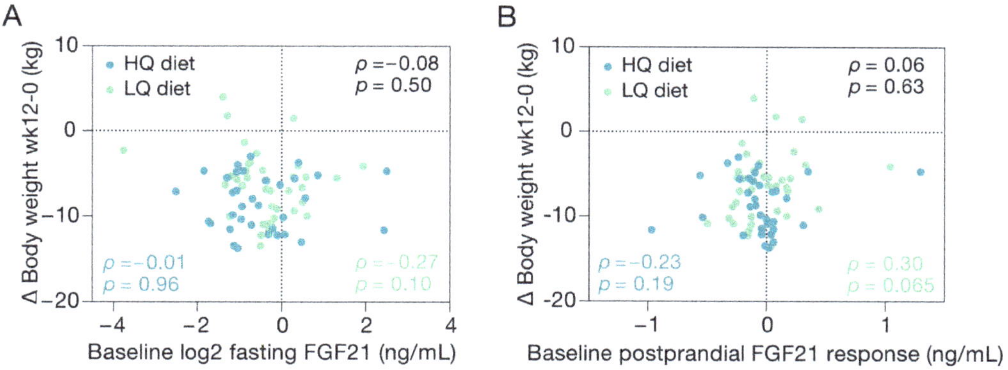

Figure 4. Scatter plots of fasting plasma FGF21 levels (**A**) and the postprandial FGF21 response (**B**) at baseline with weight change after 12 weeks of intervention on the high-nutrient-quality diet (HQ, dark green) and low-nutrient-quality diet (LQ, light green). Correlations were tested using Spearman correlation coefficients (LQ and HQ group combined in black).

4. Discussion

In this study, we investigated the effects of two 12-week energy restriction (ER) diets differing in nutrient quality on fasting and postprandial plasma FGF21 levels, and explored correlations between plasma FGF21 and markers of metabolic health. Neither overall ER nor high vs. low nutrient quality of the ER diets affected circulating fasting or postprandial FGF21 levels. Diet-induced weight loss and liver fat reduction were not accompanied by changes in fasting or postprandial plasma FGF21. Fasting plasma FGF21 was not correlated to markers of metabolic health at baseline, but the postprandial FGF21 response to the mixed meal was inversely correlated to fasting glucose, insulin, HOMA-IR, visceral AT and the liver enzyme ASAT. In addition, we assessed associations between habitual dietary intake and circulating FGF21 levels. Fasting FGF21 levels were lowest in individuals with the highest intake of polysaccharides, but did not differ according to intake of mono- and disaccharides, alcohol consumption, or sweet-taste preference.

Despite substantial weight loss of 7.3 kg on average and concomitant health improvements [32], 12 weeks of 25% energy reduction did not affect fasting FGF21 levels. Previous weight loss trials have reported conflicting findings, with some trials reporting a reduction in fasting FGF21 levels upon diet-induced weight loss [9–13], and others reporting an increase [40] or no effect on circulating FGF21 levels [14–20]. Generally, the studies that report a change in plasma fasting FGF21 were performed in individuals with more severely impaired metabolic health (e.g., T2DM, NAFLD, morbid obesity), who typically have elevated FGF21 levels and thus more room for improvement compared to individuals in this study. In addition, the degree of weight loss, as well as the content and composition of the intervention diets may contribute to disagreement between studies. Weight loss as a result of bariatric surgery, which is commonly larger than weight loss achieved by ER, such as in our study, is also not consistently accompanied by changes in FGF21 levels [41]. It thus seems that weight loss and accompanying health improvements do not consistently affect fasting FGF21 levels.

Although fasting FGF21 levels were not correlated to liver fat or markers of glucose or lipid metabolism at baseline, change in fasting plasma FGF21 levels upon the 12-week intervention was inversely correlated to change in SAT, with larger reductions in SAT being accompanied by an increase in fasting plasma FGF21. In contrast, after the exclusion of five outliers, the reductions in HOMA-IR and both fasting and postprandial plasma insulin upon the intervention were correlated to a decrease in fasting FGF21, indicating that change in fasting FGF21 may be a marker for improvement in insulin sensitivity. These correlations, however, were present only in the high-nutrient-quality diet group, and it is unclear why we did not find similar correlations in the low-nutrient-quality diet group, given that the reductions in SAT, plasma insulin, and HOMA-IR were comparable upon the two ER diets. In addition, excluding participants with deviating values from analysis may lead to bias and therefore, these results should be interpreted with caution.

At baseline, the postprandial FGF21 response was inversely correlated to insulin resistance as estimated by HOMA-IR, with more insulin resistant individuals exhibiting a larger postprandial decline in plasma FGF21 compared to insulin sensitive individuals. Circulating FGF21 levels have previously been reported to modestly decrease for 1 to 4 h after ingestion of meals containing fat, protein, or a combination of macronutrients [13,42–44]. In line with our findings, individuals with T2DM have been reported to have a more pronounced decline in postprandial FGF21 levels after a mixed meal compared to individuals with normal glucose metabolism [13]. These observations suggest that circulating FGF21 concentrations in response to mixed meals may be less well-controlled in impaired metabolic health.

The regulation of fasting and postprandial FGF21 levels in response to different nutrients and nutrient combinations is complex and not fully understood [1,2]. Overall, plasma FGF21 levels appear to display a circadian rhythm, with peak levels during fasting and lower levels during feeding [45]. During fasting, liver-derived FGF21 is primarily regulated by the transcription factor PPARα, and intake of fat, protein or a mixed meal results in diminished PPARα-mediated FGF21 secretion, possibly (partly) via a reduction in plasma FFA levels [15,45,46]. High intake of pure simple sugars or alcohol forms an exception; these nutrients acutely elevate plasma FGF21 [30,47–49], likely via activation of hepatic ChREBP [29,50]. Similar to our findings of a more pronounced postprandial response to a mixed meal in IR, plasma FGF21 excursions after pure fructose or glucose ingestion have been found to be larger in individuals with metabolic syndrome compared to healthy individuals [47]. In addition, the postprandial FGF21 response to fructose has been positively correlated to measures of hepatic and adipose tissue IR [48]. Circulating FGF21 in response to acute nutritional challenges may thus be a marker of metabolic health. Various factors including insulin, glucagon, adiponectin, and FFA appear to be involved in the regulation of FGF21 [1]. Greater FGF21 excursions in response to acute (nutritional) challenges, i.e., poor control of plasma FGF21 levels, in conditions of impaired metabolic health may reflect the disturbed control of the signals that regulate FGF21. Further research into the mechanisms that underlie altered FGF21 dynamics in impaired metabolic health is warranted.

If the postprandial FGF21 response is a marker for metabolic health, it could be expected that the substantial weight loss and concomitant health improvements after 12 weeks of ER in this study would be accompanied by a reduction in the postprandial FGF21 response. We, however, found no effects of the 12-week ER interventions on postprandial FGF21. A trial in individuals with T2DM and morbid obesity did report that weight loss of ~6.5 kg upon a 3-week very-low-calorie diet was accompanied by a less pronounced decline in postprandial in FGF21 levels up to 3 h after a mixed meal [13]. Our null findings may be due to our relatively less metabolically impaired study population and therefore less pronounced health improvements compared to the study in T2DM patients. In addition, we observed great inter-individual variation in the postprandial FGF21 response, with on average a modest decrease in plasma FGF21 levels 120 min after the mixed meal. Still, in approximately one third of the subjects, plasma FGF21 did not change or increased postprandially, which highlights the complexity of plasma FGF21 regulation and the challenge of interpreting plasma FGF21 (dynamics).

Recently, FGF21 levels have been suggested to be predictive of weight loss. We, however, did not find baseline fasting nor postprandial FGF21 concentrations to correlate with weight loss upon 12 weeks of ER. After exclusion of five outliers, we did observe that higher baseline fasting FGF21 was correlated to larger weight loss in the low- and not the high-nutrient-quality diet group, although these results should be interpreted with caution. In the DIETFITS trial, a trial in which 609 overweight or obese adults were randomized to follow a low-fat or low-carbohydrate weight-loss diet for 3 months, higher baseline

FGF21 levels were associated with larger weight loss [21]. The inconsistent findings in our study might be due to limited power. In addition, in the DIETFITS trial, participants were instructed to drastically reduce their carbohydrate or fat intake, while there were no specific instructions regarding caloric intake. As FGF21 has been suggested to regulate energy homeostasis in humans by amongst others decreasing caloric intake [1], the association between baseline FGF21 and weight loss may thus partly result from differences in FGF21-mediated caloric intake. In our study, participants were explicitly instructed and monitored to reduce caloric intake by 25%, which leaves less room for regulation of caloric intake by FGF21.

FGF21 has also been implicated in the regulation of macronutrient intake. We found that individuals with higher habitual intake of polysaccharides had lower fasting FGF21 levels, but we found no associations between FGF21 and sweet-taste preference or habitual intake of mono- and disaccharides. Previously, higher soda consumption has been associated with lower circulating FGF21 [28], and *FGF21* gene variants have been related to higher total carbohydrate intake [24–27]. The only GWAS study that made a distinction between type of carbohydrates [26], however, found that the association between *FGF21* gene variants and carbohydrate intake could be attributed solely to higher intake of mono- and disaccharides and not to higher intake of polysaccharides. Animal studies also indicate that FGF21 regulates intake of mono- and disaccharides specifically [29], so our finding of lower plasma FGF21 levels in individuals with high intake of polysaccharides remains unexplained.

Strengths of this study include its RCT design, with—next to two ER dietary intervention groups—a control group that did not receive dietary advice, which reduces bias and confounding factors. In addition, this study had relatively few drop-outs and compliance to ER was high, as is demonstrated by the substantial weight loss that participants achieved.

This was a secondary analysis of an RCT designed to study effects of ER diets differing in nutrient quality on metabolic health outcomes, and the original sample size calculation was based on the power to detect differences in IHL [32]. Given the large inter-individual variation in plasma FGF21 levels, this study may have been underpowered to detect effects on plasma FGF21. Further large trials are thus needed to confirm our findings. Another limitation may be that we measured total plasma FGF21 protein, rather than bioactive FGF21. In the circulation, FGF21 is rapidly degraded by enzymatic cleavage, rendering it inactive [51]. Measuring bioactive rather than total FGF21 concentrations may be more physiologically relevant. Furthermore, we only measured postprandial FGF21 levels at a single timepoint (2 h after consumption of the mixed meal), and do not know the plasma FGF21 levels in the time between. We, however, expect that plasma FGF21 steadily decreased throughout the 2 h after consumption, since a previous study with more frequent sampling times showed a continuous decline in plasma FGF21 up to 3 h after a mixed meal [13]. Lastly, we did not assess physical activity level and therefore cannot rule out that differences in physical activity level at baseline or follow-up may have affected plasma FGF21 levels, given that exercise modifies circulating FGF21 levels [52]. However, we consider it unlikely that the ER groups differed in physical activity level at baseline or follow-up, because (1) interventions were randomly allocated, (2) participants were unaware of the high-nutrient-quality vs. low-nutrient-quality distinction, and (3) participants were instructed to maintain their habitual physical activity level throughout the study.

5. Conclusions

In conclusion, weight loss and concomitant health improvements upon a 12-week 25% ER diet were not accompanied by changes in fasting or postprandial plasma FGF21 levels in middle-aged individuals with abdominal obesity. Neither overall ER nor nutrient quality affected plasma FGF21. In addition, we found no robust evidence that fasting plasma FGF21 is a marker for metabolic health status. We did find indications that circulating FGF21 dynamics in response to a nutritional challenge may reflect metabolic health status.

FGF21′s metabolic regulation and functions are greatly complex and further research on the potential of circulating FGF21 dynamics as a marker of metabolic health is warranted.

Supplementary Materials: The following supporting information can be downloaded at: https://www.mdpi.com/article/10.3390/nu14235061/s1, Table S1: Correlations between both fasting plasma FGF21 and the postprandial response of plasma FGF21 and markers of metabolic health; Figure S1: Scatter plots of fasting plasma FGF21 and the postprandial plasma FGF21 response upon a liquid high-fit mixed meal with markers of metabolic health; Table S2: Correlations between the change in fasting plasma FGF21 and the change in metabolic health markers upon a 12-week diet; Table S3: Correlations between the change in the postprandial plasma FGF21 response upon a liquid high-fit mixed meal and the change in metabolic health markers upon a 12-week diet; Table S4: Ranges and means of tertiles of habitual nutrient intake, alcohol consumption, and sweet-taste preference.

Author Contributions: Conceptualization and methodology, A.G., S.S., D.E., C.C.J.R.M., E.S., M.M. (Monica Mars), M.M. (Marco Mensink) and L.A.A.; investigation, S.S., D.E. and E.S.; formal analysis, visualization and writing—original draft preparation, A.G.; supervision and writing—review and editing, L.A.A. All authors have read and agreed to the published version of the manuscript.

Funding: This research was funded by the Division of Human Nutrition and Health, Wageningen University, The Netherlands and received no external funding.

Institutional Review Board Statement: The study was conducted in accordance with the Declaration of Helsinki and approved by the Medical Ethics Committee of Wageningen University (protocol code NL44614.081.13, approved on 3 June 2014). The study is registered at ClinicalTrials.gov as NCT02194504.

Informed Consent Statement: Informed consent was obtained from all subjects involved in the study.

Data Availability Statement: Data presented in this manuscript are available upon reasonable request.

Acknowledgments: We thank the volunteers that participated in this study and the Wageningen Belly Fat Study team. We thank Nhien Ly and Lisette van de Lende for technical assistance with the biochemical analyses and Suzanne de Bruijn and Fildzah Karunia Putri for assistance with the food preference ranking test.

Conflicts of Interest: The authors declare no conflict of interest.

References

1. Flippo, K.H.; Potthoff, M.J. Metabolic Messengers: FGF21. *Nat. Metab.* **2021**, *3*, 309–317. [CrossRef] [PubMed]
2. Lewis, J.E.; Ebling, F.J.P.; Samms, R.J.; Tsintzas, K. Going Back to the Biology of FGF21: New Insights. *Trends Endocrinol. Metab.* **2019**, *30*, 491–504. [CrossRef]
3. Chavez, A.O.; Molina-Carrion, M.; Abdul-Ghani, M.A.; Folli, F.; Defronzo, R.A.; Tripathy, D. Circulating fibroblast growth factor-21 is elevated in impaired glucose tolerance and type 2 diabetes and correlates with muscle and hepatic insulin resistance. *Diabetes Care* **2009**, *32*, 1542–1546. [CrossRef] [PubMed]
4. Dushay, J.; Chui, P.C.; Gopalakrishnan, G.S.; Varela-Rey, M.; Crawley, M.; Fisher, F.M.; Badman, M.K.; Martinez-Chantar, M.L.; Maratos-Flier, E. Increased fibroblast growth factor 21 in obesity and nonalcoholic fatty liver disease. *Gastroenterology* **2010**, *139*, 456–463. [CrossRef]
5. Kralisch, S.; Tönjes, A.; Krause, K.; Richter, J.; Lossner, U.; Kovacs, P.; Ebert, T.; Blüher, M.; Stumvoll, M.; Fasshauer, M. Fibroblast growth factor-21 serum concentrations are associated with metabolic and hepatic markers in humans. *J. Endocrinol.* **2013**, *216*, 135–143. [CrossRef] [PubMed]
6. Zhang, X.; Yeung, D.C.; Karpisek, M.; Stejskal, D.; Zhou, Z.G.; Liu, F.; Wong, R.L.; Chow, W.S.; Tso, A.W.; Lam, K.S.; et al. Serum FGF21 levels are increased in obesity and are independently associated with the metabolic syndrome in humans. *Diabetes* **2008**, *57*, 1246–1253. [CrossRef] [PubMed]
7. Bobbert, T.; Schwarz, F.; Fischer-Rosinsky, A.; Pfeiffer, A.F.; Möhlig, M.; Mai, K.; Spranger, J. Fibroblast growth factor 21 predicts the metabolic syndrome and type 2 diabetes in Caucasians. *Diabetes Care* **2013**, *36*, 145–149. [CrossRef]
8. Ong, K.L.; McClelland, R.L.; Allison, M.A.; Kokkinos, J.; Wu, B.J.; Barter, P.J.; Rye, K.A. Association of elevated circulating fibroblast growth factor 21 levels with prevalent and incident metabolic syndrome: The Multi-Ethnic Study of Atherosclerosis. *Atherosclerosis* **2019**, *281*, 200–206. [CrossRef]

9. Crujeiras, A.B.; Gomez-Arbelaez, D.; Zulet, M.A.; Carreira, M.C.; Sajoux, I.; de Luis, D.; Castro, A.I.; Baltar, J.; Baamonde, I.; Sueiro, A.; et al. Plasma FGF21 levels in obese patients undergoing energy-restricted diets or bariatric surgery: A marker of metabolic stress? *Int. J. Obes.* **2017**, *41*, 1570–1578. [CrossRef]

0. Gómez-Ambrosi, J.; Gallego-Escuredo, J.M.; Catalán, V.; Rodríguez, A.; Domingo, P.; Moncada, R.; Valentí, V.; Salvador, J.; Giralt, M.; Villarroya, F.; et al. FGF19 and FGF21 serum concentrations in human obesity and type 2 diabetes behave differently after diet- or surgically-induced weight loss. *Clin. Nutr.* **2017**, *36*, 861–868. [CrossRef]

1. Melhem, S.; Steven, S.; Taylor, R.; Al-Mrabeh, A. Effect of Weight Loss by Low-Calorie Diet on Cardiovascular Health in Type 2 Diabetes: An Interventional Cohort Study. *Nutrients* **2021**, *13*, 1465. [CrossRef]

2. Watanabe, M.; Risi, R.; Camajani, E.; Contini, S.; Persichetti, A.; Tuccinardi, D.; Ernesti, I.; Mariani, S.; Lubrano, C.; Genco, A.; et al. Baseline HOMA IR and Circulating FGF21 Levels Predict NAFLD Improvement in Patients Undergoing a Low Carbohydrate Dietary Intervention for Weight Loss: A Prospective Observational Pilot Study. *Nutrients* **2020**, *12*, 2141. [CrossRef]

3. Lips, M.A.; de Groot, G.H.; Berends, F.J.; Wiezer, R.; van Wagensveld, B.A.; Swank, D.J.; Luijten, A.; van Dijk, K.W.; Pijl, H.; Jansen, P.L.M.; et al. Calorie restriction and Roux-en-Y gastric bypass have opposing effects on circulating FGF21 in morbidly obese subjects. *Clin. Endocrinol.* **2014**, *81*, 862–870. [CrossRef] [PubMed]

4. Headland, M.L.; Clifton, P.M.; Keogh, J.B. Effects of Weight Loss on FGF-21 in Human Subjects: An Exploratory Study. *Int. J. Environ. Res. Public Health* **2019**, *16*, 4877. [CrossRef] [PubMed]

5. Mai, K.; Schwarz, F.; Bobbert, T.; Andres, J.; Assmann, A.; Pfeiffer, A.F.; Spranger, J. Relation between fibroblast growth factor-21, adiposity, metabolism, and weight reduction. *Metabolism* **2011**, *60*, 306–311. [CrossRef] [PubMed]

6. Telgenkamp, I.; Kusters, Y.; Schalkwijk, C.G.; Houben, A.; Kooi, M.E.; Lindeboom, L.; Bons, J.A.P.; Schaper, N.C.; Joris, P.J.; Plat, J.; et al. Contribution of Liver Fat to Weight Loss-Induced Changes in Serum Hepatokines: A Randomized Controlled Trial. *J. Clin. Endocrinol. Metab.* **2019**, *104*, 2719–2727. [CrossRef] [PubMed]

7. Tok, Ö.; Kişioğlu, S.V.; Ersöz, H.; Kahveci, B.; Göktaş, Z. Effects of increased physical activity and/or weight loss diet on serum myokine and adipokine levels in overweight adults with impaired glucose metabolism. *J. Diabetes Complicat.* **2021**, *35*, 107892. [CrossRef]

8. Xu, C.; Markova, M.; Seebeck, N.; Loft, A.; Hornemann, S.; Gantert, T.; Kabisch, S.; Herz, K.; Loske, J.; Ost, M.; et al. High-protein diet more effectively reduces hepatic fat than low-protein diet despite lower autophagy and FGF21 levels. *Liver Int.* **2020**, *40*, 2982–2997. [CrossRef]

9. Asghari, S.; Rezaei, M.; Rafraf, M.; Taghizadeh, M.; Asghari-Jafarabadi, M.; Ebadi, M. Effects of Calorie Restricted Diet on Oxidative/Antioxidative Status Biomarkers and Serum Fibroblast Growth Factor 21 Levels in Nonalcoholic Fatty Liver Disease Patients: A Randomized, Controlled Clinical Trial. *Nutrients* **2022**, *14*, 2509. [CrossRef]

0. Heinitz, S.; Hollstein, T.; Ando, T.; Walter, M.; Basolo, A.; Krakoff, J.; Votruba, S.B.; Piaggi, P. Early adaptive thermogenesis is a determinant of weight loss after six weeks of caloric restriction in overweight subjects. *Metabolism* **2020**, *110*, 154303. [CrossRef]

1. Figarska, S.M.; Rigdon, J.; Ganna, A.; Elmståhl, S.; Lind, L.; Gardner, C.D.; Ingelsson, E. Proteomic profiles before and during weight loss: Results from randomized trial of dietary intervention. *Sci. Rep.* **2020**, *10*, 7913. [CrossRef]

2. Heinitz, S.; Piaggi, P.; Yang, S.; Bonfiglio, S.; Steel, J.; Krakoff, J.; Votruba, S.B. Response of skeletal muscle UCP2-expression during metabolic adaptation to caloric restriction. *Int. J. Obes.* **2018**, *42*, 974–984. [CrossRef] [PubMed]

3. Vinales, K.L.; Begaye, B.; Bogardus, C.; Walter, M.; Krakoff, J.; Piaggi, P. FGF21 Is a Hormonal Mediator of the Human "Thrifty" Metabolic Phenotype. *Diabetes* **2019**, *68*, 318–323. [CrossRef] [PubMed]

4. Chu, A.Y.; Workalemahu, T.; Paynter, N.P.; Rose, L.M.; Giulianini, F.; Tanaka, T.; Ngwa, J.S.; Qi, Q.; Curhan, G.C.; Rimm, E.B.; et al. Novel locus including FGF21 is associated with dietary macronutrient intake. *Hum. Mol. Genet.* **2013**, *22*, 1895–1902. [CrossRef] [PubMed]

5. Frayling, T.M.; Beaumont, R.N.; Jones, S.E.; Yaghootkar, H.; Tuke, M.A.; Ruth, K.S.; Casanova, F.; West, B.; Locke, J.; Sharp, S.; et al. A Common Allele in FGF21 Associated with Sugar Intake Is Associated with Body Shape, Lower Total Body-Fat Percentage, and Higher Blood Pressure. *Cell Rep.* **2018**, *23*, 327–336. [CrossRef] [PubMed]

6. Søberg, S.; Sandholt, C.H.; Jespersen, N.Z.; Toft, U.; Madsen, A.L.; von Holstein-Rathlou, S.; Grevengoed, T.J.; Christensen, K.B.; Bredie, W.L.P.; Potthoff, M.J.; et al. FGF21 Is a Sugar-Induced Hormone Associated with Sweet Intake and Preference in Humans. *Cell Metab.* **2017**, *25*, 1045–1053.e6. [CrossRef] [PubMed]

7. Tanaka, T.; Ngwa, J.S.; van Rooij, F.J.; Zillikens, M.C.; Wojczynski, M.K.; Frazier-Wood, A.C.; Houston, D.K.; Kanoni, S.; Lemaitre, R.N.; Luan, J.; et al. Genome-wide meta-analysis of observational studies shows common genetic variants associated with macronutrient intake. *Am. J. Clin. Nutr.* **2013**, *97*, 1395–1402. [CrossRef]

8. Basolo, A.; Hollstein, T.; Shah, M.H.; Walter, M.; Krakoff, J.; Votruba, S.B.; Piaggi, P. Higher fasting plasma FGF21 concentration is associated with lower ad libitum soda consumption in humans. *Am. J. Clin. Nutr.* **2021**, *114*, 1518–1522. [CrossRef]

9. von Holstein-Rathlou, S.; BonDurant, L.D.; Peltekian, L.; Naber, M.C.; Yin, T.C.; Claflin, K.E.; Urizar, A.I.; Madsen, A.N.; Ratner, C.; Holst, B.; et al. FGF21 Mediates Endocrine Control of Simple Sugar Intake and Sweet Taste Preference by the Liver. *Cell Metab.* **2016**, *23*, 335–343. [CrossRef]

0. Søberg, S.; Andersen, E.S.; Dalsgaard, N.B.; Jarlhelt, I.; Hansen, N.L.; Hoffmann, N.; Vilsbøll, T.; Chenchar, A.; Jensen, M.; Grevengoed, T.J.; et al. FGF21, a liver hormone that inhibits alcohol intake in mice, increases in human circulation after acute alcohol ingestion and sustained binge drinking at Oktoberfest. *Mol. Metab.* **2018**, *11*, 96–103. [CrossRef]

31. Talukdar, S.; Owen, B.M.; Song, P.; Hernandez, G.; Zhang, Y.; Zhou, Y.; Scott, W.T.; Paratala, B.; Turner, T.; Smith, A.; et al. FGF21 Regulates Sweet and Alcohol Preference. *Cell Metab.* **2016**, *23*, 344–349. [CrossRef] [PubMed]
32. Schutte, S.; Esser, D.; Siebelink, E.; Michielsen, C.J.R.; Daanje, M.; Matualatupauw, J.C.; Boshuizen, H.C.; Mensink, M.; Afman, L.A.; Wageningen Belly Fat Study team. Diverging metabolic effects of 2 energy-restricted diets differing in nutrient quality: A 12-week randomized controlled trial in subjects with abdominal obesity. *Am. J. Clin. Nutr.* **2022**, *116*, 132–150. [CrossRef] [PubMed]
33. Matthews, D.R.; Hosker, J.P.; Rudenski, A.S.; Naylor, B.A.; Treacher, D.F.; Turner, R.C. Homeostasis model assessment: Insulin resistance and β-cell function from fasting plasma glucose and insulin concentrations in man. *Diabetologia* **1985**, *28*, 412–419. [CrossRef] [PubMed]
34. Gayoso-Diz, P.; Otero-Gonzalez, A.; Rodriguez-Alvarez, M.X.; Gude, F.; Cadarso-Suarez, C.; García, F.; De Francisco, A. Insulin resistance index (HOMA-IR) levels in a general adult population: Curves percentile by gender and age. The EPIRCE study. *Diabetes Res. Clin. Pract.* **2011**, *94*, 146–155. [CrossRef]
35. Szczepaniak, L.S.; Nurenberg, P.; Leonard, D.; Browning, J.D.; Reingold, J.S.; Grundy, S.; Hobbs, H.H.; Dobbins, R.L. Magnetic resonance spectroscopy to measure hepatic triglyceride content: Prevalence of hepatic steatosis in the general population. *Am. J. Physiol. Endocrinol.* **2005**, *288*, E462–E468. [CrossRef]
36. Positano, V.; Gastaldelli, A.; Sironi, A.m.; Santarelli, M.F.; Lombardi, M.; Landini, L. An accurate and robust method for unsupervised assessment of abdominal fat by MRI. *J. Magn. Reson. Imaging* **2004**, *20*, 684–689. [CrossRef]
37. Trijsburg, L.; de Vries, J.H.; Boshuizen, H.C.; Hulshof, P.J.; Hollman, P.C.; van't Veer, P.; Geelen, A. Comparison of duplicate portion and 24 h recall as reference methods for validating a FFQ using urinary markers as the estimate of true intake. *Br. J. Nutr.* **2015**, *114*, 1304–1312. [CrossRef] [PubMed]
38. Streppel, M.T.; de Vries, J.H.; Meijboom, S.; Beekman, M.; de Craen, A.J.; Slagboom, P.E.; Feskens, E.J. Relative validity of the food frequency questionnaire used to assess dietary intake in the Leiden Longevity Study. *Nutr. J.* **2013**, *12*, 75. [CrossRef]
39. de Bruijn, S.E.M.; de Vries, Y.C.; de Graaf, C.; Boesveldt, S.; Jager, G. The reliability and validity of the Macronutrient and Taste Preference Ranking Task: A new method to measure food preferences. *Food Qual. Prefer.* **2017**, *57*, 32–40. [CrossRef]
40. Mraz, M.; Bartlova, M.; Lacinova, Z.; Michalsky, D.; Kasalicky, M.; Haluzikova, D.; Matoulek, M.; Dostalova, I.; Humenanska, V.; Haluzik, M. Serum concentrations and tissue expression of a novel endocrine regulator fibroblast growth factor-21 in patients with type 2 diabetes and obesity. *Clin. Endocrinol.* **2009**, *71*, 369–375. [CrossRef]
41. Hosseinzadeh, A.; Roever, L.; Alizadeh, S. Surgery-Induced Weight Loss and Changes in Hormonally Active Fibroblast Growth Factors: A Systematic Review and Meta-Analysis. *Obes. Surg.* **2020**, *30*, 4046–4060. [CrossRef]
42. Herpich, C.; Haß, U.; Kochlik, B.; Franz, K.; Laeger, T.; Klaus, S.; Bosy-Westphal, A.; Norman, K. Postprandial dynamics and response of fibroblast growth factor 21 in older adults. *Clin. Nutr.* **2021**, *40*, 3765–3771. [CrossRef] [PubMed]
43. Schmid, A.; Leszczak, S.; Ober, I.; Karrasch, T.; Schäffler, A. Short-term and divergent regulation of FGF-19 and FGF-21 during oral lipid tolerance test but not oral glucose tolerance test. *Exp. Clin. Endocrinol. Diabetes.* **2015**, *123*, 88–94. [CrossRef] [PubMed]
44. Matikainen, N.; Taskinen, M.R.; Stennabb, S.; Lundbom, N.; Hakkarainen, A.; Vaaralahti, K.; Raivio, T. Decrease in circulating fibroblast growth factor 21 after an oral fat load is related to postprandial triglyceride-rich lipoproteins and liver fat. *Eur. J. Endocrinol.* **2012**, *166*, 487–492. [CrossRef]
45. Yu, H.; Xia, F.; Lam, K.S.; Wang, Y.; Bao, Y.; Zhang, J.; Gu, Y.; Zhou, P.; Lu, J.; Jia, W.; et al. Circadian rhythm of circulating fibroblast growth factor 21 is related to diurnal changes in fatty acids in humans. *Clin. Chem.* **2011**, *57*, 691–700. [CrossRef] [PubMed]
46. Oishi, K.; Konishi, M.; Murata, Y.; Itoh, N. Time-imposed daily restricted feeding induces rhythmic expression of Fgf21 in white adipose tissue of mice. *Biochem. Biophys. Res. Commun.* **2011**, *412*, 396–400. [CrossRef]
47. Dushay, J.R.; Toschi, E.; Mitten, E.K.; Fisher, F.M.; Herman, M.A.; Maratos-Flier, E. Fructose ingestion acutely stimulates circulating FGF21 levels in humans. *Mol. Metab.* **2015**, *4*, 51–57. [CrossRef]
48. ter Horst, K.W.; Gilijamse, P.W.; Demirkiran, A.; van Wagensveld, B.A.; Ackermans, M.T.; Verheij, J.; Romijn, J.A.; Nieuwdorp, M.; Maratos-Flier, E.; Herman, M.A.; et al. The FGF21 response to fructose predicts metabolic health and persists after bariatric surgery in obese humans. *Mol. Metab.* **2017**, *6*, 1493–1502. [CrossRef]
49. Vienberg, S.G.; Jacobsen, S.H.; Worm, D.; Hvolris, L.E.; Naver, L.; Almdal, T.; Hansen, D.L.; Wulff, B.S.; Clausen, T.R.; Madsbad, S.; et al. Increased glucose-stimulated FGF21 response to oral glucose in obese nondiabetic subjects after Roux-en-Y gastric bypass. *Clin. Endocrinol.* **2017**, *86*, 156–159. [CrossRef]
50. Iroz, A.; Montagner, A.; Benhamed, F.; Levavasseur, F.; Polizzi, A.; Anthony, E.; Régnier, M.; Fouché, E.; Lukowicz, C.; Cauzac, M.; et al. A Specific ChREBP and PPARα Cross-Talk Is Required for the Glucose-Mediated FGF21 Response. *Cell Rep.* **2017**, *21*, 403–416. [CrossRef]
51. Coppage, A.L.; Heard, K.R.; DiMare, M.T.; Liu, Y.; Wu, W.; Lai, J.H.; Bachovchin, W.W. Human FGF-21 Is a Substrate of Fibroblast Activation Protein. *PLoS ONE* **2016**, *11*, e0151269. [CrossRef] [PubMed]
52. Cuevas-Ramos, D.; Almeda-Valdés, P.; Meza-Arana, C.E.; Brito-Córdova, G.; Gómez-Pérez, F.J.; Mehta, R.; Oseguera-Moguel, J.; Aguilar-Salinas, C.A. Exercise Increases Serum Fibroblast Growth Factor 21 (FGF21) Levels. *PLoS ONE* **2012**, *7*, e38022. [CrossRef] [PubMed]

nutrients

MDPI

Article

Health Determinants Associated with the Mediterranean Diet: A Cross-Sectional Study

Nadia San Onofre Bernat [1,*], Joan Quiles i Izquierdo [2] and Eva María Trescastro-López [3]

1 Department of Community Nursing, Preventive Medicine and Public Health and History of Science, University of Alicante, 03690 Alicante, Spain
2 General Directorate of Public Health and Addictions, Department of Universal Health and Public Health, Generalitat Valenciana, Biomedical Research Consortium in Epidemiology and Public Health Network, 46021 Valencia, Spain
3 Grupo Balmis de Investigación en Historia de la Ciencia, Cuidados en Salud y Alimentación, 03690 Alicante, Spain
* Correspondence: sanonofre.nadia@gmail.com

Abstract: Introduction: The Mediterranean diet (MD) has been shown to be a good tool for the prevention of obesity and other chronic noncommunicable diseases (NCDs) and to have a low environmental impact. The aim of the present study was to evaluate the relationship between declared morbidity, lifestyles and other sociodemographic factors with high adherence to the MD (AMD) in an adult population in southeastern Spain. Material and Methods: We conducted a cross-sectional study of a sample (n = 2728) representative of a non-institutionalized population $\geq$16 years. The data corresponded to the 2010-11 Nutrition Survey of the Valencian Community. The AMD was assessed using the Mediterranean Diet Adherence Screener questionnaire. The association of variables and high AMD was assessed by univariate and multivariate logistic regression determining crude and adjusted odds ratios. Results: Multivariate analysis showed that age 45 years or older, living with a partner, eating between meals, and not smoking were associated with high AMD. The age groups 45–64 years and 65 years or older showed the strongest association with high AMD in both sexes. Conclusion: The investigation showed a generational loss of AMD. People older than 45 years and living in company are more likely to adhere to DM, the risk group being young people living alone and smokers.

Keywords: Mediterranean diet; lifestyles; health; chronic noncommunicable diseases; obesity

1. Introduction

In recent years, the Spanish population has undergone significant changes in lifestyles and, in particular, in diet, which can have a negative influence on people's state of health [1]. These changes have resulted in an increase in the rates of overweight, obesity and chronic noncommunicable diseases (NCDs), which have become an important challenge for public health as they reduce the quality of life of the people who suffer from them, as well as that of their families, and lead to an increase in healthcare expenditure [1]. On the other hand, the obesogenic environments in which the current population live have favored the development of obesity by stimulating unhealthy habits or behaviors [2,3].

For these reasons, to reduce the risk factors associated with NCDs, such as overweight and obesity, emphasis should be placed on the promotion of healthy diets, physical activity, smoking cessation, protection against alcohol consumption, as well as support for effective interventions aimed at changing environments so that the healthiest options are also the easiest [4,5]. In this contextual framework, the Mediterranean diet (MD) is presented as a healthy dietary model capable of guaranteeing adequate nutrient intake, preventing and reducing complications associated with NCDs, regulating body weight, and having a low environmental impact [6–9]. At present, numerous studies suggest that adherence to the Mediterranean Diet (AMD) plays an important role in the primary and secondary prevention of cardiovascular diseases (CVD), in addition to improving health in people with various pathologies [10]. Although it has been shown that AMD can vary according to socioeconomic characteristics of the population, as well as other determinants of health [11–14]; it is of interest to know the factors that may affect the level of adherence to this dietary pattern in a population in order to be able to carry out equitable actions that facilitate high AMD and better health for all.

For these reasons, the study of adherence to the Mediterranean dietary pattern may be relevant for public health, both in the promotion of healthy lifestyles and in the prevention of chronic diseases and obesity.

The aim of the present study was to evaluate the relationship between declared morbidity, lifestyles and other sociodemographic factors with high AMD in a sample of the adult population of southeastern Spain.

2. Materials and Methods

Description of the study: We conducted a cross-sectional population-based study of a representative sample of the adult population (16 years of age or older). The population and intake data used came from the Nutrition Survey of the Valencian Community 2010–2011 (ENCV2010-11) [15], which collects epidemiological data on the non-institutionalized population of southeastern Spain. In the ENCV2010-11, a random cluster sampling was performed, proportional to provincial demarcation and stratified by age and sex groups. The Population Information System of the Conselleria de Sanidad Universal y Salud Pública (Regional Ministry of Universal Health and Public Health) was used as the sampling frame, and the universe was the population residing in southeastern Spain over 6 years of age. The ENCV2010-11 worked with 4500 people, and the final participation rate was 68.9% (3102 individuals). The aim of the ENCV2010-11 was to find out what the eating habits of the children and adult population of southeastern Spain were and how they were related to their state of health.

For the present study, we selected all records corresponding to persons between 16 and 95 years of age who had completed the main questionnaire and the food consumption frequency questionnaire (CFQ) of the ENCV2010-11. The sample used for the analyses consisted of 2728 records corresponding to 1311 men and 1417 women.

Assessment of the AMD: To assess the AMD, the data available in the CFQ (of 142 items) of the origin survey (ENCV2010-11) were adapted to the Mediterranean Diet Adherence Screener (MEDAS) questionnaire [16,17] by converting the food consumption frequencies declared in the CFQ, expressing the results as daily servings. The conversion factors used for each category were standardized by consumption of servings per day, using the following values: less than 1 time per month (0.02 servings/day); less than 1 time per week (0.07 servings/day); 1 time per week (0.14 servings/day); 3 times per week (0.43 servings/day); between 4 and 6 times per week (0.79 servings/day); 1 time per day (1 serving/day).

In order to be able to answer all the questions in the MEDAS questionnaire, some adaptations had to be made, as was the case with the item "sofrito", which was not included in the CFQ of the ENCV2010-1. For the assessment of the item "traditional tomato sauce" (sofrito) that appears in the MEDAS questionnaire, we proceeded to adapt the variables of the CFQ used, making use of the data on the intake of onion, spring onion, garlic and fried tomato sauce reflected in the CFQ.

Each item of the MEDAS questionnaire was assigned a value of 0 if the condition was not met or a value of 1 if it was met. The criteria followed to assign a value of 1 to each item were as follows: using olive oil as the main fat; eating at least 4 tablespoons ($\geq$60 g) of olive oil throughout the day; eat at least 2 servings ($\geq$300 g) of vegetables per day; eat at least 3 servings ($\geq$360 g) of fruit per day; eat less than 1 serving (<125 g) of red meat and hamburger per day; eat less than 1 serving (<12.5 g) of butter per day; drink less than 1 serving (<250 mL) of sweetened or carbonated beverages per day; drink 7 servings

(700 mL) of wine per week or more; eat at least 3 servings (≥240 g raw or 600 g if cooked) of pulses per week; eat at least 3 servings (≥450 g) of fish per week; eat no more than 3 servings (≤150 g) per week of industrial bakery products; eat at least 3 servings (≥90 g) of nuts per week; preferably consuming more white meat than red meat; eating pasta, vegetables, rice or other dishes with soffit at least 2 times per week. Cases that did not meet these conditions were assigned a value of 0.

To estimate the degree of AMD, a sum of the score obtained in each question was made. The possible range of scores ranged from 0 to 14 points, being 0 when no condition defined in the Mediterranean dietary pattern was met and 14 when all conditions were met (14). This allowed the population to be classified into three groups according to the degree of AMD. Scores between 0–5 formed the "low adherence" group, between 6–9 "medium adherence", and scores between 10 and 14 (both included) made up the group of "high adherence" to DM [17].

For the analyses on the association between AMD and declared morbidity, lifestyles and sociodemographic factors, the population was classified into two groups according to the level of AMD (scores of 0 to 9 formed the "low-medium AMD" group, and scores of 10 to 14 formed the "high AMD" group), which allowed us to perform binomial logistic regressions.

Study variables: The variables and categories used for the analyses were as follows: sex (male or female); age groups (16–24 years, 25–44 years, 45–64 years, ≥65 years); country of birth (Spain or others); educational level (no education, primary education, secondary education or higher education); employment status (with full-time or part-time paid work or without paid work which in turn included unemployed persons, students, retired, permanently disabled, engaged in housework and other kinds of economic activity); living with a partner (yes or no); perception of health (good health, which in turn included the responses very good, good and acceptable and bad health which included bad and very bad); leisure-time physical activity (little or none or several times a week) [18]; sedentary behavior (<2 h/day or ≥2 h/day); hours of screen time per day of television, computer and Internet (>2 h/day or ≤2 h/day) [19]; smoking (yes, no or ex-smokers); snacking between hours (yes or no), alcohol consumption (no consumption–low-risk consumption, risk consumption or harmful consumption) [20], arterial hypertension (AHT) (yes or no), myocardial infarction (yes or no), neurological diseases (yes, no) hypercholesterolemia (yes or no), cancer (yes or no), diabetes (yes or no), body mass index (BMI) (underweight, normal weight, overweight or obesity) [21].

Alcohol consumption (in grams) was calculated by converting the frequency of consumption of wine, cava, beer, spirits and distillates (whiskey, gin, vodka) declared in the CFQ, to daily servings, expressing the results as grams of alcohol per day based on the following formula: grams of alcohol = [(alcohol content × volume (cl))/100] × 8. The reference alcohol content used in the conversions was 12% for wine and champagne, 5% for beer, 25% for spirits and 40% for distillates [17].The total grams of alcohol consumed per day were then summed and categorized into 3 groups: no consumption–low risk consumption (<20 g/day in women, <40 g/day in men), risk consumption (20–40 g/day in women, 40–60 g/day in men) and harmful consumption (>40 g/day in women, >60 g/day in men).

Statistical analysis: IBM® SPSS® Statistics version 27 software (IBM Corp., Armonk, New York, NY, USA) as used for statistical analysis. Quantitative variables were described by means of their mean, standard deviation and medians. The Student t test or analysis of variance (ANOVA) was used to establish differences according to sex and age group, depending on the number of categories considered. For qualitative variables, their frequencies were estimated, and the Chi-square test (X^2) was used for comparison. A *p*-value of less than 0.05 was established as the level of statistical significance.

The possible association, for the total sample and stratified by sex, between the dependent variable (AMD) and the rest of the variables was explored with the aim of making a first approximation to the estimation of the measure of association, classifying the variables according to the value of the odds ratio (OR) as a measure of the strength of association, their corresponding 95% confidence intervals and the statistical significance in the contrast to the hypothesis X^2.

To evaluate the possible association, a univariate binary logistic regression analysis was performed to explore the distribution. We worked with dichotomous categorical variables except for age groups, educational level, smoking, alcohol consumption and BMI, which were polytomous and were included in the analysis as dummy variables.

A multivariate analysis was performed for the total sample and by sex by means of logistic regression. The variables included in the analysis were those that could cause confusion according to current scientific evidence and those with $p < 0.2$ in the univariate analysis. This procedure made it possible to obtain adjusted measures of association (OR) with 95% confidence intervals and the contrast of hypotheses by means of the Wald statistical test.

3. Results

3.1. Dscriptive Analysis

Tables 1 and 2 show the distribution of the sample according to the health determinants studied based on the level of AMD.

The study showed that 18.2% of the population was classified as having high AMD, and that the AMD level of men and women was similar. No significant differences ($p > 0.05$) were found between sexes, but the level of AMD did differ between age groups.

When analyzing the proportion of the population classified as high AMD (Table 1) according to age group, it was observed that the population aged 16–24 years had the least number of respondents classified in this category. Only 6.6% ($n = 23$) of the total ($n = 352$) respondents in the 16–24 age group had high AMD. The percentages of those classified in the high AMD group increased in parallel with the age group so that 12% ($n = 113$) of the total ($n = 940$) population aged 25–44 years had high AMD; 24.6% ($n = 208$) of the total ($n = 846$) population aged 45–64 years had high AMD; 26% ($n = 153$) of the total ($n = 589$) population aged $\geq$65 years had high AMD.

Regarding the relationship between BMI and AMD, Table 3 shows the distribution of the sample according to the declared anthropometry as a function of the AMD level.

3.2. Univariate Analysis

Univariate analysis showed the association between sociodemographic factors, lifestyles and health–disease states with high AMD (Table 4).

Among the variables referring to the sociodemographic situation of the sample, it was observed that there was a positive association between age group and high AMD, and the strength of the association increased as the age of the study group increased. The group aged $\geq$65 years obtained an OR = 5.04 and 95% CI = 3.18–7.98. The variable country of birth showed significant results in the male group. It was observed that those who were not born in Spain had a negative association with high AMD (OR = 0.44; 95% CI = 0.25–0.76). Educational level also showed an association with high AMD. Having secondary and higher education levels was negatively associated with high AMD in the whole population (OR = 0.60; 95% CI = 0.42–0.86). Employment status was a variable that remained associated with high AMD. The condition of being without paid work was negatively associated with high AMD for the whole population and for men (OR = 0.70; 95% CI = 0.53–0.94). The type of cohabitation showed statistical significance in the analysis of the association with AMD. Not living with a partner was negatively associated with high AMD in all cases: in the general population (OR = 0.48; 95% CI = 0.38–0.60), in the men's group (OR = 0.39; 95% CI = 0.27–0.55) and in the women's group (OR = 0.56; 95% CI = 0.42–0.76).

Table 1. Distribution of the sample according to the determinants of health based on the level of adherence to the Mediterranean diet.

Variables	General			Men			Women		
	Adherence to the Mediterranean Diet		Total N (%)	Adherence to the Mediterranean Diet		Total N (%)	Adherence to the Mediterranean Diet		Total N (%)
	≤9 Points N (%)	10–14 Points N (%)		≤9 Points N (%)	10–14 Points N (%)		≤9 Points N (%)	10–14 Points N (%)	
Age groups [abc]									
16–24 years old	330 (14.8)	23 (4.63)	353 (12.9)	161 (14.98)	9 (3.81)	170 (13)	169 (14.6)	14 (5.36)	183 (12.9)
25–44 years old	827 (37.1)	113 (22.7)	940 (34.5)	413 (38.42)	52 (22)	465 (35.5)	414 (35.8)	61 (23.7)	475 (33.5)
45–64 years old	638 (28.6)	208 (41.9)	846 (31)	312 (29.02)	89 (37.7)	401 (30.6)	326 (28.2)	119 (45.6)	445 (31.4)
≥65 years	436 (19.5)	153 (30.8)	589 (21.6)	189 (17.58)	86 (36.4)	275 (21)	247 (21.4)	67 (25.7)	314 (22.2)
Total	2231 (100)	497 (100)	2728 (100)	1075 (100)	236 (100)	1311 (100)	1156 (100)	261 (100)	1417 (100)
Country of birth [b]									
Different from Spain	290 (13.1)	42 (8.47)	332 (12.2)	144 (13.4)	15 (6.38)	159 (12.2)	146 (12.7)	27 (10.3)	173 (12.3)
Spain	1932 (87)	454 (91.5)	2386 (87.8)	929 (86.6)	220 (93.6)	1149 (87.8)	1003 (87.3)	234 (89.7)	1237 (87.7)
Total	2222 (100)	49 (100)	2718 (100)	1073 (100)	235 (100)	1308 (100)	1149 (100)	261 (100)	1410 (100)
Level of education [ab]									
No education	203 (9.15)	63 (12.7)	266 (9.80)	72 (6.75)	31 (13.1)	103 (7.90)	131 (11.4)	32 (12.4)	163 (11.6)
Primary education	453 (20.4)	143 (28.9)	596 (22)	210 (19.7)	74 (31.4)	284 (21.8)	243 (21.1)	69 (26.6)	312 (22.1)
Secondary education	1066 (48)	197 (39.8)	1263 (46.5)	552 (51.7)	90 (38.1)	642 (49.3)	514 (44.6)	107 (41.3)	621 (44)
Higher education	497 (22.4)	92 (18.6)	589 (21.7)	233 (21.8)	41 (17.4)	274 (21)	264 (22.9)	51 (19.7)	315 (22)
Total	2219 (100)	495 (100)	2714 (100)	1067 (100)	236 (100)	1303 (100)	1152 (100)	259 (100)	1411 (100)
Employment status									
With paid work	900 (40.5)	181 (36.4)	1.081 (39.8)	576 (53.7)	147 (62.3)	585 (44.7)	745 (64.8)	169 (64.8)	496 (35.2)
No paid work	1321 (59.5)	316 (63.6)	1637 (60.2)	496 (46.3)	89 (37.7)	723 (55.3)	404 (35.2)	92 (35.3)	914 (64.8)
Total	2221 (100)	497 (100)	2718 (100)	1072 (100)	236 (100)	1308 (100)	1149 (100)	261 (100)	1410 (100)
Living together as a couple [abc]									
Yes	1256 (59.2)	353 (75.3)	1609 (62.1)	616 (60.7)	180 (80)	796 (64.2)	640 (57.8)	173 (70.9)	813 (60.2)
No	866 (40.8)	116 (24.7)	982 (37.9)	399 (39.3)	45 (20)	444 (35.8)	467 (42.2)	71 (29.1)	538 (39.8)
Total	2122 (100)	469 (100)	2591 (100)	1015 (100)	225 (100)	1240 (100)	1107 (100)	244 (100)	1351 (100)
Health perception									
Good condition	2009 (93.1)	438 (90.9)	2447 (92.7)	974 (94.3)	207 (92)	1181 (93.9)	90 (8)	26 (10.1)	1266 (91.6)
Poor condition	149 (6.90)	44 (9.13)	193 (7.31)	59 (5.71)	18 (8)	77 (6.12)	1035(92.00)	231 (89.9)	116 (8.39)
Total	2158 (100)	482 (100)	2640 (100)	1033 (100)	225 (100)	1258 (100)	1125 (100)	257 (100)	1382 (100)

Table 1. *Cont.*

Variables	General			Men			Women		
	Adherence to the Mediterranean Diet		Total N (%)	Adherence to the Mediterranean Diet		Total N (%)	Adherence to the Mediterranean Diet		Total N (%)
	≤9 Points N (%)	10–14 Points N (%)		≤9 Points N (%)	10–14 Points N (%)		≤9 Points N (%)	10–14 Points N (%)	
Leisure time physical activity									
Little or no physical activity	1934 (87.9)	440 (89.4)	2374 (88.2)	906 (85.6)	24 (10.3)	1115 (86.4)	1028(90)	231 (89.2)	1.259 (89.9)
Physical activity several times a week	266 (12.1)	52(10.6)	318 (11.8)	152 (14.4)	209 (89.7)	176 (13.6)	114 (10)	28 (10.8)	142 (10.1)
Total	2200 (100)	492 (100)	2692 (100)	1058 (100)	233 (100)	1291 (100)	1142 (100)	259 (100)	1401 (100)
Sedentary behavior									
<2 h/day	496 (22.8)	88 (18.6)	584 (22.1)	264 (25.3)	44 (19.7)	308 (24.3)	232 (20.5)	44 (17.6)	276 (20)
≥2 h/day	1679 (77.2)	385 (81.4)	2064 (78)	780 (74.7)	179 (80.3)	959 (75.7)	899 (79.5)	206 (82.4)	1105 (80)
Total	2175 (100)	473 (100)	2648 (100)	1044 (100)	223 (100)	1267 (100)	1131 (100)	250 (100)	1381 (100)
Current smoking habit									
Yes	677 (30.4)	122 (24.7)	799 (29.3)	383 (35.6)	69 (29.4)	452 (34.5)	294 (25.4)	53 (20.4)	347 (24.5)
No	1099 (49.3)	261 (52.7)	1360 (49.9)	419 (39)	94 (40)	513 (39.2)	680 (58.8)	167 (64.2)	847 (59.8)
Ex-smokers	455 (20.4)	112 (22.6)	567 (20.8)	273 (25.4)	72 (30.6)	345 (26.3)	182 (15.7)	40 (15.4)	222 (15.7)
Total	2231 (100)	495 (100)	2726 (100)	1075 (100)	235 (100)	1310 (100)	1156 (100)	260 (100)	1416 (100)
Snacking between meals [abc]									
Yes	892 (40.7)	149 (30.3)	1041 (38.8)	427 (40.8)	70 (30)	497 (38.8)	465 (40.6)	79 (30.5)	544 (38.8)
No	1300 (59.3)	343 (69.7)	1643 (61.2)	620 (59.2)	163 (70)	783 (61.2)	680 (59.4)	180 (69.5)	860 (61.3)
Total	2192 (100)	492 (100)	2684 (100)	1047 (100)	233 (100)	1280 (100)	1145 (100)	259 (100)	1404 (100)
Alcohol consumption [b]									
No consumption and low-risk consumption	2144 (96.1)	462 (93)	2606 (95.5)	1018 (94.7)	213 (90.2)	1231 (93.9)	1126 (97.4)	249 (95.4)	1375 (97)
Risky consumption	60 (2.69)	28 (5.63)	88 (3.2)	37 (3.4)	17 (7.20)	54 (4.12)	23 (2)	11 (4.22)	34 (2.40)
Harmful consumption	27 (1.21)	7 (1.41)	34 (1.3)	20 (1.9)	6 (2.54)	26 (2)	7 (0.61)	1 (0.38)	8 (0.56)
Total	2231 (100)	497 (100)	2728 (100)	1075 (100)	236 (100)	1311 (100)	1156 (100)	261 (100)	1417 (100)

[a]: p value < 0.05 in general; [b]: p value < 0.05 in men; [c]: p value < 0.05 in women.

Table 2. Distribution of the sample according to the health status based on the level of adherence to the Mediterranean diet.

Variables	General			Men			Women		
	Adherence to the Mediterranean Diet		Total N (%)	Adherence to the Mediterranean diet		Total N (%)	Adherence to the Mediterranean Diet		Total N (%)
	≤9 Points N (%)	10–14 Points N (%)		≤9 Points N (%)	10–14 Points N (%)		≤9 Points N (%)	10–14 Points N (%)	
Arterial Hypertension									
Yes	397 (17.8)	140 (28.2)	537 (19.7)	189 (17.6)	69 (29.2)	258 (19.7)	208 (18.1)	71 (27.2)	279 (19.7)
No	1828 (82.2)	357 (71.8)	2185 (80.3)	884 (82.4)	167 (70.8)	1051 (80.3)	944 (81.9)	190 (72.8)	1134 (80.3)
Total	2225 (100)	497 (100)	2.722 (100)	1073 (100)	236 (100)	1309 (100)	1152 (100)	261 (100)	1413 (100)
Infarction									
Yes	45 (2.02)	22 (4.43)	67 (2.46)	32 (3)	18 (7.63)	50 (3.82)	13 (1.13)	4 (1.53)	17 (1.20)
No	2181 (98)	475 (95.6)	2656 (97.5)	1042 (97)	218 (92.4)	1260 (96.2)	1139 (98.9)	257 (98.5)	1396 (98.8)
Total	2226 (100)	497 (100)	2723 (100)	1074 (100)	236 (100)	1310 (100)	1152 (100)	261 (100)	1413 (100)
Diabetes									
Yes	162 (7.27)	46 (9.26)	208 (7.64)	79 (7.36)	28 (11.9)	107 (8.17)	83 (7.20)	18 (6.90)	101 (7.14)
No	2065 (92.7)	451 (90.7)	2516 (92.4)	995 (92.6)	208 (88.1)	1203 (91.8)	1070 (92.8)	243 (93.1)	1313 (92.9)
Total	2227 (100)	497 (100)	2724 (100)	1074 (100)	236 (100)	1310 (100)	1153 (100)	261 (100)	1414 (100)
Neurological disease									
Yes	76 (3.41)	12 (2.42)	88 (3.23)	27 (2.52)	9 (3.81)	36 (2.75)	49 (4.25)	3 (1.15)	52 (3.68)
No	2151 (96.6)	484 (97.6)	2635 (96.8)	1046 (97.5)	227 (96.2)	1273 (97.2)	1105 (95.8)	257 (98.8)	1362 (96.32)
Total	2227 (100)	496 (100)	2723 (100)	1073 (100)	236 (100)	1309 (100)	1154 (100)	260 (100)	1414 (100)
Hypercholesterolemia									
Yes	322 (14.5)	120 (24.1)	442 (16.2)	143 (13.3)	56 (23.7)	199 (15.2)	179 (15.5)	64 (24.5)	243 (17.2)
No	1904 (85.5)	377 (75.9)	2281 (83.8)	930 (86.7)	180 (76.3)	1110 (84.8)	974 (84.5)	197 (75.5)	1171 (82.8)
Total	2226 (100)	497 (100)	2723 (100)	1073 (100)	236 (100)	1309 (10)	1153 (100)	261 (100)	1414 (100)
Cancer									
Yes	52 (2.34)	15 (3.02)	67 (2.46)	17 (1.58)	6 (2.54)	23 (1.76)	35 (3.04)	9 (3.45)	44 (3.11)
No	2173 (97.7)	482 (97)	2655 (97.5)	1056 (98.4)	230 (97.5)	1286 (98.2)	1117 (97)	252 (96.6)	1369 (96.9)
Total	2225 (100)	497 (100)	2722 (100)	1073 (100)	236 (100)	1309 (100)	1152 (100)	261 (100)	1413 (100)
Body mass index (kg/m^2)									
Underweight (<18.5 kg/m^2)	58 (2.81)	13 (2.86)	71 (2.82)	11 (1.08)	0 (0,00)	11 (0.89)	47 (4.50)	13 (5.60)	60 (4.70)
Normal weight (18.5–24.99 kg/m^2)	973 (47.2)	181 (39.8)	1154 (45.8)	408 (40.1)	78 (35)	486 (39.2)	565 (54.1)	103 (44.4)	668 (52.4)
Overweight (25–30 kg/m^2)	710 (34.4)	381 (83.7)	1091 (43.3)	436 (42.8)	107 (48)	543 (43.8)	274 (26.3)	76 (32.8)	350 (27.4)
Obesity (>30 kg/m^2)	321 (15.6)	78 (17.1)	399 (15.8)	163 (16)	38 (17)	201 (16.2)	158 (11.1)	40 (17.2)	198 (15.5)
Total	2063 (100)	455 (100)	2518 (100)	1018 (100)	223 (100)	1241 (100)	1044(100)	232(100)	1276 (100)

Table 3. Adherence to the Mediterranean diet in an adult population of southeastern Spain according to body mass index.

MEDAS * Score	N	Median BMI †	Standard Deviation	Standard Error	95% Confidence Interval for the Mean		*p*-Value
					Lower Limit	Upper Limit	
2	5	22.21	4.368	1.95	16.79	27.64	
3	18	24.20	4.98	1.17	21.72	26.68	
4	60	23.57	4.38	0.56	22.44	24.70	
5	183	24.65	5.27	0.39	23.89	25.42	
6	312	25.23	4.94	0.28	24.69	25.79	
7	484	26.08	9.14	0.42	25.26	26.89	
8	565	26.19	5.19	0.22	25.76	26.62	0.002
9	436	26.06	4.79	0.23	25.61	26.51	
10	300	26.29	4.99	0.29	25.73	26.86	
11	124	26.48	3.53	0.32	25.85	27.11	
12	27	24.93	3.30	0.64	23.62	26.24	
13	5	25.77	1.52	0.68	23.89	27.65	
Total	2519	25.84	5.98	0.12	25.61	26.08	

* MEDAS: Mediterranean Diet Adherence Screener. † BMI: Body Mass Index

Lifestyle variables were also associated with high AMD. Smoking was significantly associated with high AMD, with a negative association between smoking and high AMD in the whole population (OR = 0.76; 95% CI = 0.60–0.96). Eating between meals was also negatively associated with high AMD in the whole population (OR = 0.63; 95% CI = 0.51–0.78), in men (OR = 0.62; 95% CI = 0.46–0.85) and in women (OR = 0.64; 95% CI = 0.48–0.86). Risky alcohol consumption was positively associated in all cases with high AMD (OR = 2.17; 95% CI = 1.37–3.43) but not with harmful consumption (OR = 1.20; 95% CI = 0.52–2.78). The practice of leisure-time physical activity and sedentary behavior did not obtain statistically significant results in the study of the association with high AMD.

Health–disease status was also associated with high AMD. Having HT was positively associated with high AMD in the general population (OR = 1.81; 95% CI = 1.44–2.26), in men (OR = 1.93; 95% CI = 1.40–2.67), and in women (OR = 1.70; 95% CI = 1.24–2.32). Hypercholesterolemia was positively associated with high AMD in the general population (OR = 1.88; 95% CI = 1.49–2.39), in men (OR = 2.02; 95% CI = 1.43–2.87), and in women (OR = 1.77; 95% CI = 1.28–2.44). Having diabetes was also positively associated with high AMD in men (OR = 1.70; 95% CI = 1.07–2.68). Having suffered a myocardial infarction was positively associated with high AMD in the general population (OR = 2.25; 95% CI = 1.34–3.77) and in men (OR = 2.69; 95% CI = 1.48–4.88). Suffering from neurological diseases was negatively associated with high AMD in women (OR = 0.26; 95% CI = 0.08–0.85). The perception of health status did not show statistical significance in the study of the association with high AMD.

3.3. Multivariate Analysis

Multivariate analysis (Tables 5–7) showed the association between the study variables and high AMD by means of adjusted ORs and their 95% CIs.

The variables included in the model for the general population are shown in Table 5, of which age group, cohabitation with a partner and snacking between meals were statistically significant ($p < 0.05$). The results of the multivariate analysis for men are shown in Table 6. In the men's group, the variables of age group, cohabitation and smoking were significantly associated with high AMD. In the women's group, the variables of age group and cohabitation were statistically significant, as shown in Table 7.

Table 4. Univariate analysis of risk factors related to high adherence to the Mediterranean diet in the adult population of southeastern Spain.

Univariate	General		Men		Women	
Variables	**p-Value**	**Odds Ratio (95% Confidence Interval)**	**p-Value**	**Odds Ratio (95% Confidence Interval)**	**p-Value**	**Odds Ratio (95% Confidence Interval)**
Sex						
Men		1 (ref.)				
Women	0.78	1.03 (0.85–1.25)				
Age groups						
16–24 years old		1 (ref.)		1 (ref.)		1 (ref.)
25–44 years old	0.01	1.96 (1.23–3.13)	<0.01	2.25 (1.09–4.68)	<0.01	1.78 (0.97–3.27)
45–64 years old	<0.01	4.68 (2.98–7.34)	<0.01	5.10 (2.51–10.39)	<0.01	4.41 (2.46–790)
≥65 years	<0.01	5.04 (3.18–7.98)	<0.01	8.14 (3.97–16.69)	0.13	3.27 (1.78–6.02)
Country of birth						
Different from Spain	0.57	0.95 (0.78–1.15)	<0.01	0.44 (0.25–0.76)	0.29	1.26 (0.82–1.95)
Spain		1 (ref.)		1 (ref.)		1 (ref.)
Level of education						
No education		1 (ref.)		1 (ref.)	0.21	1 (ref.)
Primary education	0.92	1.02 (0.72–1.43)	<0.01	0.82 (0.50–1.35)	0.05	1.16 (0.73–1.86)
Secondary education	<0.01	0.60 (0.43–82)	<0.01	0.38 (0.24–0.61)	0.33	0.85 (0.55–1.33)
Higher education	0.01	0.60 (0.42–0.86)	<0.01	0.41 (0.24–0.70)	0.26	0.79 (0.49–1.29)
Employment status						
With paid work		1 (ref.)		1 (ref.)		1 (ref.)
No paid work	0.09	0.84 (0.69–1.03)	0.02	0.70 (0.53–0.94)	0.98	1.00 (0.76–1.33)
Living together as a couple						
Yes		1 (ref.)		1 (ref.)		1 (ref.)
No	<0.01	0.48 (0.38–0.60)	<0.01	0.39 (0.27–0.55)	<0.01	0.56 (0.42–0.76)
Health perception						
Good condition		1 (ref.)		1 (ref.)		1 (ref.)
Poor condition	0.09	1.35 (0.95–1.93)	0.20	1.44 (0.83–2.49)	0.27	1.29 (0.82–2.05)
Leisure time physical activity						
Little or no physical activity	0.34	1.16 (0.85–1.59)	0.10	1.46 (0.93–2.31)	0.69	0.92 (0.59–1.42)
Physical activity several times a week		1 (ref.)		1 (ref.)		1 (ref.)
Sedentary behavior						
<2 h/day		1 (ref.)		1 (ref.)		1 (ref.)
≥2 h/day	0.05	1.29 (1.00–1.66)	0.08	1.38 (0.96–1.97)	0.30	1.21 (0.85–1.73)
Current smoking habit					0.19	
Yes	0.01	0.76 (0.60–0.96)	0.07	1.33 (0.98–1.81)	0.09	1.73 (0.52–1.03)
No		1 (ref.)		1 (ref.)		1 (ref.)
Ex-smokers	0.04	1.04 (0.81–1.33)	0.10	0.80 (0.57–1.13)	0.89	0.90 (0.61–1.31)

Table 4. *Cont.*

Univariate	General		Men		Women	
Variables	***p*-Value**	**Odds Ratio (95% Confidence Interval)**	***p*-Value**	**Odds Ratio (95% Confidence Interval)**	***p*-Value**	**Odds Ratio (95% Confidence Interval)**
Snacking between meals						
Yes	<0.01	0.63 (0.51–0.78)	<0.01	0.62 (0.46–0.85)	<0.01	0.64 (0.48–0.86)
No		1 (ref.)		1 (ref.)		1 (ref.)
Alcohol consumption						
No consumption–low-risk consumption		1 (ref.)		1 (ref.)		1 (ref.)
Risky consumption	<0.01	2.17(1.37–3.43)	0.01	2.20 (1.21–3.97)	0.03	2.16 (1.04–4.50)
Harmful consumption	0.72	1.20 (0.52–2.78)	0.50	1.43 (0.57–3.61)	0.67	0.65 (0.08–5.27)
Arterial hypertension (AHT)						
Yes	<0.01	1.81 (1.44–2.26)	<0.01	1.93 (1.40–2.67)	<0.01	1.70 (1.24–2.32)
No		1 (ref.)		1 (ref.)		1 (ref.)
Hypercholesterolemia						
Yes	<0.01	1.88 (1.49–2.39)	<0.01	2.02 (1.43–2.87)	<0.01	1.77 (1.28–2.44)
No		1 (ref.)		1 (ref.)		1 (ref.)
Diabetes						
Yes	0.13	1.30 (0.92–1.83)	0.02	1.70 (1.07–2.68)	0.86	0.96 (0.56–1.62)
No		1 (ref.)		1 (ref.)		1 (ref.)
Myocardial infarction						
Yes	<0.01	2.25 (1.34–3.77)	<0.01	2.69 (1.48–4.88)	0.59	1.36 (0.44–4.22)
No		1 (ref.)		1 (ref.)		1 (ref.)
Neurological diseases						
Yes	0.26	0.70 (0.38–1.30)	0.27	1.54 (0.71–3.31)	0.03	0.26 (0.08–0.85)
No		1 (ref.)		1 (ref.)		1 (ref.)
Cancer						
Yes	0.38	1.30 (0.73–2.33)	0.32	1.62 (0.63–4.16)	0.73	1.14 (0.54–2.40)
No		1 (ref.)		1 (ref.)		1 (ref.)
Body mass index (BMI)	0.03		0.49		0.06	
Normal Weight				1 (ref.)		1 (ref.)
Underweight	0.56	1.21 (0.65–2.24)	0.99	1 (0.00-)	0.21	1.52 (0.79–2.90)
Overweight	<0.01	1.39 (1.10–1.74)	0.12	1.28 (0.93–1.77)	0.01	1.52 (1.09–2.12)
Obesity	0.07	1.31 (0.97–1.75)	0.36	1.22 (0.79–1.87)	0.11	1.39 (0.93–2.08)

Table 5. Multivariate analysis of risk factors related to high adherence to the Mediterranean diet in the adult population of southeastern Spain.

General Multivariate Model			
Variables	* Raw **RO**	Adjusted **OR (** 95% CI)**	***p*-Value**
Age groups			
16–24 years old	1 (ref.)	1 (ref.)	<0.01
25–44 years old	1.96	1.98 (1.10–3.59)	
45–64 years old	4.68	4.23 (2.33–7.70)	
≥65 years	5.04	3.61 (1.91–6.80)	
Employment status			
With paid work	1 (ref.)	1 (ref.)	0.29
No paid work	0.84	0.87 (0.66–1.13)	
Living together as a couple			
Yes	1 (ref.)	1 (ref.)	0.02
No	0.48	0.65 (0.50–0.85)	
Health perception			
Good condition	1 (ref.)		0.87
Poor condition	1.35	0.97 (0.62–1.49)	
Snacking between meals			
No	1 (ref.)	1 (ref.)	0.03
Yes	0.63	0.77 (0.59–0.98)	
Sedentary behavior			
<2 h/day	1 (ref.)	1 (ref.)	0.25
≥2 h/day	1.29	1.18 (0.89–1.58)	
Current smoking habit			
No	1 (ref.)	1 (ref.)	0.24
Yes	0.76	0.83 (0,62–1.11)	
Ex-smokers	1.04	0.81 (0.61–1.07)	
Alcohol consumption			
No consumption–low-risk consumption	1 (ref.)	1 (ref.)	0.42
Risky consumption	2.17	1.44 (0.83–2.49)	
Harmful consumption	1.20	1.12 (0.44–2.85)	
Arterial hypertension (AHT)			
No	1 (ref.)	1 (ref.)	0.29
Yes	1.81	1.18 (0.87–1.59)	
Hypercholesterolemia			
No	1 (ref.)	1 (ref.)	0.06
Yes	1.88	1.32 (0.98–1.76)	
Diabetes			
No	1 (ref.)	1 (ref.)	0.50
Yes	1.30	0.86 (0.56–1.33)	
Myocardial infarction			
No	1 (ref.)	1 (ref.)	0.83
Yes	2.25	1.08 (0.54–2.16)	
Body mass index (BMI)			
Normal Weight	1 (ref.)	1 (ref.)	0.09
Underweight	1.21	2.16 (1.07–4.34)	
Overweight	1.39	1.02 (0.79–1.33)	
Obesity	1.31	0.85 (0.60–1.18)	

* OR = odds ratio, ** IC = confidence interval.

Table 6. Multivariate analysis of risk factors related to high adherence to the Mediterranean diet in adult men in southeastern Spain.

Multivariate Model Men			
Variables	*** Raw RO**	**Adjusted OR (** CI 95%)**	***p*-Value**
Age groups			
16–24 years old	1 (ref.)	1 (ref.)	<0.01
25–44 years old	2.25	2.97 (1.10–8.06)	
45–64 years old	5.10	6.16 (2.25–16.9)	
≥65 years	8.14	8.16 (2.89–23.1)	
Employment status			
With paid work	1 (ref.)	1 (ref.)	0.19
No paid work	0.70	0.77 (0.52–1.14)	
Living together as a couple			
Yes	1 (ref.)	1 (ref.)	0.01
No	0.39	0.59 (0.40–0.90)	
Snacking between meals			
No	1 (ref.)		0.33
Yes	0.62	0.84 (0.59–1.19)	
Leisure time physical activity			
Physical activity several times a week	1 (ref.)	1 (ref.)	0.85
Little or no physical activity	1.46	0.95 (0.58–1.57)	
Sedentary behavior			
<2 h/day	1 (ref.)	1 (ref.)	0.46
≥2 h/day	1.29	1.16 (0.78–1.73)	
Current smoking habit			
No	1 (ref.)	1 (ref.)	
Yes	1.33	0.60 (0.40–0.89)	0.03
Ex-smokers	0.80	0.71 (0.48–1.04)	
Alcohol consumption			
No consumption–low-risk consumption	1 (ref.)	1 (ref.)	
Risky consumption	2.20	1.72 (0.89–3.32)	0.24
Harmful consumption	1.43	1.35 (0.47–3.90)	
Arterial hypertension (AHT)			
No	1 (ref.)	1 (ref.)	0.95
Yes	1.93	1.04 (0.70–1.53)	
Hypercholesterolemia			
No	1 (ref.)	1 (ref.)	0.08
Yes	2.02	1.41 (0.95–2.10)	
Diabetes			
No	1 (ref.)	1 (ref.)	0.71
Yes	1.70	0.90 (0.54–1.53)	
Myocardial infarction			
No	1 (ref.)	1 (ref.)	0.60
Yes	2.69	1.21 (0.60–2.44)	

* OR = odds ratio, ** IC = confidence interval.

Table 7. Multivariate analysis of risk factors related to high adherence to the Mediterranean diet in adult women in southeastern Spain.

Multivariate Model Women			
Variables	* $_{\text{Raw}}$ **RO**	$_{\text{Adjusted}}$ **OR (** 95% CI)**	***p*-Value**
Age groups			
16–24 years old	1 (ref.)	1 (ref.)	
25–44 years old	1.78	1.55 (0.76–3.13)	<0.01
45–64 years old	4.41	3.55 (1.76–7.18)	
≥65 years	3.27	2.04 (0.94–4.45)	
Living together as a couple			
Yes	1 (ref.)	1 (ref.)	0.03
No	0.56	0.68 (0.48–0.97)	
Snacking between meals			
No	1 (ref.)		0.07
Yes	0.64	0.74 (0.53–1.02)	
Alcohol consumption			
No consumption–low-risk consumption	1 (ref.)	1 (ref.)	
Risky consumption	2.16	1.20 (0.48–2.96)	0.79
Harmful consumption	0.65	0.54 (0.06–4.62)	
Arterial hypertension (AHT)			
No	1 (ref.)	1 (ref.)	0.11
Yes	1.70	1.41 (0.93–2.14)	
Hypercholesterolemia			
No	1 (ref.)	1 (ref.)	0.18
Yes	1.77	1.31 (0.88–1.95)	
Neurological diseases			
No	1 (ref.)	1 (ref.)	0.81
Yes	0.26	0.19 (0.05–0.82)	
Body mass index (BMI)			
Normal Weight	1 (ref.)	1 (ref.)	
Underweight	1.52	2.43 (1.20–4.92)	0.09
Overweight	1.52	1.04 (0.72–1.50)	
Obesity	1.39	0.93 (0.59–1.45)	

* OR = odds ratio, ** IC = confidence interval.

4. Discussion

The present study evaluated the risk factors associated with adherence to the Mediterranean dietary pattern in the adult population of southeastern Spain. The results provide a clearer view of the sociodemographic factors, lifestyles, and health–disease states associated with high AMD in order to propose interventions to promote well-being at different stages of life and reduce morbidity and premature mortality due to NCDs, which is one of the Sustainable Development Goals [22].

The results obtained indicated that less than one-fifth of the population followed traditional, healthy, and sustainable MD, which is in agreement with the results of other studies performed in the general Spanish population [23]. Apart from the low proportion of the population classified at a high level of AMD, the results of the present study also showed that the younger population had the highest proportion of those classified in the low AMD group and the lowest proportion of those classified in the high AMD group. The results of the present work show how the older age groups, which are those that experienced the Spanish epidemiological–nutritional transition in the 1960s and 1970s [24], have a higher AMD. The progressive incorporation of dietary patterns typical of Western countries, which fundamentally affect younger groups, distances the young Spanish population from the traditional MD. This study highlights the generational loss of the MD and the shift away from the high AMD that is occurring in younger age groups. It would therefore be necessary to direct MD promotion and adherence actions to the groups with the lowest adherence as a public health strategy and for the prevention of overweight and obesity.

In recent years, the prevalence of overweight and obesity along with NCDs has steadily increased worldwide and the *European Regional Obesity Report 2022* [25] points out that Spain is one of the European countries with the highest prevalence of childhood obesity. The World Health Organization (WHO) [26] explains that unhealthy dietary patterns and sedentary lifestyles could be some of the causes of weight gain in the population. Actions should therefore be promoted in this regard. There is an urgent need to promote dietary patterns that guarantee the well-being of people and planetary health (as is the case with the Mediterranean diet). The results of this research show that the young population of southeastern Spain is the segment of the population that most departs from the Mediterranean dietary pattern, and this departure can lead to health problems (as explained by the WHO). The predominance of Westernized dietary patterns in the general population and more specifically among the young population is no coincidence. Rather, it is a combination of factors that have resulted in the deterioration of the quality of the population's diet. In recent decades, as a result of changes in the global food supply [27], high and middle income countries have seen food environments saturated with unhealthy, highly accessible, relatively cheap and highly promoted foods, with easy access to foods high in sodium, saturated fats and/or added sugars [28]. These obesogenic environments encourage overconsumption of energy-dense, nutrient-poor foods. Given this situation, it is recommended at the global level to favour regulations to restrict exposure of children in terms of marketing unhealthy foods, better labelling of products and policies that encourage the consumption of healthy and sustainable foods [29].

The sociodemographic and economic changes that occurred from the mid-20th century to the present also favored the change in the pattern of food consumption in Mediterranean areas [24], the shift away from the Mediterranean dietary pattern and the increase in NCDs and rates of overweight and obesity [30,31]. The present study detected the association between sociodemographic factors with high AMD. On the one hand, the condition of living in a couple was positively associated with high AMD. Previous research [32] had already detected that people living alone were more likely to have deficient intakes of staple foods such as fruits, vegetables, and fish compared to those living with a partner. On the other hand, it was observed that male smokers had a negative association with high AMD, i.e., they had a higher risk of having a low AMD. This same phenomenon was already observed in other studies in which smokers had a low AMD [33]. As a consequence of the results obtained in the present study, as well as the data available in the scientific literature, it would be of interest to study the level of AMD in individuals with toxic habits (such as the consumption of legal and illegal drugs) in order to explain the observed phenomenon in greater detail, since smoking is a toxic habit that should be adequately controlled through the application of effective actions [34]. Despite the advances that have been made [35], smoking continues to be an important public health problem that causes cancer and respiratory and cardiovascular diseases and is one of the main causes of preventable death [36].

Snacking between meals was also negatively associated with high AMD. In a first estimation of the association, it showed statistical significance for the whole population and in both sexes. After adjusting the analysis in the multivariate model, the variable showed statistical significance in the general population, and it was observed that snacking between meals was associated with lower AMD. Dietary guidelines recommend eating three main meals a day [37] to promote dietary balance. However, snacking between meals implies an alteration of the usual eating schedules, an increase in daily food intake and therefore an alteration of circadian rhythms with possible harmful consequences for health [38]. Apart from the negative impact on health of altered mealtimes, in the present study we observed a shift away from MD that may be a consequence of the nutritional quality of the foods chosen for these snacks. If highly processed foods are introduced during snacking, the quality of the diet will be diminished [39] because they are usually products that induce excessive intake of free sugar [40], low-quality fats and, in short, foods that are nutritionally uninteresting and dispensable in a healthy diet [41]. All this is closely related to body weight, since the recurrent intake of this type of products favors an increase in dietary energy, which can result in excess body weight [42]. In any case, there is a clear need to prioritize fresh and plant-based foods and to promote eating habits that emphasize quality, quantity and meal times, as three fundamental aspects to achieve healthy lifestyles [43,44].

It is noteworthy that variables such as educational level, physical activity, sedentary lifestyle, hypercholesterolemia and BMI, did not obtain statistical significance in the multivariate model in any of the cases since scientific evidence closely relates them to AMD.

In the present study, in a first estimation of risk, an association was observed between health–disease status and high AMD, in both men and women. The population with chronic health problems showed a positive association with high AMD, although when the analysis was adjusted, the statistical significance of the observed phenomenon disappeared. Some studies explain the phenomenon that the majority of people with these pathologies present a moderate AMD and associate it with sociodemographic factors and health status [45–47]. Likewise, other studies indicate that dietary recommendations play an important role in the prevention of certain diseases and that MD should be promoted among the population with cardiovascular pathologies [48]. Therefore, it is not surprising that those who suffer from CVD or related health problems have a higher AMD than those who do not, although it would be of interest to find out when this change in diet occurred. Due to the typology of the study (an official survey of a public health agency and endorsed by the Department of Health and the General Directorate of Public Health, with a scope of 4500 people), we could not add an additional questionnaire to solve the dilemma, but we can explain and justify it with the scientific literature and propose that for future occasions this section be considered. The authors point out the importance of carrying out further research that contemplates people with pathologies in order to provide an answer to the unknown. However, it is to be expected that in the population with CVD, cancer and other chronic NCDs, a change in dietary pattern will occur after their detection and diagnosis, since diet plays a very important role in the prevention of these pathologies, and specifically the MD is referenced in many medical guides as a recommended dietary pattern [49–51].

Improving diet is a public health priority that can lead to a significant reduction in CVD morbidity and mortality [52]. It is therefore important for healthcare providers to understand current dietary practice guidelines and to apply evidence-based dietary counseling to persons at high risk for CVD. In addition, there is evidence demonstrating that a change in dietary pattern after the diagnosis of some disease or pathology can be explained by the "health belief model" [53]. This model pays preferential attention to the role of the individual's perception or belief about his or her vulnerability to a disease that threatens his or her health and the actions he or she can take to prevent that threat and avoid the possible disease. According to this model, the person has to feel threatened by his or her previous or current pattern of behavior (in this case a poor diet) in order to make the change towards healthier actions (in this case, the MD) [54].

In view of the above, in our study sample we observed participants modifying their diet towards a Mediterranean dietary pattern to improve their health when confronted with disease diagnoses. It would be interesting to conduct future cohort studies along these lines that would allow us to confirm these observations.

Limitations

The present investigation was able to use data from a regional nutrition and health survey to assess AMD using the validated MEDAS questionnaire, although not all available survey data could be used due to the lack of responses from participants.

Regarding the methodology and instruments used, the choice of the diet quality index is one of the most relevant aspects of the study since it establishes the cut-off points on which the conclusions will be drawn. Although diet quality indices are very useful for assessing adherence to dietary patterns in specific populations [18], there is no universal indicator that can be extrapolated to all populations.

In relation to the study sample, the present study evaluated the quality of the diet in relation to the pattern of MD and the factors associated with its practice in the adult population of southeastern Spain but did not consider the population under 16 years of age.

For future lines of research, it would be of interest to observe whether changes in dietary patterns and other lifestyles occur after the diagnosis of CVD and whether these are associated with the traditional Mediterranean pattern. Moreover, as this is a cross-sectional epidemiological study, the results obtained do not allow us to affirm that those with CVD have always had a high AMD. It would be of interest to analyze this phenomenon by means of different surveys (past and future) to be able to observe this change in the pattern of food consumption and corroborate the hypothesis. It would also be of interest to know how the elements of the food and physical environment favor or hinder high AMD and other healthy lifestyles. It would also be interesting to widen the study area to have a clearer and more detailed view of AMD, making use of the different nutrition and health surveys available.

5. Conclusions

The present study evaluated the relationship between declared morbidity, lifestyles, and other sociodemographic factors associated with high AMD in a sample of the adult population of southeastern Spain. Age, type of cohabitation, and smoking habit were found to be related to the level of AMD.

Evidence suggests that MD has salutogenic effects in healthy populations, preventing overweight and obesity and other NCDs, and that it has a lower environmental footprint than the current dietary pattern of the Spanish and Western population [55]. Therefore, it is a priority for public health to promote MD adherence. Likewise, public health actions and policies should focus their efforts on promoting MD in younger groups living alone and on maintaining adherence in older groups. This association should be analyzed in depth, and priority should be given to interventions aimed at the most vulnerable groups in order to facilitate the adoption of healthy lifestyles among the entire population. Likewise, health interventions with a multifactorial approach, including diet and smoking, can be positive in improving lifestyles.

Author Contributions: Conceptualization, N.S.O.B., J.Q.i.I. and E.M.T.-L.; methodology, N.S.O.B., J.Q.i.I. and E.M.T.-L.; software, N.S.O.B.; validation, E.M.T.-L. and J.Q.i.I.; formal analysis, N.S.O.B.; investigation, N.S.O.B.; data curation, N.S.O.B.; writing—original draft preparation, N.S.O.B.; writing—review and editing, N.S.O.B., J.Q.i.I. and E.M.T.-L.; visualization, N.S.O.B., J.Q.i.I. and E.M.T.-L.; supervision, J.Q.i.I. and E.M.T.-L. All authors have read and agreed to the published version of the manuscript.

Funding: This research received no external funding.

Institutional Review Board Statement: Not applicable.

Informed Consent Statement: Not applicable.

Data Availability Statement: Not applicable.

Acknowledgments: We would like to thank all those who participated in the regional survey.

Conflicts of Interest: The authors declare no conflict of interest.

References

1. World Health Organization. *Combating NCDs: "Best Investments" and Other Recommended Interventions for the Prevention and Control of Noncommunicable Diseases*; World Health Organization: Geneva, Switzerland, 2017; Available online: https://extranet.who.int/iris/restricted/handle/10665/259351 (accessed on 15 August 2022).
2. Gómez, S.F.; Rajmil, L. Advertising, obesity and child health: The case of Spain. *BMJ Paediatr. Open* **2022**, *6*, e001482. [CrossRef]

3. Muzenda, T.; Dambisya, P.M.; Kamkuemah, M.; Gausi, B.; Battersby, J.; Oni, T. Mapping food and physical activity environments in low- and middle-income countries: A systematized review. *Health Place* **2022**, *75*, 102809. [CrossRef]
4. Massimo, F.P.; Arno, W.H.; Stefan, A.; Christian, A.; Carlos, B.; Alberico, L.; Cooney, M.T.; Corrà, U.; Cosyns, B.; Deaton, C.; et al. 2016 European Guidelines on cardiovascular disease prevention in clinical practice. *Rev. Esp. Cardiol.* **2016**, *69*, 939.
5. Ministry of Health, Consumer Affairs and Social Welfare. Public Health Strategy 2022 Improving the Health and Well-Being of the Population. 2022. Available online: https://www.sanidad.gob.es/ciudadanos/pdf/Estrategia_de_Salud_Publica_2022___Pendiente_de_NIPO.pdf (accessed on 10 September 2022).
6. Barrea, L.; Muscogiuri, G.; Pugliese, G.; de Alteriis, G.; Colao, A.; Savastano, S. Metabolically Healthy Obesity (MHO) vs. Metabolically Unhealthy Obesity (MUO) Phenotypes in PCOS: Association with Endocrine-Metabolic Profile, Adherence to the Mediterranean Diet, and Body Composition. *Nutrients* **2021**, *13*, 3925. [CrossRef]
7. Scannell, N.; Moran, L.; Mantzioris, E.; Cowan, S.; Villani, A. Efficacy, Feasibility and Acceptability of a Mediterranean Diet Intervention on Hormonal, Metabolic and Anthropometric Measures in Overweight and Obese Women with Polycystic Ovary Syndrome: Study Protocol. *Metabolites* **2022**, *12*, 311. [CrossRef] [PubMed]
8. AlAufi, N.S.; Chan, Y.M.; Waly, M.I.; Chin, Y.S.; Mohd Yusof, B.-N.; Ahmad, N. Application of Mediterranean Diet in Cardiovascular Diseases and Type 2 Diabetes Mellitus: Motivations and Challenges. *Nutrients* **2022**, *14*, 2777. [CrossRef] [PubMed]
9. Galiuto, L.; Patrono, C. Efficacy of a Mediterranean diet for the secondary prevention of cardiovascular disease. *Eur. Heart J.* **2022**, *43*, 2727–2728. [CrossRef]
10. Franquesa, M.; Pujol-Busquets, G.; García-Fernández, E.; Rico, L.; Shamirian-Pulido, L.; Aguilar-Martínez, A.; Medina, F.X.; Serra-Majem, L.; Bach-Faig, A. Mediterranean Diet and Cardiodiabesity: A Systematic Review through Evidence-Based Answers to Key Clinical Questions. *Nutrients* **2019**, *11*, 655. [CrossRef]
11. Alonso-Cabezas, M.; Pollán, M.; Alonso-Ledesma, I.; Fernández de Larrea-Baz, N.; Lucas, P.; Sierra, Á.; Castelló, A.; Pino, M.N.; Pérez-Gómez, B.; Martínez-Cortés, M.; et al. Sociodemographic and Lifestyle Determinants of Adherence to Current Dietary Recommendations and Diet Quality in Middle-Aged Spanish Premenopausal Women. *Front. Nutr.* **2022**, *14*, 904330. [CrossRef]
12. Tong, T.Y.N.; Imamura, F.; Monsivais, P.; Brage, S.; Griffin, S.J.; Wareham, N.J.; Forouhi, N.G. Dietary cost associated with adherence to the Mediterranean diet, and its variation by socio-economic factors in the UK Fenland Study. *Br. J. Nutr.* **2018**, *119*, 685–694. [CrossRef]
13. Bibiloni, M.d.M.; Gallardo-Alfaro, L.; Gómez, S.F.; Wärnberg, J.; Osés-Recalde, M.; González-Gross, M.; Gusi, N.; Aznar, S.; Marín-Cascales, E.; González-Valeiro, M.A.; et al. Determinants of Adherence to the Mediterranean Diet in Spanish Children and Adolescents: The PASOS Study. *Nutrients* **2022**, *14*, 738. [CrossRef]
14. Mattavelli, E.; Olmastroni, E.; Bonofiglio, D.; Catapano, A.L.; Baragetti, A.; Magni, P. Adherence to the Mediterranean Diet: Impact of Geographical Location of the Observations. *Nutrients* **2022**, *14*, 2040. [CrossRef] [PubMed]
15. Quiles, J.; Jiménez, R.; Marín, S.; Rizk, J.; Zubeldía, L. *Nutrition Survey of the Valencian Community 2010–2011: Reduced Report*; Generalitat Valenciana, Conselleria de Sanitat: Valencia, Spain, 2013.
16. Schröder, H.; Fitó, M.; Estruch, R.; Martínez-González, M.A.; Corella, D.; Salas-Salvadó, J.; Lamuela-Raventós, R.; Ros, E.; Salaverría, I.; Fiol, M.; et al. A short screener is valid for assessing Mediterranean diet adherence among older Spanish men and women. *J. Nutr.* **2011**, *141*, 1140–1145. [CrossRef]
17. Martínez-González, M.A.; García-Arellano, A.; Toledo, E.; Salas-Salvadó, J.; Buil-Cosiales, P.; Corella, D.; Covas, M.I.; Schröder, H.; Arós, F.; Gómez-Gracia, E.; et al. A 14-Item Mediterranean Diet Assessment Tool and Obesity Indexes among High-Risk Subjects: The PREDIMED Trial. *PLoS ONE* **2012**, *7*, e43134. [CrossRef]
18. San Onofre Bernat, N.; Trescastro-López, E.M.; Quiles, J. Different classification of a population by two validated indices of adherence to Mediterranean diet. *Nutr. Hosp.* **2019**, *36*, 1116–1122. [CrossRef] [PubMed]
19. Ministry of Health, Consumer Affairs and Social Welfare. Strategy for Health Promotion and Prevention in the SNS. 2014. Available online: https://www.mscbs.gob.es/profesionales/saludPublica/prevPromocion/Estrategia/docs/EstrategiaPromocionSaludyPrevencionSNS.pdf (accessed on 15 August 2022).
20. Anderson, P.; Gual, A.; Colon, J. *Alcohol and Primary Health Care: Basic Clinical Information for the Identification and Management of Risks and Problems*; Pan American Health Organization: Washington, DC, USA, 2008. Available online: www.who.int/substance_abuse/publications/alcohol_atencion_primaria.pdf (accessed on 16 August 2022).
21. World Health Organization. *Obesity: Preventing and Managing the Global Epidemic*; Report of a WHO Consultation; WHO Technical Report Series 894; World Health Organization: Geneva, Switzerland, 2000.
22. United Nations, General Assembly. *Draft Outcome Document of the United Nations Summit for the Adoption of the Post-2015 Development Agenda*; United Nations: New York, NY, USA, 2015. Available online: https://www.cooperacionespanola.es/sites/default/files/agenda_2030_desarrollo_sostenible_cooperacion_espanola_12_ago_2015_es.pdf (accessed on 12 August 2022).
23. González, I.; Torres, M.; Martínez, C.A.; Luque, T. The Mediterranean diet in different age groups. *Eur. J. Health Res.* **2016**, *2*, 73–81. [CrossRef]
24. Trescastro-López, E.M.; Galiana-Sánchez, M.E.; Bernabeu-Mestre, J. Epidemiological-nutritional transition and demographic changes in contemporary Spain. *Soc. Panor.* **2016**, *23*, 63–71.
25. WHO. *European Regional Obesity Report 2022*; WHO Regional Office for Europe: Copenhagen, Denmark, 2022.
26. WHO. Obesity and Overweight. Available online: https://www.who.int/es/news-room/fact-sheets/detail/obesity-and-overweight (accessed on 20 September 2022).

27. White, M.; Aguirre, E.; Finegood, D.T.; Holmes, C.; Sacks, G.; Smith, R. What role should the commercial food system play in promoting health through better diet? *BMJ* **2020**, *368*, m545. [CrossRef] [PubMed]
28. Swinburn, B.A.; Sacks, G.; Hall, K.D.; McPherson, K.; Finegood, D.T.; Moodie, M.L.; Gortmaker, S.L. The global obesity pandemic: Shaped by global drivers and local environments. *Lancet* **2011**, *378*, 804–814. [CrossRef]
29. Swinburn, B.A.; Kraak, V.I.; Allender, S.; Atkins, V.J.; Baker, P.I.; Bogard, J.R.; Brinsden, H.; Calvillo, A.; De Schutter, O.; Devarajan, R.; et al. The global syndemic of obesity, undernutrition, and climate change: The Lancet Commission report. *Lancet* **2019**, *393*, 791–846. [CrossRef]
30. Varela-Moreiras, G.; Ávila, J.M.; Cuadrado, C.; del Pozo, S.; Ruiz, E.; Moreiras, O. Evaluation of food consumption and dietary patterns in Spain by the Food Consumption Survey: Updated information. *Eur. J. Clin. Nutr.* **2010**, *64*, 37–43. [CrossRef]
31. Partearroyo, T.; Laja, A.; Varela-Moreiras, G. Strengths and weaknesses of nutrition in the Spanish population of the 21st century. *Nutr. Hosp.* **2019**, *36*, 3–6. [CrossRef] [PubMed]
32. Hanna, K.L.; Collins, P.F. Relationship between living alone and food and nutrient intake. *Nutr. Rev.* **2015**, *73*, 594–611. [CrossRef]
33. Zaragoza, A.; Ferrer, R.; Cabañero, M.J.; Hurtado, J.A.; Laguna, A. Adherence to the Mediterranean diet and its relationship with nutritional status in the elderly. *Nutr. Hosp.* **2015**, *31*, 1667–1674. [CrossRef]
34. Fernández, E.; Peruga, A. Tobacco control in the 21st century: A global and local perspective. *Med. Clin.* **2022**, *8*, S0025-7753(22)00370-0.
35. Córdoba-García, R. Fourteen years of tobacco control law in Spain. *Current situation and proposals. Aten. Primaria* **2020**, *52*, 563–569. [CrossRef] [PubMed]
36. World Health Organization. *Report on the Global Tobacco Epidemic, 2017: Monitoring Tobacco Use and Prevention Policies*; World Health Organization: Geneva, Switzerland, 2017.
37. Bach-Faig, A.; Berry, E.M.; Lairon, D.; Reguant, J.; Trichopoulou, A.; Dernini, S.; Medina, F.X.; Battino, M.; Belahsen, R.; Miranda, G.; et al. Mediterranean diet pyramid today. Science and cultural updates. *Public Health Nutr.* **2011**, *14*, 2274–2284. [CrossRef]
38. Lopez-Minguez, J.; Gómez-Abellán, P.; Garaulet, M. Timing of Breakfast, Lunch, and Dinner. Effects on Obesity and Metabolic Risk. *Nutrients* **2019**, *11*, 2624. [CrossRef]
39. Martini, D.; Godos, J.; Bonaccio, M.; Vitaglione, P.; Grosso, G. Ultra-Processed Foods and Nutritional Dietary Profile: A Meta-Analysis of Nationally Representative Samples. *Nutrients* **2021**, *13*, 3390. [CrossRef]
40. Machado, P.P.; Steele, E.M.; Louzada, M.L.D.C.; Levy, R.B.; Rangan, A.; Woods, J.; Gill, T.; Scrinis, G.; Monteiro, C.A. Ultra-processed food consumption drives excessive free sugar intake among all age groups in Australia. *Eur. J. Nutr.* **2020**, *59*, 2783–2792. [CrossRef]
41. Monteiro, C.A.; Cannon, G.; Lawrence, M.; Costa Louzada, M.L.; Pereira, P. *Ultraprocessed Foods, Diet Quality, and Health Using the NOVA Classification System*; FAO: Rome, Italy, 2019.
42. Mendonça, R.D.; Pimenta, A.M.; Gea, A.; de la Fuente-Arrillaga, C.; Martinez-Gonzalez, M.A.; Lopes, A.C.; Bes-Rastrollo, M. Ultraprocessed food consumption and risk of overweight and obesity: The University of Navarra Follow-Up (SUN) cohort study. *Am. J. Clin. Nutr.* **2016**, *104*, 1433–1440. [CrossRef]
43. Manoogian, E.N.C.; Chaix, A.; Panda, S. When to Eat: The Importance of Eating Patterns in Health and Disease. *J. Biol. Rhythms* **2019**, *34*, 579–581. [CrossRef]
44. Serra-Majem, L.; Tomaino, L.; Dernini, S.; Berry, E.M.; Lairon, D.; Ngo de la Cruz, J.; Bach-Faig, A.; Donini, L.M.; Medina, F.X.; Belahsen, R.; et al. Updating the Mediterranean Diet Pyramid towards Sustainability: Focus on Environmental Concerns. *Int. J. Environ. Res. Public Health* **2020**, *17*, 8758. [CrossRef] [PubMed]
45. Magriplis, E.; Panagiotakos, D.; Kyrou, I.; Tsioufis, C.; Mitsopoulou, A.V.; Karageorgou, D.; Dimakopoulos, I.; Bakogianni, I.; Chourdakis, M.; Micha, R.; et al. Presence of Hypertension Is Reduced by Mediterranean Diet Adherence in All Individuals with a More Pronounced Effect in the Obese: The Hellenic National Nutrition and Health Survey (HNNHS). *Nutrients* **2020**, *12*, 853. [CrossRef] [PubMed]
46. Azorín, M.; Martínez, M.; Sánchez, A.B.; de la Ossa, M.; Hernández, I.; Tello Nieves, G.M. Adherence to the Mediterranean diet in hypertensive patients in Primary Care. *Rev. Clin. Med. Fam.* **2018**, *11*, 15–22. Available online: http://www.revclinmedfam.com/PDFs/85422afb467e9456013a2a51d4dff702.pdf (accessed on 16 August 2022).
47. Menotti, A.; Puddu, P.E.; Maiani, G.; Catasta, G. Lifestyle behaviour and lifetime incidence of heart diseases. *Int. J. Cardiol.* **2015**, *201*, 293–299. [CrossRef]
48. Lönnberg, L.; Ekblom-Bak, E.; Damberg, M. Improved unhealthy lifestyle habits in patients with high cardiovascular risk: Results from a structured lifestyle programme in primary care. *Ups. J. Med. Sci.* **2019**, *124*, 94–104. [CrossRef]
49. Tang, C.; Wang, X.; Qin, L.-Q.; Dong, J.-Y. Mediterranean Diet and Mortality in People with Cardiovascular Disease: A Meta-Analysis of Prospective Cohort Studies. *Nutrients* **2021**, *13*, 2623. [CrossRef]
50. Prieto-González, P.; Sánchez-Infante, J.; Fernández-Galván, L.-M. Association between Adherence to the Mediterranean Diet and Anthropometric and Health Variables in College-Aged Males. *Nutrients* **2022**, *14*, 3471.
51. Barrea, L.; Pugliese, G.; Laudisio, D.; Colao, A.; Savastano, S.; Muscogiuri, G. Mediterranean diet as medical prescription in menopausal women with obesity: A practical guide for nutritionists. *Crit. Rev. Food Sci. Nutr.* **2021**, *61*, 1201–1211. [CrossRef]
52. Pallazola, V.A.; Davis, D.M.; Whelton, S.P.; Cardoso, R.; Latina, J.M.; Michos, E.D.; Sarkar, S.; Blumenthal, R.S.; Arnett, D.K.; Stone, N.J.; et al. A Clinician's Guide to Healthy Eating for Cardiovascular Disease Prevention. *Mayo Clin. Proc. Innov. Qual. Outcomes* **2019**, *3*, 251–267. [CrossRef]

53. Khani Jeihooni, A.; Hidarnia, A.; Kaveh, M.H.; Hajizadeh, E. The effect of a prevention program based on health belief model on osteoporosis. *J. Res. Health Sci.* **2015**, *15*, 47–53.
54. Green, L. The health belief modeland personal health behavior. *Health Educ. Monogr.* **1974**, *2*, 324–325. [CrossRef]
55. Bôto, J.M.; Rocha, A.; Miguéis, V.; Meireles, M.; Neto, B. Sustainability Dimensions of the Mediterranean Diet: A Systematic Review of the Indicators used and Its Results. *Adv. Nutr.* **2022**, *13*, 2015–2038. [CrossRef] [PubMed]

nutrients

Article

Proposal of a Mathematical Model to Monitor Body Mass over Time in Subjects on a Diet

Jose M. Soriano [1,2,*], Giovanna Sgambetterra [3] and Pietro Marco Boselli [3]

1 Food & Health Lab, Institute of Materials Science, University of Valencia, 46980 Valencia, Spain
2 Joint Research Unit on Endocrinology, Nutrition and Clinical Dietetics, University of Valencia-Health Research Institute La Fe, 46026 Valencia, Spain
3 Departament de Biosciencies, University of Milan, 20122 Milan, Italy
* Correspondence: jose.soriano@uv.es

Abstract: Nowadays, slimming diet methodology works within a reduction of body mass using a decrease of dietary energy intake. However, there is no suitable method for understanding the dynamic process of body mass metabolic transformation over time. In the present paper, we have developed a biomathematic model to explain the temporal trend of body mass and its variations of people who have undergone a change in their diet using the solving equation of the model. Data relating to sex, age, body mass, and BMI were collected, and the compartmental model used to interpret the body mass trends was constructed by assuming that the mass results from the sum of the metabolic processes: catabolic, anabolic, distributive. The validation of the model was carried out by variance analysis both on the total and individual data sets. The results confirm that the trend of body mass and its variations over time depends on metabolic rates. These are specific to each individual and characterize the distribution of nutritional molecules in the various body districts and the processes catabolic, anabolic, distributive. Body mass and its variations are justified by the metabolic transformations of the nutritional quantities. This would explain why energetically equal diets can correspond to people of different body mass and that energy-different diets can correspond to people of body mass at all similar.

Keywords: BMI cut-offs; BMI; body fat; pseudothickness; obesity; BMI-BFMNU; anthropometric indices

1. Introduction

Every biological phenomenon, including the dynamic processes regarding the absorption, distribution, metabolism and excretion of molecules obtained from the diet, should be interpreted as a function of time. In fact, the rule applied in the slimming diet is derived from the estimation of the energy content of the lost weight but ignores the dynamic physiological adaptations that arise during the change of weight, which lead to changes both in the basal metabolic rate and in energy expenditure for physical activity. Several models have been developed to verify changes in body mass over time. They have incorporated metabolic adjustment and a nonlinear resting metabolic rate (RMR) term [1], the use of a one-dimensional differential equation [2], the application of a multiplier for the adaptation of dietary-induced thermogenesis [3], the calculation of a new parameter that considers the energy expended to store energy during weight gain [4], the development of a differential equation model based on the first law of thermodynamics that incorporates all three adjustments along with the natural age-related reduction in the resting metabolic rate [5] and mechanism-based model spanning full individual life and capturing changes in body weight, composition and height [6]. However, no suitable method exists to describe trends in body mass over time; at best, a broken line fits individual instantaneous data related to mass, as in a discontinuous process. Therefore, interpolating and extrapolating data as a function of time is difficult because each situation was considered static and detached [5]. Predictive equations [7–9] combined with anthropometric parameters or not [10–15], have been applied to calculate the resting metabolic rate. It is therefore important to find a model whose solving equation can interpret the temporal trend of body mass in any environmental, physiological and/or pathological condition.

The aim of this study is to propose a mathematic model that explains trends in body mass and its variations using a continuous function, valid in any physiological and pathological condition.

2. Materials and Methods

For this study, we selected 374 patients of both sexes, aged between 7 and 73 years, with different pathophysiological conditions who came to our university laboratory, and at least four controls were performed during the nutritional pathway using the Biological-Physiological Model of Human Nutrition (BFMNU) method, which is a mathematical formula applicable in any physiological and pathological condition. The criterion was to motivate them to voluntarily join the research first of all to take advantage of the benefits of the new diet protocol, as well as to collaborate to improve the health service of prevention and treatment through nutrition. We decided to collect the data in a single broad set to stay consistent for the purpose of the work. Of course, the probability of finding a template for each of the endless categories of belonging of the people tested may be higher than finding one that applies to everyone. However, it would be better to find one of general meaning, valid for everyone regardless of age, sex, muscle activity and pathologies. The choice to consider only those who had had at least four check-ups was mandatory. In fact, checking a curvilinear pattern with two or three experimental points makes no sense.

The number of experimental samples was adequate to calculate the statistical analysis. In order to obtain a dataset suitable for the analysis of variance, only subjects who had performed no less than four direct measurements of body mass over the entire transition period of initial body mass to the final one was admitted to the study. The size of the sample thus selected largely guaranteed the applicability of the statistical analysis. In fact, the distribution of variance indicates that a set of data pairs that has at least 240 degrees of freedom is congruous. Since only volunteers who had carried out at least four experimental checks would have been admitted to the study, 60 patients would have been enough (however, we worked with 374 patients). Anthropometric and weight measurements were carried out in the clinic by qualified personnel. The complete set of results was evaluated with variance analysis. This formula was considered an alternative to energy-based methods that enable the prediction of changes in body composition in response to energy intake through food, a crucial factor in the management of diet therapy. This method was devised by Boselli [16,17] with the objective of proposing a new nutritional intervention method different from the existing methods, which was able to systemically interpret the metabolic processes of mass and energy and to overcome the many and obvious contradictions of the methods already in use. The technical error of measurement (TEM), which is an accuracy index that represents the measurement quality and control dimension, was determined according to Perini et al. [18].

The Ethical Committee approved the study of the University of Milan (Milan, Italy) (Ethical Committee Number UnivMil-1-2014). All subjects provided written informed consent before study entry.

3. Results

The BFMNU model assumes that body mass results from the sum of three contributions from the catabolic, anabolic, and redistributive phases:

Catabolic phase

$$V(t) \xrightarrow{K_V}$$

with $K_V > 0$

$$\frac{dV(t)}{dt} = -K_V V(t)$$

initial conditions:

$$V(0) = M_i$$

final conditions:

$$V(t \to \infty) = 0$$

$$dV(t)/V(t) = -k_v\, dt; \int dV(t)/V(t) = -k_v \int dt; \ln V(t) = -k_v\, t + \text{cost.};$$

$$\text{per } t = 0 \text{ cost.} = \ln V(0) = \ln M_i; \ln V(t) = \ln M_i - k_v\, t;$$

$$\ln V(t) - \ln M_i = -k_v\, t; \ln[V(t)/M_i] = -k_v\, t; V(t)/M_i = e^{-k_v t};$$

$$M_{old}(t) = Mi\, e^{-k_v t}$$

Anabolic phase

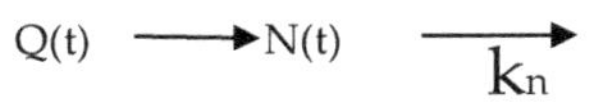

with $Q(t) > 0$, $k_n > 0$
initial conditions:

$$N(0) = 0;$$

final conditions:

$$N(t \to \infty) = M_f$$

the model is described by the following equation:

$$dN(t)/dt = -k_n\, N(t) + Q(t)$$

how transformed is:

$$s\, n + k_n\, n = q/s; n = q/s\, (s + k_n);$$

we get A and B from the identity:

$$q/s\, (s + k_n) = A/s + B/(s + k_n); A = q/k_n; B = -q/k_n$$

leading to the following solution:

$$N(t) = (Q/k_n)\, (1 - e^{-knt})$$

that because of

$$t \to \infty, N(t \to \infty) = M_f,$$

can be written as:

$$M_{new}(t) = M_f\, (1 - e^{-k_n t})$$

Redistributive phase

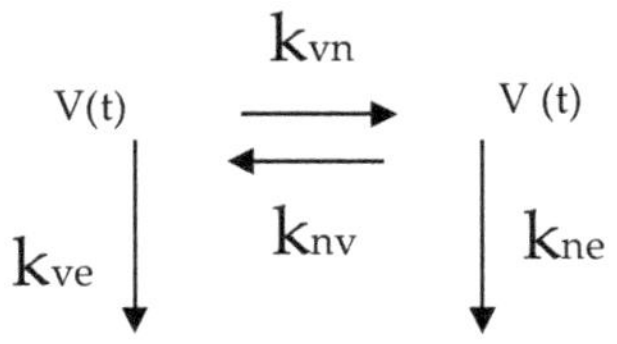

with: k_{vn}, k_{nv}, k_{ve}, $k_{ve} > 0$

with: $\mathbf{k_e} = k_{ve} = k_{ne}$; $\mathbf{k_v} = k_{vn} + k_{ve}$; $\mathbf{k_n} = k_{nv} + k_{ne}$
where: $k_v - k_{vn} = k_n - k_{nv}$ and $k_v + k_{nv} = k_n + k_{vn} = \mathbf{K}$

And since the transition phase is intermediate between the initial phase and the final phase, we must bear in mind that for $0 < t < \infty$, V $(0 < t < \infty)$ = Vx yN $(0 < t < \infty)$ = Nx.

The system of differential equations that the model describes is:

$$dV(t)/dt = -k_v V(t) + k_{nv} N(t)$$

$$dN(t)/dt = -k_n N(t) + k_{vn} V(t)$$

with the Laplace-transform:

$$s\,v + k_v\,v - k_{nv}\,n = V_x$$

$$s\,n + k_n\,n - k_{vn}\,v = N_x$$

$$(s + k_v)\,v - k_{nv}\,n = V_x$$

$$-k_{vn}\,v + (s + k_n)\,n = N_x$$

v	n	Known
$(s + k_v)$	$-k_{nv}$	V_x
$-k_{vn}$	$(s + k_n)$	N_x

$D_t = (s + k_v)\,(s + k_n) - k_{nv}\,k_{vn} = (s + \alpha)\,(s + \beta)$; (the roots of the equation in s^2 are α, β)

$$D_v = V_x\,(s + k_n) + N_x\,k_{nv}$$

$$D_n = N_x\,(s + k_v) + V_x\,k_{vn}$$

where:

$$v = V_x\,(s + k_n)/(s + \alpha)(s + \beta) + N_x\,k_{nv}/(s + \alpha)(s + \beta)$$

$$n = N_x\,(s + k_v)/(s + \alpha)(s + \beta) + V_x\,k_{vn}/(s + \alpha)(s + \beta)$$

Since the writing of the two previous equations is analogous, it is enough to find the constants A, B, C, F of the first two identities (only of the first equation because those of the second are analogous):

$$V_x\,(s + k_n)/(s + \alpha)(s + \beta) = A/(s + \alpha) + B/(s + \beta)$$

$$N_x\,k_{nv}/(s + \alpha)(s + \beta) = C/(s + \alpha) + F/(s + \beta)$$

$$V_x\,(s + k_n) = A\,(s + \beta) + B\,(s + \alpha) = s(A + B) + A\,\beta + B\,\alpha$$

where:

$$A + B = V_x, \quad \text{and} \quad V_x\,k_n = A\,\beta + B\,\alpha$$

$$A = V_x - B$$

so what:

$$V_x\,k_n = V_x\,\beta - B\,\beta + B\,\alpha = V_x\,\beta - B\,(\beta - \alpha)$$

$$V_x\,(k_n - \beta) = -B\,(\beta - \alpha)$$

thus

$$B = -V_x(k_n - \beta)/(\beta - \alpha)$$

and, in consequence:

$$A = V_x - B = V_x + V_x\,(k_n - \beta)/(\beta - \alpha)$$

i.e.,:

$$A = V_x(k_n - \alpha)/(\beta - \alpha)$$

$$N_x\,k_{nv} = C\,(s + \beta) + F\,(s + \alpha) = s\,(C + F) + C\,\beta + F\,\alpha$$

where:

$$C + F = 0, \quad e \quad N_x\,k_{nv} = C\,\beta + F\,\alpha$$
$$C = -F$$

so what:

$$N_x\,k_{nv} = -F\,\beta + F\,\alpha = -F\,(\beta - \alpha);$$

thus:

$$F = -N_x\,k_{nv}/(\beta - \alpha)$$

and, in consequence:

$$C = N_x\,k_{nv}/(\beta - \alpha)$$

The following equations:

$$v = V_x\,(s + k_n)/(s + \alpha)(s + \beta) + N_x\,k_{nv}/(s + \alpha)(s + \beta)$$

$$n = N_x\,(s + k_v)/(s + \alpha)(s + \beta) + V_x\,k_{vn}/(s + \alpha)(s + \beta)$$

can be written:

$$V(t) = \frac{Vx(kn-\alpha)}{(\beta-\alpha)(s+\alpha)} - Vx(kn - \beta)/(\beta - \alpha)(s + \beta) + Nx\,knv/(\beta - \alpha)(s + \alpha) - Nx\,knv/(\beta - \alpha)(s + \beta)$$
$$N(t) = Nx(kv - \alpha)/(\beta-\alpha)(s + \alpha) - Nx(kv - \beta)/(\beta-\alpha)(s + \beta) + Vx\,kvn/(\beta-\alpha)(s + \alpha) - Vx\,kvn/(\beta-\alpha)(s + \beta)$$

Of which, we obtain:

$$\mathbf{V(t)} = V_x(k_n - \alpha)e^{-\alpha t}/(\beta - \alpha) - V_x(k_n - \beta)e^{-\beta t}/(\beta - \alpha) + N_x\,k_{nv}\,e^{-\alpha t}/(\beta - \alpha) - N_x\,k_{nv}\,e^{-\beta t}/(\beta - \alpha)$$
$$\mathbf{N(t)} = N_x(k_v - \alpha)e^{-\alpha t}/(\beta - \alpha) - N_x(k_v - \beta)e^{-\beta t}/(\beta - \alpha) + V_x\,k_{vn}\,e^{-\alpha t}/(\beta - \alpha) - V_x\,k_{vn}\,e^{-\beta t}/(\beta - \alpha)$$

Given that

$$M(t) = V(t) + N(t)$$

then:

$$M(t) = V_x(k_n - \alpha + k_{vn})e^{-\alpha t}/(\beta - \alpha) + N_x(k_v - \alpha + k_{nv})e^{-\alpha t}/(\beta - \alpha) +$$
$$-V_x(k_n - \beta + k_{vn})e^{-\beta t}/(\beta - \alpha) - N_x(k_v - \beta + k_{nv})e^{-\beta t}/(\beta - \alpha)$$
$$M(t) = [V_x(k_n - \alpha + k_{vn}) + N_x(k_v - \alpha + k_{nv})]\,e^{-\alpha t}/(\beta - \alpha) +$$
$$-[V_x(k_n - \beta + k_{vn}) + N_x(k_v - \beta + k_{nv})\,]\,e^{-\beta t}/(\beta - \alpha)$$

and remembering that

$$k_e = k_v - k_{vn} = k_n - k_{vn};\; k_v + k_{vn} = k_n + k_{vn} = K$$

then:

$$M(t) = [V_x(K - \alpha) + N_x(K - \alpha)]\,e^{-\alpha t}/(\beta - \alpha) - [V_x(K - \beta) + N_x(K - \beta)]\,e^{-\beta t}/(\beta - \alpha)$$

$$M_{redistributive}\,(t) = (V_x + N_x)(K - \alpha)\,e^{-\alpha t}/(\beta - \alpha) - (V_x + N_x)(K - \beta)\,e^{-\beta t}/(\beta - \alpha)$$

Finally how $(K - \alpha) \sim (K - \beta) \sim (\beta - \alpha)$, can be approximated:

$$M_{redistributive}(t) = (M_i + M_f)\,(e^{-\alpha t} - e^{-\beta t})$$

that in the initial and final conditions:

$$\text{for } t = 0 \; M_{redistributive}\,(0) = 0$$

$$\text{and for } t \to \infty \; M_{redistributive}\,(t \to \infty) = 0$$

Finally, the solution of the model is given by the sum of the three solving equations of the catabolic, anabolic, and distributive processes:

$$M_c(t) = M_i\, e^{-kvt} + M_f\,(1 - e^{-knt}) + (M_i + M_f)(e^{-\alpha t} - e^{-\beta t})$$

Since the metabolic rate constant of the "old" mass is substantially the initial metabolic constant and that of the "new" mass is defined as the final or final, the above equation becomes:

$$M_c(t) = M_i\, e^{-kmit} + M_f\,(1 - e^{-kmft}) + (M_i + M_f)(e^{-\alpha t} - e^{-\beta t})$$

where M_c is the body mass at time t, M_i the body mass at the beginning of the observations, M_f the body mass at the end, respectively, and α and β are the constants controlling the distributive process. To facilitate the calculations necessary to obtain the numerical solution of the model on the experimental data set, specially compiled software (Dies4) was used. Body mass values were measured monthly by means of an electronic balance (sensitivity of 0.1 kg). The metabolic rate constants were calculated with the following formula:

$$k_m\,[h^{-1}] = -(1/24)\ln\,[(M_c - M_a)/M_c]$$

where M_c (kg) is the body mass and M_a (kg) the daily food mass.

If this equation is applied to all the pairs of values for M_C and M_a, the metabolic constants of the body mass can be calculated at any time. A balanced diet was assigned for each of the patients with the aim of making the patients tend toward normal with respect to their BMI interval. Body mass was measured initially and then subsequently at each control. The initial food mass was reported by the patients through the food diary and subsequently replaced by the dietary mass of the assigned diet. Patients were required to follow the diet scrupulously and to maintain the same lifestyle at least as long as necessary to carry out the checks. For each of the patients, the metabolic constants were calculated during the control visits using the same formula with which the initial values were calculated. Therefore, the constants varied because the body mass, not the food mass, varied over time. The metabolic constants are stable when body mass stabilizes. Considering body mass as a result of the three catabolic, anabolic, and redistributive phases for each patient, a temporal trend was constructed by inserting the initial, intermediate, and final constants into the formal solution of the model. The expected body masses were calculated, whereas the observed values were measured experimentally during the control visits. At every time on the curve, each patient was characterized by a couple of expected–observed values. A database was constructed by randomly inserting the following parameters for each patient: sex, age, initial body mass, body mass index (BMI), initial k_m, final body mass, final k_m, number of control visits, deviance, and variance. Figure 1 shows an example of fitting a patient's body mass.

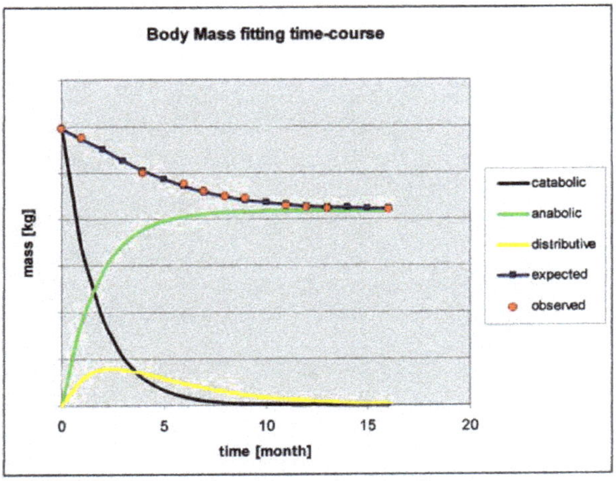

Figure 1. An example of fitting a patient's body mass. The expected body mass (blue line and points) is the sum of three contributions from the catabolic (dark line), anabolic (green line), and redistributive phases (yellow line).

Deviance is the sum of the squares of the differences between the calculated (expected) data and the experimentally measured (observed) data: Dev = $\sum_1^n = (Y_{\text{observed}} - Y_{\text{expected}})^2$. The variance is Var = $\frac{\text{Dev}}{\text{DF}}$, where Dev = deviance and DF = degrees of freedom. Table S1 shows all values obtained for the studied subjects and Table S2 reflects all values with statistical analysis.

4. Discussion

The logical sequence of the phases that lead to the realization of a biomathematic model such as the one proposed in this research are: (i) draw one or more block diagrams that have biological sense and, above all, indicate the connections and direction of matter transfers, (ii) describe the scheme with a system of differential equations (Formal model), (iii) solve the system of differential equations to obtain the integral equation (Formal solution of the model), (iv) calculate, from the formal solution, the values that the dependent variable (in our case the Body Mass) takes in correspondence with the independent variable (time), (v) analyze all pairs of values calculated and measured experimentally to understand if there are significant differences (validation process) and (vi) the model is valid to interpret the experimental data only if the variance, calculated on the total set of value pairs and/or on the subgroups tends to zero (at 240 degrees of freedom it is sufficient that it is less than 1).

All mean variances of the pathophysiological groups are less than 1 and are no different from the total variance. The model is validated. However, if we compare the mean variances of the individual pathological groups with the group of healthy people, it is observed that the model applied to the groups of anorexia and tumors (much more evident in anorexia) proves to be valid but at the limit of significance. This is due to the insufficient number of samples. A more in-depth investigation, which could remove any doubt about the validity of the model also in these two groups, is desirable and to be carried out in future research. In fact, the variance analysis carried out on the results showed that no significant differences existed between the expected and the experimental data; therefore, we concluded that the model was suitable for interpreting trends in body mass over time. In our viewpoint, the limits of this study are determined by the purpose of the research itself and therefore by the consequent experimental plan. No other result, obtained outside the experimental plan, can be considered valid. If by limits we mean the critical elements then it can be said that the random choice of the sample guarantees the statistical representativeness of the population but cannot guarantee in the same way the comparison between those groups, internal to the sample, which have lower degrees of freedom. For example, in this study, the comparison between anorexic and oncological groups with healthy people could be questioned for the low number of degrees of freedom at stake (37 and 43 respectively). On the other hand, it should be considered that the analysis of variance on partial sets and on the whole set cannot be misunderstood. We are not demonstrating the equality between pathophysiological situations, which obviously does not exist and cannot be there. Instead, we are evaluating whether, in each pathophysiological situation, the model can interpret the experimental data.

In the future, the research could be extended to each single metabolic compartment (protein, aqueous, glucose, and lipid). Metabolic constants are specific to the subject and are the result of the functional state of the subject, and do not depend on whether they belong to a particular pathophysiological class. Our results confirm that body mass and its variation do not depend on energy but on the metabolic speed constants [19] where the body mass of an individual is determined by mass balance, regulated by corresponding metabolic rate, calculated by the BFMNU method, thanks to which the macronutrients in the diet are absorbed, redistributed and eliminated. In fact, this study reflected that a significant correlation, although not straight, is demonstrated between Δ% of food energy, supplied after processing through the dietary BFMNU method, and the Δ% of body mass, obtained following the dietetic path. Furthermore, this tool was applied in university students [20]. Currently, the clinical application of predictive equations [2–10] is useful for calculating the resting metabolic rate. However, the best fit allows us to predict body mass instantaneously as well as throughout life, providing the significant advantage of control over the whole process.

Currently, the diet methodology is premised on energy and tends to understand body mass as a result of dietary energy contained in the diet. It is said that body mass is related to introduced food energy, but the correlation between the two is so low as to be considered casual and not significant. Within the same patient, starting from a steady state, the only method to determine the end point is to evaluate the percentage variation of the energy contained in the assigned diet with respect to the previous diet. This is correlated, but not in a straight line, to the percentage change in the body mass [5]. The overall process that leads to the formation of body mass is the sum of partial dynamic processes: catabolic, anabolic, and distributive. These processes are contemporary and occur throughout life, even if at different rates depending on age and pathophysiological conditions. The modelling approach allows us to determine the speed constants that regulate these three processes. Body mass depends on the diet mass and mainly on the speed constants (k) with which the mass is transformed, which depends on metabolism [7]. The calculation of speed constants indicates the space–time context of the biological process and predicts its progress and possible outcomes. Therefore, if nutritional needs can be determined on the basis of metabolic constants, then optimal and specific diets can be formulated. The main purpose of the method is to optimize health with proper nutrition, which means finding a diet that is able to produce a combined change in body mass and composition and provide useful energy to the body to improve its performance [8]. Several authors have examined the importance of other factors on resting metabolic rate and energy expenditure, including specific behaviors [21] and environmental factors [22,23]. The literature indicates that measured RMR (mRMR) is positively correlated with BMI, total fat mass, and fat-free mass [24–26]. In longitudinal studies, animal models were used to understand and examine individual variation in resting metabolic rate. Krom et al. [27] used model components from obesogenic environments when using animal models to elucidate aspects of human obesity. The advantage of animal models is that rats can be selected, placed in a well-controlled environment, and followed throughout the development, treatment, and relapse of nutritional diseases [28–31]. Unlike humans, the behavior of rats is not influenced by peer pressure, the concept of an ideal physique, or other societal factors that provide the motivation to alter behavior [28]. Recently, the applicability of BFMNU with the BMI has been used to define a new formula called BMI-BFMNU where it is possible to obtain an indication of the body structure related to the amount of fat [32].

5. Conclusions

In summary, the use of BFMNU is useful to systemically determine the metabolic processes of mass and energy and to overcome the many contradictions of the methods already in use. It is a phenomenological and mathematical method applicable to any individual in any pathophysiological condition, and its primary objective is to determine the optimal diet for producing a synergistic change in body mass, body composition, and energy to improve the functionality of the body with the smallest possible variation in comparison to previous eating habits. The promotion of this study reflected that the BFMNU method is a model that can help describe trends in body mass and its variations over time using a continuous function that is useful in daily clinical work. Together with the advantages, however, it is necessary to highlight some limitations that derive precisely from the very nature of the method. The collection of data, information, direct measurements, processing and calculations takes time on the part of specialists.

Supplementary Materials: The following supporting information can be downloaded at: https://www.mdpi.com/article/10.3390/nu14173575/s1, Table S1: Body Mass fitting time course. Table S2: Database manuscript.

Author Contributions: Conceptualization, methodology, validation, formal analysis, investigation and data curation, J.M.S., G.S. and P.M.B.; writing—original draft preparation, J.M.S. and P.M.B.; writing—review and editing, G.S. All authors have read and agreed to the published version of the manuscript.

Funding: This research received no external funding.

Institutional Review Board Statement: The study was conducted in accordance with the Declaration of Helsinki, and approved by the Ethics Committee of University of Milan (Milan, Italy) (Ethical Committee Number UnivMil-1-2014) for studies involving humans.

Informed Consent Statement: Informed consent was obtained from all subjects involved in the study.

Data Availability Statement: Not applicable.

Conflicts of Interest: The authors declare no conflict of interest.

References

1. Kozusko, F.P. Body weight, setpoint, metabolic adaptation and human starvation. *Bull. Math. Biol.* **2001**, *63*, 393–403. [CrossRef]
2. Chow, C.C.; Hall, K.D. The dynamics of human weight change. *PLoS Comp. Biol.* **2008**, *4*, e1000045. [CrossRef]
3. Hall, K.D.; Jordan, P.N. Modeling weight-loss maintenance to help prevent body weight regain. *Am. J. Clin. Nutr.* **2008**, *88*, 1495–1503. [CrossRef] [PubMed]
4. Christiansen, E.; Garby, L.; Srensen, T.I.A. Quantitative analysis of the energy requirements for development of obesity. *J. Theor. Biol.* **2005**, *234*, 99–106. [CrossRef]
5. Thomas, D.M.; Ciesla, A.; Levine, J.A.; Stevens, J.G.; Martin, C.K. A mathematical model of weight change with adaptation. *Math. Biosci. Eng.* **2009**, *6*, 873–887. [CrossRef] [PubMed]
6. Rahmandad, H. Human growth and body weight dynamics: An integrative systems model. *PLoS ONE* **2014**, *9*, e114609. [CrossRef] [PubMed]
7. Ferrannini, E. The theoretical bases of indirect calorimetry: A review. *Metabolism* **1988**, *37*, 287–301. [CrossRef]
8. Frankenfield, D.C.; Rowe, W.A.; Smith, J.S.; Cooney, R.N. Validation of several established equations for resting metabolic rate in obese and nonobese people. *J. Am. Diet. Assoc.* **2003**, *103*, 1152–1159. [CrossRef]
9. Frankenfield, D.; Roth-Yousey, L.; Compher, C. A mathematical model of weight change with adaptation. *J. Am. Diet. Assoc.* **2005**, *105*, 775–789. [CrossRef]
10. Achamrah, N.; Jésus, P.; Grigioni, S.; Rimbert, A.; Petit, A.; Déchelotte, P.; Folope, V.; Coëffier, M. Validity of predictive equations for resting energy expenditure developed for obese patients: Impact of body composition method. *Nutrients* **2018**, *10*, 63. [CrossRef]
11. Pinho, C.P.S.; Diniz, A.D.S.; de Arruda, I.K.G.; Leite, A.P.D.L.; Petribú, M.M.V.; Rodrigues, I.G. Predictive models for estimating visceral fat: The contribution from anthropometric parameters. *PLoS ONE* **2017**, *12*, e0178958. [CrossRef] [PubMed]

2. Verbraecken, J.; van de Heyning, P.; de Backer, W.; van Gaal, L. Body surface area in normal-weight, overweight, and obese adults. A comparison study. *Metabolism* **2006**, *55*, 515–524. [CrossRef]
3. Bonora, E.; Micciolo, R.; Ghiatas, A.A.; Lancaster, J.L.; Alyassin, A.; Muggeo, M.; DeFronzo, R.A. Is it possible to derive a reliable estimate of human visceral and subcutaneous abdominal adipose tissue from simple anthropometric measurements? *Metabolism* **1995**, *44*, 1617–1625. [CrossRef]
4. Ramírez-Vélez, R.; García-Hermoso, A.; Prieto-Benavides, D.H.; Correa-Bautista, J.E.; Quino-Ávila, A.C.; Rubio-Barreto, C.M.; González-Ruíz, K.; Carrillo, H.A.; Correa-Rodríguez, M.; González-Jiménez, E.; et al. Muscle mass to visceral fat ratio is an important predictor of the metabolic syndrome in college students. *Br. J. Nutr.* **2019**, *121*, 330–339. [CrossRef]
5. Lahav, Y.; Epstein, Y.; Kedem, R.; Schermann, H. A novel body circumferences-based estimation of percentage body fat. *Br. J. Nutr.* **2018**, *119*, 720–725. [CrossRef] [PubMed]
6. Boselli, P.M. *Fenomenologia della Nutrizione*; Raffaelo Cortina Editore: Milano, Italy, 2011.
7. Boselli, P.M. *El método BFMNU: Interpretación Modelo-Fenomenológica de la Nutrición*; Ediciones Mónsul: Valencia, Spain, 2020.
8. Perini, T.A.; Oliveira, G.L.D.; Ornellas, J.D.S.; Oliveira, F.P.D. Technical error of measurement in anthropometry. *Rev. Bras. Med. Esporte* **2005**, *11*, 81–85. [CrossRef]
9. Rondini, G.; Olearo, B.; Soriano, J.M.; Boselli, P.M. The BFMNU method as an alternative to the methods in use based on energy: Study of the correlation between food energy and body mass. *Nutr. Hosp.* **2018**, *35*, 346–350. [CrossRef] [PubMed]
0. Olearo, B.; Soriano, J.M.; Boselli, P.M.; Pascual, L.M. Assessment of body composition, through anthropometric and non-anthropometric methods, of university students from Valencia. *Nutr. Hosp.* **2014**, *30*, 911–918. [CrossRef]
1. Crawford, D.; Ball, K. Behavioural determinants of the obesity epidemic. *Asia Pac. J. Clin. Nutr.* **2002**, *11*, S718–S721. [CrossRef]
2. Goran, M.I.; Weinsier, R.L. Role of environmental vs. metabolic factors in the etiology of obesity: Time to focus on the environment. *Obes. Res.* **2000**, *8*, 407–409. [CrossRef]
3. Ravussin, E.; Bogardus, C. Energy balance and weight regulation: Genetics versus environment. *Br. J. Nutr.* **2000**, *83*, S17–S20. [CrossRef]
4. Weyer, C.; Snitker, S.; Rising, R.; Bogardus, C.; Ravussin, E. Determinants of energy expenditure and fuel utilization in man: Effects of body composition, age, sex, ethnicity and glucose tolerance in 916 subjects. *Int. J. Obes. Relat. Metab. Disord.* **1999**, *23*, 715–722. [CrossRef] [PubMed]
5. Bogardus, C.; Lillioja, S.; Ravussin, E.; Abbott, W.; Zawadzki, J.K.; Young, A.; Knowler, W.C.; Jacobowitz, R.; Moll, P.P. Familial dependence of the resting metabolic rate. *N. Engl. J. Med.* **1986**, *315*, 96–100. [CrossRef] [PubMed]
6. Reneau, J.; Obi, B.; Moosreiner, A.; Kidambi, S. Do we need race-specific resting metabolic rate prediction equations? *Nutr. Diabetes* **2019**, *9*, 21. [CrossRef] [PubMed]
7. Krom, M.; Bauer, F.; Collier, D.; Adan, R.A.H.; la Fleur, S.E. Genetic variation and effects on human eating behavior. *Annu. Rev. Nutr.* **2009**, *29*, 283–304. [CrossRef]
8. MacLean, P.S.; Higgins, J.A.; Johnson, G.C.; Fleming-Elder, B.K.; Donahoo, W.T.; Melanson, E.L.; Hill, J.O. Enhanced metabolic efficiency contributes to weight regain after weight loss in obesity-prone rats. *Am. J. Physiol. Regul. Integr. Comp. Physiol.* **2004**, *287*, R1306–R1315. [CrossRef]
9. Chang, S.; Graham, B.; Yakubu, F.; Lin, D.; Peters, J.C.; Hill, J.O. Metabolic differences between obesity-prone and obesity-resistant rats. *Am. J. Physiol. Regul. Integr. Comp. Physiol.* **1990**, *259*, R1103–R1110. [CrossRef]
0. Cheng, H.S.; Ton, S.H.; Phang, S.C.W.; Tan, J.B.L.; Kadir, K.A. Increased susceptibility of post-weaning rats on high-fat diet to metabolic syndrome. *J. Adv. Res.* **2017**, *8*, 743–752. [CrossRef] [PubMed]
1. Pagliassotti, M.J.; Gayles, E.C.; Hill, J.O. Fat and energy balance. *Ann. N. Y. Acad. Sci.* **1997**, *827*, 431–448. [CrossRef]
2. Sechi, P.; Soriano, J.M.; Boselli, P.M. BMI-BFMNU: A structural index linked to fat mass. *Rev. Esp. Nutr. Hum. Diet.* **2021**, *25*, 104–110. [CrossRef]

nutrients

MDPI

Article

Interplay between Intestinal Bacterial Communities and Unicellular Parasites in a Morbidly Obese Population: A Neglected Trinomial

Jana Caudet [1,2,†], María Trelis [2,3,*,†], Susana Cifre [2], José M. Soriano [2,4,*], Hortensia Rico [2,5] and Juan F. Merino-Torres [1,2,6]

1 Department of Endocrinology and Nutrition, University and Polytechnic Hospital La Fe, 46026 Valencia, Spain
2 Joint Research Unit on Endocrinology, Nutrition and Clinical Dietetics, University of Valencia-Health Research Institute La Fe, 46026 Valencia, Spain
3 Parasite & Health Research Group, Area of Parasitology, Department of Pharmacy and Pharmaceutical Technology and Parasitology, University of Valencia, 46010 Valencia, Spain
4 Food & Health Lab, Institute of Materials Science, University of Valencia, 46980 Valencia, Spain
5 Area of Microbiology, Department of Microbiology and Ecology, University of Valencia, 46010 Valencia, Spain
6 Department of Medicine, Faculty of Medicine, University of Valencia, 46010 Valencia, Spain
* Correspondence: maria.trelis@uv.es (M.T.); jose.soriano@uv.es (J.M.S.)
† These authors contributed equally to this work.

Abstract: Obesity is an epidemic causing a metabolic health crisis. Herein, the interactions between the gut prokaryotic and eukaryotic communities, metabolic comorbidities and diet were studied. Stool samples from 56 subjects, 47 with type III obesity and 9 with type II obesity and cardiovascular risk or metabolic disease, were assessed for the richness, diversity and ecology of the bacterial gut community through metagenomics, together with the study of the presence of common unicellular eukaryote parasites (*Blastocystis* sp., *Dientamoeba fragilis* and *Giardia intestinalis*) by qPCR. Clinical information regarding metabolic comorbidities and non-alcoholic hepatic fatty liver disease was gathered. To assess the quality of the patients' diet, each participant filled in three dietary questionnaires. The most prevalent parasite *Blastocystis* sp. (46.4%), together with *D. fragilis* (8.9%), was found to be associated with higher mean diversity indexes regarding non-colonized subjects; the opposite of that which was observed in those with *G. intestinalis* (16.1%). In terms of phyla relative abundance, with *Blastocystis* sp. and *D. fragilis*, very slight differences were observed; on the contrary, *G. intestinalis* was related to an increase in Bacteroidetes and Proteobacteria, and a decrease in Firmicutes and Actinobacteria, presenting the lowest Firmicutes/Bacteroidetes ratio. At genus level, *Blastocystis* sp. and/or *D. fragilis* was accompanied with an increase in *Lactobacillus* spp., and a decrease in *Akkermansia* spp., *Bifidobacterium* spp. and *Escherichia* spp., while *G. intestinalis* was associated with an increase in *Bacteroides* spp., and a decrease in *Faecalibacterium* spp., *Prevotella* spp. and *Lactobacillus* spp., and the highest *Bacteroides* spp./*Prevotella* spp. ratio. Participants with non-alcoholic hepatic fatty liver presented a higher Firmicutes/Bacteroidetes ratio, and those with type 2 diabetes displayed a significantly lower *Faecalibacterium* spp./*Escherichia* spp. ratio, due to an overrepresentation of the genus *Escherichia* spp. The presence of parasites was associated with variations in the richness, diversity and distribution of taxa in bacterial communities, confirming a gain in diversity associated with *Blastocystis* sp. and providing different functioning of the microbiota with a potential positive effect on comorbidities such as type 2 diabetes, insulin resistance and metabolic syndrome. Future basic and clinical studies should assess the beneficial or pathogenic effect of these eukaryotes on obese subjects and focus on deciphering whether they may imply a healthier metabolic profile.

Keywords: obesity; eukaryotic microbiota; *Blastocystis* sp.; *Giardia intestinalis*; *Dientamoeba fragilis*; metabolic markers; diet

1. Introduction

Human gut microbiota encompasses millions of different microbes, including bacteria, archaea, fungi, viruses, helminths and protozoans, which are harboured by the human gastrointestinal tract in a symbiotic relationship. They carry a vast collection of genes referred to as the microbiome [1] and constitute an intestinal community that is stable over time, highly dissimilar and specific between subjects. Its functions are diverse in nature, ranging from metabolic and energy harvesting [2,3], to anti-infective and immunomodulatory [4,5].

Various studies have comprehensively described the bacterial composition of the gut microbiota, both in healthy and unhealthy subjects, even though there is still a lack of thorough understanding of its interactions with the human host. It is hypothesized that modifications in the western lifestyle (e.g., the practical disappearance of helminthic and protozoan infections, the incorporation of processed foods and the generalized use of antibiotics) have contributed to changes in the composition of the intestinal communities towards a decrease in the levels of prokaryotic and eukaryotic diversity [6–8]. This fact has altered the bidirectional relationship between microbiota and host, and a growing number of diseases have been suggested to be linked to this phenomenon, including obesity [9–12].

Although less abundant, unicellular eukaryotic microorganisms represent an on-topic component of the gut microbiota, but their significance within the microbial ecology remains largely unknown. Their presence has not been clearly defined as pathogenic or commensal, and knowledge about their impact on the composition of microbiota and host homeostasis remains limited. *Giardia intestinalis* is one of the most prevalent and studied parasites in this area. The establishment of *G. intestinalis* has been suggested to be conditioned by the microbiota composition of the host [7], modulating susceptibility and allowing the progression to a clinically significant infection. Furthermore, numerous studies indicate that this protozoan has the potential to reconfigure the structure of the gut ecosystem and cause a dysbiotic condition that persists even after its eradication [13–17].

On the other hand, *Blastocystis* sp. is one of the most common intestinal parasites isolated in human faeces, usually as an incident finding. The exposure to the parasite is insufficient to develop intestinal colonization, since its clearance depends on the resident microorganisms and the interactions between them, and with the host's immune system. Once the parasite is established, it can exist for more than ten years, thereby becoming a stable member of the gut ecosystem and modulating its structure [11,18]. However, its role as a pathogenic organism in humans remains speculative [19], since a link with intestinal pathology has not been unequivocally demonstrated. Additionally, high bacterial diversity and richness are traits of a healthy human microbiota [20], and their loss has been linked to several disorders [21]; in this sense, the presence of *Blastocystis* sp. in the gut has been associated with a higher biodiversity and better functionality of the microbiota [22,23], and could, therefore, be considered beneficial instead of harmful. Additionally, several descriptive studies reveal a protective role of this microorganism in obesity [18,21,23].

Dientamoeba fragilis is another protozoan that has been neglected for decades [24]. Virtually since its discovery, there has been controversy in the scientific community about its pathogenic role, since it is common to find asymptomatic parasitized subjects [25,26]. Research regarding its impact on intestinal microbial structure is scarce, and no differences in composition or diversity have been found when comparing the intestinal communities of subjects with and without the parasite [27].

According to this current state of the art, a study on morbidly obese residents in Spain was designed to further address the interactions between these three unicellular eukaryotic parasites and the richness, diversity and ecology of the intestinal bacterial community.

2. Materials and Methods

2.1. Design of the Study

This research is part of a larger single-centre and cross-sectional study conducted from August 2018 to February 2020, in obese subjects attending the Endocrinology and Nutrition Service of University and Polytechnic Hospital La Fe (Valencia, Spain).

The main aims of this study were to describe the presence of three common enteric parasites, *Giardia intestinalis*, *Dientamoeba fragilis* and *Blastocystis* sp., and analyse their occurrence with the metagenomics results of the bacterial community analysis, outlining any differences concerning richness, diversity and ecology. A secondary objective of the study was to ascertain the differences in microbiota composition with regard to metabolic comorbidities and diet composition.

Confusing factors previously described as modifiers of the composition of human gut microbiota were registered, namely: smoking status, regular use of Proton Pump Inhibitors (PPI), *Helicobacter pylori* colonization and history of a cholecystectomy.

Informed consent was obtained from all participants, after being informed about the aim of the study, risks, and implications of their participation in it, as well as the treatment and confidentiality of the data. This study was approved by the Ethics Committee for Drug Research of the University and Polytechnic Hospital La Fe, ensuring that the fundamental principles established by the Helsinki Declaration, data protection and bioethics were respected.

2.2. Study Population

Data from 56 subjects were gathered. Mean age was 48.1 $\pm$ 9.8 years, with 36 women and 20 men. The individuals included in the study were mostly patients with type III (n = 47) obesity, but also a few with type II (n = 9) and comorbidities of cardiovascular risk or metabolic disease were included. Fifty participants were Spanish, while the remainder were of Bulgarian (2), Colombian (1), German (1), Dominican (1) and Honduran (1) nationality.

Inclusion criteria were: (a) age: 18–65 years old; (b) Body Mass Index (BMI): >40 kg/m^2, or >35 kg/m^2 in coexistence with significant comorbidity; (c) no sustained weight loss with non-surgical measures. Exclusion criteria were: (a) diagnosis of oncologic disease or active oncologic process in the last 5 years; (b) autoimmune or chronic gut inflammatory diseases; (c) history of intestinal intervention that may alter the intestinal secretion dynamics; and (d) consumption of any oral or parenteral antibiotic during the six weeks prior to faecal sampling.

Every participant put on a standard hypocaloric diet, defined as a caloric input between 20–25 kcal/kg total weight/day [28]. Additionally, patients who were close to bariatric surgery were encouraged to progressively introduce commercial hypocaloric-hyperproteic meal replacements to enhance weight loss before surgery. To this end, either Optisource® (Nestlé Health Science, Vevey, Switzerland) or Vegestart Complet® (Vegenat Health Care, Badajoz, Spain) products were prescribed.

2.3. Clinical Interview

Every patient had interviews with an endocrinologist and a nutritionist, in which relevant information was recorded regarding medical history, epidemiological data and regular drug consumption. To assess the quality of the diet followed during the previous months, each participant completed the following tools: (i) a short 14-item questionnaire of adherence to the Mediterranean diet (validated in a Spanish population and used by the PREDIMED group) [29,30]; (ii) a validated Spanish food frequency questionnaire [31]; (iii) a 24 h recall questionnaire conducted in quintuplicate, according to the European recommendations [32] and methodology [33]. The evaluation of the nutritional composition of meals and the estimation of the daily intake of energy, macro- and micronutrients was carried out using the DIAL 3.0.0.5 software [34]. The cut-offs were applied as a reference to consider whether the participants fulfilled the daily nutritional requirements or not [35].

Furthermore, the patients were categorized according to the following metabolic comorbidities: hypertension, type 2 diabetes (T2D) or pre-diabetes, dyslipidaemia and hyperuricemia. Metabolic syndrome was diagnosed according to the National Cholesterol Education Program (NCEP) Adult Treatment Panel III (ATP III) definition [36]. An insulin cut-off point of >3.8, previously validated in our population [37], was established as indicative of insulin resistance. The presence of hepatic steatosis suggestive of Non-Alcoholic Hepatic Fatty Liver Disease (NAFLD) was assessed by means of ultrasonography.

Finally, anthropometric measurements were obtained after an overnight fast to gather information concerning weight and height. A multi-frequency bioelectrical impedance analysis (InBody 770®, Biospace Co., Ltd., Seoul, Korea); Frequencies: 1, 5, 250, 500 and 1000 kHz) [38] and a wall height rod were employed for every participant. Body Mass Index (BMI) was calculated as kg/m^2.

2.4. Stool Sampling, DNA Extraction and Parasitological Analysis

Each patient provided three stool samples collected on alternate days in REAL Mini-Systems with Total-fix fixative (Durviz, Valencia, Spain) for conservation and concentration by centrifugation. Stool DNA was extracted from 200 µL of the concentrate with the QIAamp DNA Stool Mini Kit (QIAGEN, Hilden, Germany) according to the manufacturer's instructions. Extracted DNA was stored at −20 °C until its use in parasitological and microbiological analysis.

Multiplex PCR for the detection and identification of intestinal parasites was performed using a commercially available kit, *Allplex GI-Parasite Assay* (GIPPA) (Seegene, Seoul, South Korea) for common human unicellular parasites such as *Giardia duodenalis, Entamoeba histolytica, Cryptosporidium* spp., *Blastocystis hominis, Dientamoeba fragilis* and *Cyclospora cayetanensis* [39–41]. Amplification was performed on the CFX96 Real Time PCR System (Bio-Rad, Marnes-la-Coquette, France), and managed with CFX Manager IVD 1.6 software, in a 25 µL reaction volume containing 20 µL reaction mix (5 µL Primers Mom, 5 µL Anyplex PCR MM (EM2), 8 µL of DNase/RNase-free water and 2 µL of internal control) and 5 µL of DNA. Negative (DNase/RNase-free water) and positive controls were included in each assay. Results were analysed and interpreted using the Seegene Viewer V3 software optimized for multiplex assays. Samples were considered positive for specific parasites if the cycle threshold (Ct) was $\leq$43 cycles, according to the manufacturer's instructions.

2.5. Microbiota Analysis by Next Generation Sequencing and Interpretation

Metagenomics analysis of the intestinal bacterial community was obtained from stool DNA as described in the previous section, which was delivered to the Sequencing and Bioinformatics Service of the Foundation for the Promotion of Health and Biomedical Research of Valencia Region (FISABIO).

For the study of the intestinal microbiome, the bacterial gene coding for the *16S* rDNA was analysed according to the Illumina MiSeq *16S* Metagenomics Sequencing Library Preparation protocol (Cod. 15044223 Rev. A). The pair of primers used for the PCR was suggested by Klindworth et al. (2013) [42]. Bacterial genomic DNA (5 ng/µL in 10 mM Tris pH 8.5) was used to initiate the protocol. After *16S* rDNA gene amplification, the multiplexing step was performed using Nextera XT Index Kit (FC-131-1096). One µL of the PCR product was run on a Bioanalyzer DNA 1000 chip to verify the expected size (~550 bp). After size verification, the libraries were sequenced using a 2 × 300 pb paired-end run (MiSeq Reagent kit v3 (MS-102-3001)) on a MiSeq Sequencer according to the manufacturer's instructions (Illumina, San Diego, CA, USA). Quality assessment was performed using the "prinseqlite" program [43], applying the following parameters: min_length: 50; trim_qual_right: 30; trim_qual_type: mean; trim_qual_window: 20.

Meta-taxonomy assessment was performed using some of QIIME2 (Quantitative Insights into Microbial Ecology) plugins. Denoising, paired-ends joining and chimera depletion were performed, starting from paired ends data using DADA2 pipeline [44]. Taxonomic affiliations were assigned using the Naïve Bayesian classifier integrated in QIIME2 plugins. The database used for this taxonomic assignation was the SILVA_release_132 [45]. The sequence data were analysed using QIIME2 pipeline, as originally cited in Caporaso (2010) [46]. The sequences are available in the ENA public repository (https://www.

ebi.ac.uk/ena/browser/view/PRJEB51819 accesion number: ERA10729632) (accessed on 25 March 2022).

Microbiome diversity is typically described in terms of within (i.e., alpha) and between samples (i.e., beta) diversities. Alpha diversity of the microbiota from each sample was determined by means of Chao1 and Shannon indexes. The Chao1 index assesses the bacterial richness within a community, whereas the Shannon index evaluates the diversity in a community based on the distribution of taxa abundances within a sample. Beta diversity was analysed with Jaccard and Sorensen indexes, the most widely used in ecology and evolution, which express the similarity or dissimilarity of microbial community composition between samples. Likewise, Principal Coordinate Analyses (PCoA) were plotted against samples as a summary of the beta diversity.

Secondly, the different taxonomic categories were explored, describing the following relative abundances and ratios: (i) relative abundance of the human main intestinal phyla (Firmicutes, Bacteroidetes, Proteobacteria and Actinobacteria); (ii) Firmicutes/Bacteroidetes ratio; (iii) relative abundance of genera described as beneficial [47–51]: *Akkermansia* spp., *Faecalibacterium* spp., *Roseburia* spp., *Bifidobacterium* spp., and *Lactobacillus* spp.; (iv) *Bacteroides* spp./*Prevotella* spp. ratio, whose relative abundances are usually inversely correlated [52,53]; and (v) *Faecalibacterium* spp./*Escherichia* spp. ratio, which has been previously used as a dysbiosis index caused by parasitic colonization [14].

2.6. Statistical Analysis

Data obtained are shown as absolute frequency (%) in qualitative variables and as mean $\pm$ standard deviation or median (Q1, Q3) in quantitative variables. To compare the differences between groups, the Chi2 test for qualitative variables and Wilcoxon rank sum test with continuity correction for quantitative variables were performed. A p value < 0.05 was considered to indicate statistical significance when comparing clinical variables. All analyses were performed using the statistical software R (4.0 version) [54].

2.7. Ethical Statement

Informed consent was obtained from all participants after being informed about the aim of the study, risks and implications of their participation in it, as well as the treatment and confidentiality of the data.

This study was approved by the Biomedical Research Ethics Committee of University and Polytechnic Hospital La Fe on 1 July 2019 (Project identification code: 2017/0486), respecting the fundamental principles of the Declaration of Helsinki, of the Council of Europe Convention in relation to Human Rights and Biomedicine of the UNESCO Declaration.

3. Results

3.1. Studied Population Description

In terms of the WHO classification [55], mean BMI of the participants was 45.6 $\pm$ 6.5 kg/m^2 and mean waist circumference 129.9 $\pm$ 13.5 cm. Active smoking was present in 25.0% of the participants, and 14.3% regularly consumed PPI. Five patients (8.9%) had a history of cholecystectomy. Up to 22 (42.3%) were taking at least one meal replacement per day during the month before faecal sampling.

The most frequent metabolic comorbidities were dyslipidaemia (73.2%), hypertension (53.6%), hyperuricemia (46.4%) and T2D (33.9%). Metabolic syndrome (ATP-III diagnostic criteria) was diagnosed in 51.7% of cases; 61.2% were insulin resistant, and 71.2% presented hepatic steatosis (US assessment).

Thirty-one participants (55.4%) were demonstrated to be colonized for intestinal unicellular parasites by multiplex qPCR. The most frequent species were *Blastocystis* sp. (46.4%), *Giardia intestinalis* (16.1%) and *Dientamoeba fragilis* (8.9%), with 5 cases combining *Blastocystis* sp./*G. intestinalis*, 2 cases of *Blastocystis* sp./*D. fragilis* and 1 case colonized by the three species. No cases of *Cryptosporidium* spp., *Entamoeba histolytica*, or *Cyclospora cayetanensis* species included in the same multiplex assay was detected.

The group of subjects colonized by a unicellular eukaryote (n = 31) was comparable with the non-colonized group (n = 25) in terms of age, gender, metabolic comorbidities, meal replacement consumption and smoking condition (Table 1). However, colonized participants were significantly more obese (mean BMI 47.3 vs. 43.4 kg/m^2; $p = 0.025$).

Table 1. Comparison between sociodemographic, anthropometric and clinical variables categorized by colonization status.

	Colonized	Non-Colonized
Female n (%)	19 (*61.3*)	17 (*68.0*)
Male n (%)	12 (*38.7*)	8 (*32.0*)
Age (years) mean (SD)	47.8 (*10.3*)	48.6 (*9.3*)
BMI (kg/m^2) mean (SD)	**47.3 (6.7)**	**43.4 (5.8)**
Abdominal circumference (cm) mean (SD)	132.4 (*11.6*)	126.9 (*15.4*)
Type II obesity n (%)	3 (*9.7*)	6 (*24.0*)
Type III obesity n (%)	28 (*90.3*)	19 (*76.0*)
Smokers n (%)	11 (*35.5*)	4 (*16.0*)
Meal replacement consumption n (%)	11 (*35.5*)	11 (*44.0*)
PPI regular use n (%)	3 (*9.7*)	5 (*20.0*)
History of a cholecystectomy n (%)	1 (*3.2*)	4 (*16.0*)
Hypertension n (%)	14 (*45.2*)	16 (*64.0*)
Dyslipidaemia n (%)	25 (*80.6*)	16 (*64.0*)
T2D n (%)	8 (*25.8*)	11 (*44.0*)
Hepatic steatosis n (%)	10 $^+$ (*37.0*)	5 (*20.0*)
Hyperuricemia n (%)	15 (*48.4*)	11(*44.0*)
Metabolic syndrome n (%)	15 (*48.4*)	14 (*56.0*)
Insulin resistance n (%)	17 (*56.7*)	12 (*63.2*)

BMI: Body Mass Index; PPI: Proton Pump Inhibitors; T2D: Type 2 Diabetes. Numbers in bold indicate significance at the 0.05 level between groups. $^+$ Missing data from 4 subjects.

3.2. *Metagenomics Analysis of the Intestinal Bacterial Community*

3.2.1. Reads by Sample

Among all stool samples, the mean number of raw sequences found was 188,847. After the quality assessment protocol included in the DADA2 pipeline (initial quality filtering, denoising, paired-ends joining and chimera filtering), the mean number of reads was reduced to 136,840 (73.1% of non-chimeric inputs). The final dataset produced 3783 Amplicon Single Variants (ASV), distributed into 13 phyla, 96 families, 330 genera and 668 known species. Supplementary tables show individual results regarding reads by count clustered by phylum (Table S1) and genus (Table S2).

A trend towards a higher number of reads was found in subjects colonized with parasites, which resulted as statistically significant in the subgroup of the *Blastocystis* positives (mean number of reads: 136,282 vs. 118,070; $p = 0.038$). In addition, a significantly lower recount of sequences was identified among participants suffering from Non-Alcoholic Hepatic Fatty Liver Disease (NAFLD) (mean number of reads: 118,374 vs. 140,395; $p = 0.002$).

3.2.2. Alpha and Beta Diversity

Chao1 and Shannon indexes were used at genus level to assess the intestinal bacterial structure in terms of alpha diversity. When comparing these indexes between subjects with or without intestinal parasites, higher alpha diversity was observed in *Blastocystis* sp. and/or *D. fragilis* positive ones, compared to those colonized by *G. intestinalis* (Table 2) (Figure 1); however, the differences were not significant.

Table 2. Alpha and beta diversity mean indexes at genus level categorized by colonization status and parasitic species.

	Non-Colonized (n = 25)	*B/DF* (n = 22)	*G. intestinalis* (n = 9)
Chao 1	109.8	119.1	103.3
Shannon	2.89	2.94	2.72
Jaccard	0.443	0.477	0.376
Sorensen	0.599	0.632	0.520

B/DF = *Blastocystis* sp. and/or *D. fragilis* positives after excluding co-infections with *G. intestinalis*.

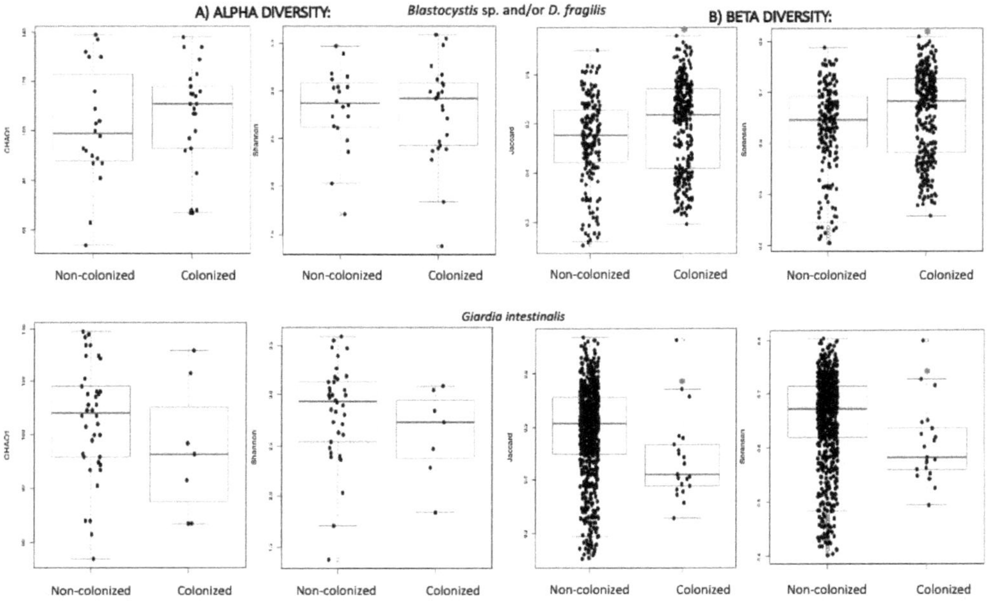

Figure 1. (**A**) Alpha diversity distances boxplots for comparison of genus richness (Chao1) and diversity (Shannon) between subjects regarding colonization status and parasitic species. (**B**) Beta diversity distances boxplots for comparison of microbial community composition at genus level (Jaccard and Sorensen) between the subjects clustered by colonization status and parasitic species. Horizontal lines indicate medians. * denotes $p < 0.05$ compared to the non-colonized group.

The same trend was observed when analysing beta diversity (Jaccard and Sorensen indexes) and significant differences in the community structure were detected (Figure 1), with a higher variability of genera among participants colonized by *Blastocystis* sp. and/or *D. fragilis*, and lower in those colonized by *G. intestinalis* (Table 2). The divergence on the structure of the bacterial community when comparing *Blastocystis* sp. and/or *D. fragilis* cases and non-colonized subjects is reflected in Figure S1, which shows the PCoA charts of both conditions.

Evidence points to an unhealthier microbiome in subjects suffering from metabolic syndrome [20,56]. Therefore, for a more complete analysis of the alpha diversity, patients were grouped according to two variables: the colonization with parasites, and the presence of metabolic syndrome. In this combined study, the higher values of microbial diversity were found among metabolically healthy participants who harboured *Blastocystis* sp. and/or *D. fragilis* (Table 3).

Table 3. Mean alpha diversity indexes at genus level categorized by the presence of metabolic syndrome or NAFLD and colonization by *Blastocystis* sp. and/or *D. fragilis*.

	Metabolic syndrome		*Metabolically healthy*	
	Non-colonized	*B/DF*	Non-colonized	*B/DF*
Chao 1	104.9	112.5	116.3	124.5
Shannon	2.86	2.74	2.94	3.09
	NAFLD positives		***NAFLD negatives***	
	Non-colonized	*B/DF*	Non-colonized	*B/DF*
Chao 1	107.4	110.9	120.0	129.6
Shannon	2.90	2.75	2.89	3.09

B/DF = *Blastocystis* sp. and/or *D. fragilis* positives after excluding co-infections with *G. intestinalis*.

On the contrary, the lowest indexes corresponded to those with metabolic syndrome and *G. intestinalis* (Figure 2).

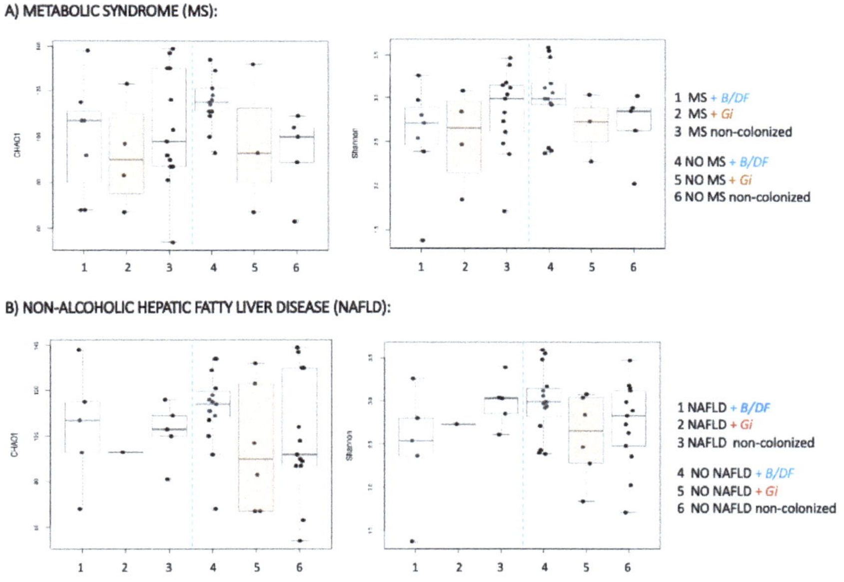

Figure 2. Alpha diversity distances boxplots for comparison of genus richness (Chao1) and diversity (Shannon) between subjects regarding metabolic and colonization status. (**A**) Comparison among patients regarding the colonization with parasites and the presence of metabolic syndrome. (**B**) Comparison among patients regarding the colonization with parasites and the presence of Non-alcoholic hepatic fatty liver disease. Horizontal lines indicate medians.

A similar combined sub-analysis was carried out, regarding suffering from NAFLD. Consistently with the previous results, the highest diversity was obtained in NAFLD-negatives harbouring *Blastocystis* sp. and/or *D. fragilis* (Table 3) (Figure 2). After clustering according to the presence of parasites and the other metabolic comorbidities, no significant differences in alpha diversity indexes were uncovered. However, a common diversity pattern associated with parasite species was identified among patients with dyslipidaemia, hepatic steatosis, insulin resistance and T2D (Figure S2) those individuals with *Blastocystis* sp. and/or *D. fragilis* showed the greatest alpha diversity, and those with *G. intestinalis* the lowest, while non-colonized subjects displayed an intermediate situation between them. Similar results in terms of beta diversity were obtained when comparing bacterial communities at genus level with regard to metabolic comorbidities and parasitic species. Significant differences existed between non-colonized subjects and those with *Blastocystis* sp. and/or *D. fragilis*, and also with *G. intestinalis*-positive ones (Table 4).

Table 4. Beta diversity mean indexes at genus level regarding metabolic comorbidities and colonization.

	Jaccard			*Sorensen*		
	Nc	*B/DF*	*G. intestinalis*	Nc	*B/DF*	*G. intestinalis*
Metabolic syndrome	0.429	0.400	0.320 *	0.582	0.542	0.445 *
Dyslipidaemia	0.459	0.475 *	0.384 *	0.610	0.622 *	0.522 *
Hepatic steatosis	0.430	0.425	0.331 *	0.579	0.567	0.459 *
Insulin resistance	0.444	0.481 *	0.320 *	0.598	0.627 *	0.445 *
Type II diabetes mellitus	0.412	0.341	0.279 *	0.559	0.451	0.393 *

Nc= Non-colonized; *B/DF* = *Blastocystis* sp. and/or *D. fragilis* positives after excluding co-infections with *G. intestinalis*; * paired-test statistics with $p < 0.05$ when compared mean indexes of colonized with the non-colonized.

In an attempt to analyse the differences observed in bacterial diversity with the metabolic profile of the patients, the frequency of metabolic comorbidities in the patients depending on whether or not they were colonized by *Blastocystis* sp. and/or *D. fragilis* is shown in Figure 3. As can be observed in the figure, the prevalence of metabolic syndrome, insulin resistance and T2D are lower in colonized patients. On the contrary, the prevalence of hepatic steatosis and dyslipidaemia are higher in association with colonization, although these differences are not significant in any case.

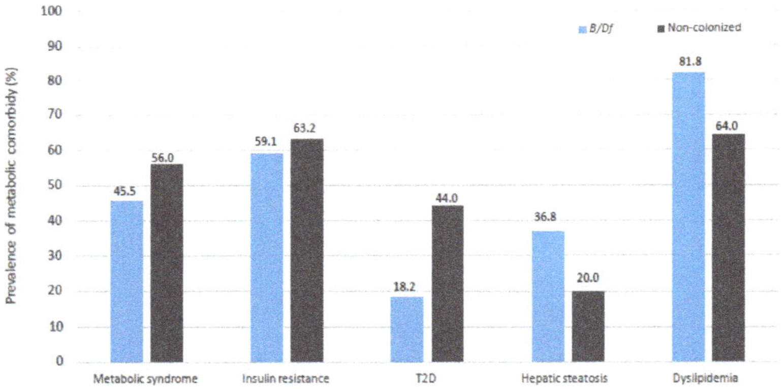

Figure 3. Comparison of prevalence of metabolic comorbidities in subjected enrolled regarding colonization status by *Blastocystis* sp. and/or *Dientamoeba fragilis*.

3.2.3. Relative Abundance of Taxa

The most abundant phyla in the studied population were: Bacteroidetes (50.0%), Firmicutes (40.1%), Proteobacteria (6.6%), Actinobacteria (1.2%) and Verrucomicrobia (1.2%). The mean Firmicutes/Bacteroidetes ratio was 0.95. For each subject enrolled, a quantitative representation of the individual relative abundance of the bacterial phyla is reported in Figure S3.

A comparative analysis regarding the presence/absence of unicellular eukaryotes was performed, obtaining similar relative abundances of the dominating phyla between both groups. Considering that dissimilar effects may have been generated by the different parasitic species, the results were reanalysed with regard to specific parasite clusters. In case of *G. intestinalis*, an increase in Bacteroidetes and Proteobacteria relative abundance was observed compared to the other situations. The opposite occurred for Firmicutes and Actinobacteria, for which a considerable decrease was observed with respect to the non-colonized population. Regarding the Firmicutes/Bacteroidetes ratio, participants with *G. intestinalis* showed the lowest value, driven by both lower abundances of Firmicutes and higher ones of Bacteroidetes. For individuals with *Blastocystis* sp. and/or *D. fragilis*, very slight differences were observed in terms of main phyla distribution with respect to negative subjects, as shown in Table 5.

Table 5. Relative abundance (%) of the main phyla clustered by colonization.

	Non-Colonized	*B/DF*	*G. intestinalis*
Phyla			
Firmicutes	40.1	42.2	35.0
Bacteroidetes	49.8	48.6	53.8
Proteobacteria	6.2	6.5	8.1
Actinobacteria	1.6	0.9	0.8
Verrucomicrobia	1.4	1.0	1.1
Ratio (mean ± S.D.)			
Firmicutes/Bacteroidetes	0.97 ± 0.8	1.0 ± 0.7	0.68 ± 0.2

B/DF = *Blastocystis* sp. and/or *D. fragilis* positives after excluding co-infections with *G. intestinalis*.

When comparing the relative abundance of taxa at genus level and sub-analysing the presence of a specific parasite, significant differences were identified with respect to non-colonized subjects. *Blastocystis* sp.-positives presented higher relative abundances of *Pyramidobacter* spp. (p = 0.022), *Peptococcus* spp. (p = 0.027), *Anaerofilum* spp. (p = 0.037) and *Negativibacillus* spp. (p = 0.04), and lower abundances of *Citrobacter* spp. (p = 0.034), *Enorma* spp. (p = 0.04) and *Ezakiella* spp. (p = 0.04). Subjects colonized by *D. fragilis* showed a higher relative abundance of *Aggregatibacter* spp. (p = 0.0031), *Brachyspira* spp. (p = 0.0075), *Phocea* spp. (p = 0.012), *Butyrivibrio* spp. (p = 0.017), *Pseudoflavonifractor* spp. (p = 0.01), *Saccharimonas* spp. (p = 0.02) and *Adlercreutzia* spp. (p = 0.04), and a lower frequency of *Papilibacter* spp. (p = 0.008), *Paraprevotella* spp. (p = 0.035) and *Snegalimassilia* spp. (p = 0.04). Finally, the presence of *G. intestinalis* displayed a higher relative abundance of *Murdochiella* spp. (p = 0.0009), *Finegolia* spp. (p = 0.0009), *Eubacterium* spp. (p = 0.005), *Flavonifractor* spp. (p = 0.008), *Sarcina* spp. (p = 0.01), *Succiniclasticum* spp. (p = 0.02), *Paraeggerthella* spp. (p = 0.02), *Oscilibacter* spp. (p = 0.03), *Campylobacter* spp. (p = 0.03), *Synergistes* spp. (p = 0.04) and *Ezakiella* spp. (p = 0.04).

Regarding a few selected genera frequently analysed in the scientific literature (Table 6), it was observed that in the group colonized by *Blastocystis* sp. and/or *D. fragilis*, there was a slight increase in *Roseburia* spp. and *Lactobacillus* spp. were prominent, and a decrease in *Akkermansia* spp., *Bifidobacterium* spp. and *Escherichia* spp. was also found. The presence of *G. intestinalis* was associated with a different genus-level pattern, with an increase in *Bacteroides* spp. and a decrease in *Faecalibacterium* spp., *Prevotella* spp. and *Lactobacillus* spp.

Table 6. Relative abundance (%) of selected genera clustered by colonization.

	Non-Colonized	*B/DF*	*G. intestinalis*
Faecalibacterium spp.	3.6	3.8	2.0
Roseburia spp.	2.9	3.6	2.2
Akkermansia spp.	1.3	0.9	1.1
Bacteroides spp.	21.3	20.5	27.1
Prevotella spp.	11.5	11.0	10.5
Lactobacillus spp.	0.09	0.82	0.03
Bifidobacterium spp.	0.68	0.28	0.51
Escherichia spp.	0.68	0.25	0.67

B/DF = *Blastocystis* sp. and/or *D. fragilis* positives after excluding co-infections with *G. intestinalis*.

With respect to the *Bacteroides* spp./*Prevotella* spp. and the *Faecalibacterium* spp./*Escherichia* spp. ratios (Table 7), they globally showed no significant differences between subjects with and without parasites. However, *G. intestinalis* positives presented the highest median *Bacteroides* spp./*Prevotella* spp. ratio, and positives with *Blastocystis* sp. and/or *D. fragilis* the lowest. In relation to these results, it can be stated that the presence of *G. intestinalis* may be associated with higher abundances of the genus *Bacteroides*, which is the main representative of the phylum Bacteroidetes, in accordance with the data shown in Tables 5 and 6. In case of the *Faecalibacterium* spp./*Escherichia* spp. ratio, the presence of parasites, either *Blastocystis* sp. and/or *D. fragilis* or *G. intestinalis* increased, which was more evident for the data with *G. intestinalis*.

Table 7. Comparison of main genus ratios clustered by colonization.

	Non-Colonized	*B/DF*	*G. intestinalis*
	Median [Q1, Q2]	Median [Q1, Q2]	Median [Q1, Q2]
Bacteroides spp./*Prevotella* spp.	460 [0.3, 11.300]	200 [0.3, 4.681]	1.625.0 [0.9, 3.687.1]
Faecalibacterium spp./*Escherichia* spp.	40.6 [9.0, 107.6]	63.5 [1.9, 277.8]	84.6 [0.9, 345.0]

B/DF = *Blastocystis* sp. and/or *D. fragilis* positives after excluding co-infections with G. *intestinalis*.

Considering metabolic comorbidities, subjects suffering from NAFLD displayed significantly different gut microbial profiles with higher ratios of Firmicutes/Bacteroidetes (1.4 vs. 0.8; $p = 0.041$); a lower relative abundance of Bacteroidetes (43.5 vs. 52.9; $p = 0.031$) and a higher one of Firmicutes (47.5 vs. 37.1; $p = 0.031$). All this related to a significant increase in the genus *Faecalibacterium* spp. (4.3 vs. 3.1; $p = 0.037$) and *Clostridium* spp. (0.5 vs. 0.08; $p = 0.002$), both representatives of the predominant phylum. The condition of insulin resistance was associated with a significantly lower frequency of the genus *Blautia* spp. (0.38% vs. 0.89%; $p = 0.015$) and a higher one of *Desulfovibrio* spp. (1.0% vs. 0.2%; $p = 0.032$). Participants with T2D displayed a *Faecalibacterium* spp./*Escherichia* spp. ratio that was significantly lower ($p = 0.01$), due to an overrepresentation of the genus *Escherichia* spp., along with a trend towards a lower representation of *Akkermansia* spp. (0.5% vs. 1.3%, in non-diabetics). No differences in the composition of the microbiota at genus level were detected in relation to the presence of dyslipidaemia, hyperuricemia, hypertension or metabolic syndrome.

Finally, the structure of the microbiota regarding other variables registered during the clinical interview showed some significant results. Cholecystectomy was related at phylum level to a lower relative frequency of *Proteobacteria* ($p = 0.02$), and at genus level with a higher relative presence of *Roseburia* ($p = 0.02$) and *Blautia* ($p = 0.03$) and underrepresented genera such as *Proteus* ($p = 0.001$), *Peptoclostridium* ($p = 0.001$), *Epulopiscium* ($p = 0.001$), *Enorma* ($p = 0.01$), *Romboutsia* ($p = 0.01$,) and *Anaerostipes* ($p = 0.02$). Secondly, the individuals who were consuming meal replacements displayed a lower relative abundance of *Clostridium* ($p = 0.007$), and the presence of rare genera such as *Fusecatenibacter* ($p < 0.001$) and *Ralstonia* ($p < 0.01$).

Another variable that provided significant results was taking proton pump inhibitors regularly, with higher relative frequency of the genus *Parabacteroides* ($p = 0.02$) and overrepresentation of infrequent genera such as: *Neisseria* ($p < 0.001$), *Brachyspira* ($p = 0.01$), *Fructobacillus* ($p = 0.01$), *Peptosclostridium* ($p = 0.01$) and *Oscillospira* ($p = 0.03$). Active colonization with *H. pylori* was coupled with a lower relative abundance of the genera *Akkermansia* ($p = 0.02$), *Collinsella* ($p = 0.02$), *Coprobacter* ($p = 0.03$) and *Bifidobacterium* ($p = 0.04$). Finally, smoking condition conferred a lower relative amount of the genera *Barnesiella* ($p = 0.01$) and *Haemophilus* ($p = 0.04$).

3.3. Dietary Results

Considering the information gathered from dietary questionnaires and registers, adherence to the dietetic recommendations provided by the healthcare team was, globally, extremely low. Less than one-third of the subjects ingested an optimal amount of kcal (20–25 kcal/kg adjusted weight/day), the rest either exceeding or not reaching the international recommendations. Only 14.6% were considered adherent to the Mediterranean diet, determined by a score of ≥10 points obtained in the validated questionnaire. Furthermore, fulfilment of dietary recommended daily intakes was only occasional, thus implying a very poor quality of the diet among participants: over-ingestion of simple sugars was present in 95%, of lipids in 54% and of proteins in 10%, while none of the subjects met the daily recommended intake of fibres. Insufficient dietary intake was frequently present for omega-6 (54.0%), vitamin A (80.0%), vitamin B6 (66.0%), vitamin C (49.0%) and almost in every patient for vitamin E, vitamin D, copper, zinc and iron.

A comparative metagenomics analysis of the microbiota was performed regarding the following dietary variables: total caloric intake, fulfilment of the recommended intake for the three main macronutrients and fulfilment of the daily intake of micronutrient requirements. After analysing these variables regarding the presence of parasites in a combined way, no significant difference was obtained to point to an influence of diet on microbiota diversity and parasitic colonization. However, results depending on the parasitic species in those patients with a correct daily intake of macronutrient were much appreciated. With an adequate consumption of carbohydrates, greater diversity was observed among the colonized, highlighting those of *Blastocystis* sp. and/or *D. fragilis*. Additionally, it is also interesting that when fat intake is adequate, the diversity of those colonized with *G. intestinalis* is greater than expected according to the previously detected patterns (Figure S4).

Regarding the relative abundance of the bacteria of interest, a trend to a lower relative abundance of *Faecalibacterium* spp. among omega-3-deficient subjects ($p = 0.024$) and to a lower relative abundance of Actinobacteria among omega-6-deficient ones ($p = 0.026$) was detected. Furthermore, among vitamin-A-deficient subjects, a lower abundance of *Parabacteroides* spp. ($p = 0.029$), *Lactobacillus* spp. ($p = 0.008$) and *Colinsella* spp. ($p = 0.012$), together with a lower abundance of *Lactobacillus* spp. among B12-deficient ones ($p = 0.029$), was observed.

4. Discussion

Several studies assessing the composition and diversity of gut microbiota have been carried out, both in healthy and unhealthy obese subjects. However, it is surprising how the literature, thus far, lacks consistent data on the interactions between eukaryotic colonization and gut microbial profiles, particularly among obese subjects. In our previous studies, a high prevalence of gut colonization with common intestinal parasites (51.0%) was detected in a population of type II and type III obese subjects [56,57]. Consequently, it was believed that exploring these interactions merited further study and the present investigation was conceived, which jointly analyses the metagenomics analysis with the presence of these microorganisms in an obese population.

The relationship between unicellular eukaryotes and prokaryotes ecology and diversity has been previously assessed and recently reviewed [58]. Several researchers have demonstrated that hosting one of these parasitic species was associated with a richer and more diverse bacterial microbiome [22,23,59–61]. A study by Krogsgaard et al. [62] specifically evaluated this aspect in a relatively large population, assessing the presence of *D. fragilis* and *Blastocystis* sp. via molecular analysis. A high global prevalence of parasites (47.0%) and a more diverse and richer bacterial microbiome in colonized versus non-colonized subjects was observed, supporting our results. Accordingly, we found higher richness (assessed by the number of reads) among *Blastocystis*-positive subjects. Conversely, an inverse effect between the bacterial community diversity and the presence of *G. intestinalis* was stated in the study by Mejía et al. [63], and it was suggested that this relationship may depend upon the specific parasite colonizing the gut, as well as the intensity of infection it causes. According to recent articles reviewing studies on the association between single-celled intestinal parasites and microbial communities, a differential effect could be expected depending on the species considered [64]. We assessed alpha diversity indexes in our population, comparing the parasitic species independently, and although the differences were not significant, trends described previously were confirmed, such as higher alpha and beta diversity at genus level in *Blastocystis* and/or *D. fragilis*-positive samples, and lower in *G. intestinalis*-positives.

Furthermore, we analysed whether *Blastocystis* sp. and/or *D. fragilis* were associated with higher microbiota diversity in different metabolic conditions, considering the presence of metabolic syndrome and NAFLD. The presence of these parasites was coincident with higher diversities when compared with their negative counterparts. Although we could not confirm differences attributable to the colonization, this finding seems to suggest a healthier microbiome structure in agreement with some published data [22,23,58]. We have already described, in the same obese population as the one presented here, a lower frequency of insulin resistance among subjects harbouring these unicellular eukaryotes [56]. In the present research, the greatest alpha diversity was shown by subjects colonized with *Blastocystis* sp. and/or *D. fragilis*, and without metabolic syndrome. In this context, the outcomes reported may point towards a beneficial effect of the gut colonization with *Blastocystis* sp., in agreement with recent studies, which demonstrated, in an experimental model, that long-term exposition to the parasite prior to the induction of colitis promotes a faster recovery in a protective manner, with a significant reduction in inflammatory markers [65].

Secondly, the intestinal microbiota composition was analysed with regard to the presence of intestinal parasites. At phylum level, we were not able to establish clear differences between groups, which suggests that interactions with the bacterial intestinal community are determined at a lower level (genus, species), probably related to functional niche specialization, and are also dependent on other factors. At genus level, several differences were detected regarding the occurrence of a specific parasite, but they were not consistent between parasitic species and generally affected low prevalent bacterial members. It is probable that unicellular eukaryotes display a variety of effects in shaping the gut microbiome that differ widely among each kind, which could explain the discrepancies found in the effects on microbiome composition. Additionally, considering that we compared bacterial relative abundances, the differences observed between groups may have reflected modifications in the absolute levels of a specific taxonomic category, as well as changes in other components of the microbiome. Finally, numerous factors have the potential to affect the microbiome composition, allowing confounding variables to prevent us from obtaining a clear differential pattern in colonized subjects.

The presence of *G. intestinalis* in the gut ecosystem has been related to a dysbiotic condition in several studies [13,14,66,67]. Its presence was related to a significant lower *Faecalibacterium* spp./*Escherichia* spp. ratio compared to *Blastocystis*-positive individuals [14]; the same low trend was demonstrated with the presence of other pathogenic protozoa, such as *Cryptosporidium* spp. and *Cyclospora cayetanensis* [67]. However, the prevalence of *G. intestinalis* in the studied population was too low to allow us to perform significant comparisons. Therefore, further research is needed to shed more light on the significance of this parasite in the human gut ecosystem.

Regarding *Blastocystis* sp., the results obtained in previously published metagenomics studies differ widely in the relative abundances of different taxa. A consistent finding has been a microbiome less dominated by the genus *Bacteroides* spp. in subjects harbouring this parasite [13,22,58,59], which we were not able to reproduce in the present study. Additionally, some other studies reported [22,58] a higher relative quantity of *Faecalibacterium* spp. and *Roseburia* spp., two genera considered beneficial in the gut ecosystem for their short-chain-fatty-acids production potential. We could not find any difference in the relative abundance of these genera, neither of Archaea, which has also been reported as more abundant by Beghini's group [17], who performed the largest investigation to date on the prevalence of this parasite in human samples. They were able to identify microbiome signatures (distinguishable features that were consistent across populations) in the intestinal ecology linked to the presence of *Blastocystis* sp. On the other hand, Principal Coordinate Analysis charts reflecting beta diversity of microbial communities allowed us to establish phylogenetic distances between samples when comparing the diversity of genera with regard to the presence of *Blastocystis* sp. and/or *D. fragilis* in agreement with a previous study [61].

Additionally, we analysed the metagenomics, considering several metabolic comorbidities. An inverse relationship between the abundance of *Akkermansia muciniphila* and the BMI has been broadly described in the literature, along with a direct relationship with insulin sensitivity [68–72]. In this study, we observed differences in the relative abundance of other genera with regard to insulin sensitivity, such as *Blautia* spp. and *Desulfovibrio* spp. Conversely, despite the amount of evidence providing pathogenic links between the development of NAFLD and the structure of gut microbiota, human studies describing its composition in this situation are scarce and sometimes contradictory [73,74]. In our population, we detected a higher relative frequency of Firmicutes (and specifically of the genera *Faecalibacterium* spp. and *Clostridium* spp.) and a lower relative frequency of Bacteroidetes, thus causing a lower Firmicutes/Bacteroidetes ratio. Similar results in subjects suffering from NASH were found by some researchers, while other studies found the opposite alteration of the ratio [75,76]. Still unknown factors probably interfere in driving the direction of this ratio and may be determinant of the development of hepatic inflammation and fibrosis.

On the other hand, cholecystectomy is known to alter the bile flow into the intestine and therefore modify the enterohepatic circulation of bile salts, which has the potential to disrupt the structure of gut microbiota. In a case–control study [77], a higher relative abundance of two bacterium species (*Blautia obeum* and *Veillonella parvula*) was detected in subjects after cholecystectomy. In our study, we also noticed a higher relative abundance of *Blautia* spp., along with differences in the abundance of Proteobacteria (previously not reported). The meaning of these changes into the microbiome composition remains to be elucidated.

Finally, from the information gathered in this is study, it was remarkable that the participants kept to a diet of extremely poor quality, despite being in an intensive nutritional re-education programme, prior to bariatric surgery. The diet followed was considered of a western pattern in every subject, thus hindering the identification of differences in the gut microbiome structure or diversity that could have been related to this variable. Globally, it strengthens the idea of obesity as a chronic disease, and reinforces the need of preventive measures, to avoid its development from its very beginning.

A strength in our study was the number of patients on whom we performed metagenomics analysis, including subjects from different social environments. Another interesting point was the faecal samples collection, since each patient delivered three samples collected on alternating days, thereby increasing the sensitivity for detecting the genes of any intestinal unicellular eukaryotic parasite. There are some limitations of the present study that warrant consideration. First, the possibility that faecal sampling may have not been completely representative of the microbiota composition from the upper gastrointestinal tract has to be considered; thus, false negative results for some intestinal parasites may have occurred. Likewise, we cannot rule out a former infection with an intestinal parasite that had been spontaneously cleared from the intestinal ecosystem at the time of study, and hence yielded a negative result in PCR analysis. This condition may have left alterations in the composition of gut microbiota, since, as described by Beatty (2016) [15], a persistent intestinal dysbiosis-induced state is possible after infection and clearance of *G. intestinalis*, causing long-term changes in microbiota composition. Finally, we are aware that the structure and function of human intestinal microbiota is altered by a myriad of factors, many of them still unknown, which may have interfered with the results of our study.

This study provides additional data of the effects of unicellular eukaryotes on the diversity and ecology of human gut microbiota on obese subjects. The presence of *Blastocystis* sp. and/or *D. fragilis* was associated with the highest values for the mean indexes analysed, for both alpha and beta diversity, while the opposite is observed in the presence of *G. intestinalis*. The richness and diversity of the microbiota detected in association with

Blastocystis sp. and/or *D. fragilis* could be related to a healthier metabolic profile in patients, since cases of comorbidities such as metabolic syndrome, insulin resistance and T2D are less frequent among those patients.

In terms of relative abundance of taxa, differences in bacterial community composition have been evidenced regarding parasitic species; at phylum level, in the presence of *G. intestinalis*, there was an increase in Bacteroidetes and Proteobacteria along with the lowest Firmicutes/Bacteroidetes ratio, and conversely, individuals with *Blastocystis* sp. and/or *D. fragilis* displayed a pattern similar to non-colonized subjects. At genus level, *Blastocystis* sp. and/or *D. fragilis* colonization was accompanied by a prominent increase in *Lactobacillus* spp., and a decrease in *Akkermansia* spp., *Bifidobacterium* spp. and *Escherichia* spp., while *G. intestinalis* was associated with a different genus-level pattern, with an increase in *Bacteroides* spp. and a decrease in *Faecalibacterium* spp., *Prevotella* spp. and *Lactobacillus* spp., along with the highest *Bacteroides* spp./*Prevotella* spp. ratio. Considering metabolic comorbidities, subjects suffering from NAFLD displayed significantly higher ratios of Firmicutes/Bacteroidetes, and a significant increase in the genera *Faecalibacterium* spp. and *Clostridium* spp. Participants with T2D displayed a *Faecalibacterium* spp./*Escherichia* spp. ratio that was significantly lower, due to an overrepresentation of the genus Escherichia spp., along with a trend towards a lower representation of *Akkermansia* spp.

Considering the globally high prevalence of these parasites in the human gut ecosystem, research efforts should focus on further describing the interplay with the microbiota and the host immune system. Based on our findings, we recommend designing basic and clinical studies to address the possible beneficial or pathogenic effect of these eukaryotes on shaping the bacterial community of obese subjects, and to decipher whether it may imply a healthier metabolic profile. Hopefully, future evidence on this field will provide us with new opportunities for therapeutic interventions against the development of obesity and its comorbidities.

5. Conclusions

This study provides additional data on the effects of unicellular eukaryotes on the diversity and composition of human gut microbiota of obese subjects. The cases of *Blastocystis* sp. and/or *Dientamoeba fragilis* presented the richest and most diverse bacterial communities according to metagenomics data. No clear patterns in the relative frequency of taxa were identified in regards of parasitic status, even though the occurrence of *Giardia intestinalis* and *D. fragilis* among participants was low. Considering the globally high prevalence of these parasites within the human gut ecosystem, research efforts should focus on further describing the interplay with the microbiota and the host immune system. Based on our findings, we recommend designing basic and clinical studies to address the possible beneficial effect of *Blastocystis* sp. on shaping the bacterial community of obese subjects, and to decipher whether it may imply a healthier metabolic profile. Hopefully, future evidence on this field will provide us with new opportunities for therapeutic interventions against the development of obesity and its comorbidities.

Supplementary Materials: The following supporting information can be downloaded at: https://www.mdpi.com/article/10.3390/nu14153211/s1, Figure S1: The community structures of gut microbiota were analysed by principal coordinates analysis (PCoA). Each point corresponds to a subject where the colour indicates its category. PCO1 and PCO2 are shown, with the percentage variation explained for each axis, Figure S2: Alpha diversity distances boxplots for comparison of genus richness (Chao1) between subjects with a metabolic comorbidity: (A) dyslipidaemia; (B) insulin resistance; (C) hepatic steatosis and (D) Type 2 diabetes regarding colonization status. Horizontal lines indicate medians, Figure S3: Relative abundance of phyla in the studied population for each subjected enrolled, Figure S4: Alpha diversity distances boxplots for comparison of genus richness (Chao1) between subjects with correct daily intake of macronutrients regarding colonization status: (A) carbohydrates; (B) proteins; (C) fats. Horizontal lines indicate median, Table S1: Number of reads by count according to the phyla for each sample, Table S2: Number of reads by count according to the genus for each sample.

Author Contributions: Conceptualization, M.T., J.M.S., H.R. and J.F.M.-T.; Data curation, J.C. and M.T.; Formal analysis, J.C. and M.T.; Funding acquisition, M.T.; Investigation, J.C., M.T. and S.C.; Methodology, J.C., M.T., S.C. and J.M.S.; Project administration, M.T. and J.F.M.-T.; Resources, J.F.M.-T.; Supervision, M.T., J.M.S. and J.F.M.-T.; Validation, M.T., J.M.S., H.R. and J.F.M.-T.; Visualization, M.T., J.M.S., H.R. and J.F.M.-T.; Writing—original draft, J.C.; Writing—review and editing, M.T., J.M.S., H.R. and J.F.M.-T. All authors have read and agreed to the published version of the manuscript.

Funding: This study was supported by the Health Research Institute Hospital La Fe (award number: 2017/0486).

Institutional Review Board Statement: The study was conducted in accordance with the Declaration of Helsinki, and approved by the Biomedical Research Ethics Committee of University and Polytechnic Hospital La Fe on 1 July 2019 (protocol code 2017/0486) for studies involving humans.

Informed Consent Statement: Informed consent was obtained from all subjects involved in the study.

Data Availability Statement: The sequences generated after metagenomics are available in the ENA public repository (https://www.ebi.ac.uk/ena/browser/view/PRJEB51819 accesion number: ERA10729632) (accessed on 25 Mach 2022).

Acknowledgments: We acknowledge Gabriela Elizabeth Tapia Veloz for analysing the nutritional composition of the diets from the information gathered from the dietary questionnaires and registers. We are grateful to Health Research Institute La Fe for supporting our research team and this specific project. We are grateful to Health Research Institute La Fe for supporting our research team and this specific project. Thanks are extended to the Biostatistics and Bioinformatics at Health Research Institute La Fe.

Conflicts of Interest: The authors declare no conflict of interest. The funder had no role in the design of the study; in the collection, analysis, or interpretation of data; in the writing of the manuscript; or in the decision to publish the results.

References

1. Yatsunenko, T.; Rey, F.E.; Manary, M.J.; Trehan, I.; Dominguez-Bello, M.G.; Contreras, M.; Magris, M.; Hidalgo, G.; Baldassano, R.N.; Anokhin, A.P.; et al. Human gut microbiome viewed across age and geography. *Nature* **2012**, *486*, 222–227. [CrossRef] [PubMed]
2. Cani, P.D.; Delzenne, N.M. The role of the gut microbiota in energy metabolism and metabolic disease. *Curr. Pharm. Des.* **2009**, *15*, 1546–1558. [CrossRef] [PubMed]
3. Heiss, C.N.; Olofsson, L.E. Gut microbiota-dependent modulation of energy metabolism. *J. Innate Immun.* **2018**, *10*, 163–171. [CrossRef] [PubMed]
4. Lin, L.; Zhang, J. Role of intestinal microbiota and metabolites on gut homeostasis and human diseases. *BMC Immunol.* **2017**, *18*, 2. [CrossRef]
5. Ratajczak, W.; Rył, A.; Mizerski, A.; Walczakiewicz, K.; Sipak, O.; Laszczyńska, M. Immunomodulatory potential of gut microbiome-derived short-chain fatty acids (SCFAs). *Acta Biochim. Pol.* **2019**, *66*, 1–12. [CrossRef]
6. Burgess, S.L.; Gilchrist, C.A.; Lynn, T.C.; Petri, W.A. Parasitic protozoa and interactions with the host intestinal microbiota. *Infect. Immun.* **2017**, *85*, e00101–e00117. [CrossRef]
7. Bär, A.; Phukan, N.; Pinheiro, J.; Simoes-Barbosa, A. The interplay of host microbiota and parasitic protozoans at mucosal interfaces: Implications for the outcomes of infections and diseases. *PLoS Negl. Trop. Dis.* **2015**, *9*, e0004176. [CrossRef]
8. Stensvold, C.R.; van der Giezen, M. Associations between gut microbiota and common luminal intestinal parasites. *Trends Parasitol.* **2018**, *34*, 369–377. [CrossRef]
9. Ley, R.E.; Bäckhed, F.; Turnbaugh, P.; Lozupone, C.A.; Knight, R.D.; Gordon, J.I. Obesity alters gut microbial ecology. *Proc. Natl. Acad. Sci. USA* **2005**, *102*, 11070–11075. [CrossRef]
10. Turnbaugh, P.J.; Hamady, M.; Yatsunenko, T.; Cantarel, B.L.; Duncan, A.; Ley, R.E.; Sogin, M.L.; Jones, W.J.; Roe, B.A.; Affourtit, J.P.; et al. A core gut microbiome in obese and lean twins. *Nature* **2009**, *457*, 480–484. [CrossRef]
11. Clemente, J.C.; Ursell, L.K.; Parfrey, L.W.; Knight, R. The impact of the gut microbiota on human health: An integrative view. *Cell* **2012**, *148*, 1258–1270. [CrossRef]
12. Joyce, S.A.; Gahan, C.G.M. The gut microbiota and the metabolic health of the host. *Curr. Opin. Gastroenterol.* **2014**, *30*, 120–127. [CrossRef]
13. Allain, T.; Amat, C.B.; Motta, J.-P.; Motta, J.-P.; Manko, A.; Buret, A.G. Interactions of Giardia sp. with the intestinal barrier: Epithelium, mucus, and microbiota. *Tissue Barriers* **2017**, *5*, e1274354. [CrossRef]

14. Iebba, V.; Santangelo, F.; Totino, V.; Pantanella, F.; Monsia, A.; Di Cristanziano, V.; Di Cave, D.; Schippa, S.; Berrilli, F.; D'Alfonso, R. Gut microbiota related to Giardia duodenalis, Entamoeba spp. and Blastocystis hominis infections in humans from Côte d'Ivoire. *J. Infect. Dev. Ctries.* **2016**, *10*, 1035–1041. [CrossRef]
15. Beatty, J.K.; Akierman, S.V.; Motta, J.-P.; Muise, S.; Workentine, M.L.; Harrison, J.J.; Bhargava, A.; Beck, P.L.; Rioux, K.P.; McKnight, G.W.; et al. Giardia duodenalis induces pathogenic dysbiosis of human intestinal microbiota biofilms. *Int. J. Parasitol.* **2017**, *47*, 311–326. [CrossRef]
16. Fekete, E.; Allain, T.; Siddiq, A.; Sosnowski, O.; Buret, A.G. Giardia spp. and the gut microbiota: Dangerous liaisons. *Front. Microbiol.* **2021**, *11*, 618106. [CrossRef]
17. Scanlan, P.D.; Stensvold, C.R.; Rajilić-Stojanović, M.; Heilig, H.G.; De Vos, W.M.; O'Toole, P.W.; Cotter, P.D. The microbial eukaryote Blastocystis is a prevalent and diverse member of the healthy human gut microbiota. *FEMS Microbiol. Ecol.* **2014**, *90*, 326–330. [CrossRef]
18. Beghini, F.; Pasolli, E.; Truong, T.D.; Putignani, L.; Cacciò, S.M.; Segata, N. Large-scale comparative metagenomics of Blastocystis, a common member of the human gut microbiome. *ISME J.* **2017**, *11*, 2848–2863. [CrossRef]
19. Tan, K.S.; Mirza, H.; Teo, J.D.; Wu, B.; Macary, P.A. Current views on the clinical relevance of *Blastocystis* spp. *Curr. Infect. Dis. Rep.* **2010**, *12*, 28–35. [CrossRef]
20. Bäckhed, F.; Fraser, C.M.; Ringel, Y.; Sanders, M.E.; Sartor, R.B.; Sherman, P.M.; Versalovic, J.; Young, V.; Finlay, B.B. Defining a healthy human gut microbiome: Current concepts, future directions, and clinical applications. *Cell Host Microbe* **2012**, *12*, 611–622. [CrossRef]
21. Le Chatelier, E.; Nielsen, T.; Qin, J.; Prifti, E.; Hildebrand, F.; Falony, G.; Almeida, M.; Arumugam, M.; Batto, J.M.; Kennedy, S.; et al. Richness of human gut microbiome correlates with metabolic markers. *Nature* **2013**, *500*, 541–546. [CrossRef]
22. Audebert, C.; Even, G.; Cian, A.; Blastocystis Investigation Group; Loywick, A.; Merlin, S.; Viscogliosi, E.; Chabe, M. Colonization with the enteric protozoa Blastocystis is associated with increased diversity of human gut bacterial microbiota. *Sci. Rep.* **2016**, *6*, 25255. [CrossRef]
23. Andersen, L.O.; Bonde, I.; Nielsen, H.B.; Stensvold, C.R. A retrospective metagenomics approach to studying Blastocystis. *FEMS Microbiol. Ecol.* **2015**, *91*, fiv072. [CrossRef]
24. Garcia, L.S. Dientamoeba fragilis, one of the neglected intestinal protozoa. *J. Clin. Microbiol.* **2016**, *54*, 2243–2250. [CrossRef]
25. Knoll, E.W.; Howell, K.M. Studies on Dientamoeba fragilis: Its incidence and possible pathogenicity. *Am. J. Clin. Pathol.* **1945**, *15*, 178–183. [CrossRef]
26. Wong, Z.; Faulder, K.; Robinson, J.L. Does Dientamoeba fragilis cause diarrhea? A systematic review. *Parasitol. Res.* **2018**, *117*, 971–980. [CrossRef]
27. van Kalleveen, M.W.; Budding, A.E.; Benninga, M.A.; Savelkoul, P.H.M.; van Gool, T.; van Maldeghem, I.; Dorigo-Zetsma, J.W.; Bart, A.; Plötz, F.B.; de Meij, T.G. Intestinal microbiota in children with symptomatic Dientamoeba fragilis infection: A case-control study. *Pediatr. Infect. Dis. J.* **2020**, *40*, 279–283. [CrossRef]
28. Garvey, W.T.; Mechanick, J.I.; Brett, E.M.; Garber, A.J.; Hurley, D.L.; Jastreboff, A.M.; Nadolsky, K.; Pessah-Pollack, R.; Plodkowski, R. American association of clinical endocrinologists and American college of endocrinology comprehensive clinical practice guidelines for medical care of patients with obesity. *Endocr. Pract.* **2016**, *22* (Suppl. S3), 1–203. [CrossRef]
29. Martínez-González, M.A.; García-Arellano, A.; Toledo, E.; Salas-Salvadó, J.; Buil-Cosiales, P.; Corella, D.; Covas, M.I.; Schröder, H.; Arós, F.; Gómez-Gracia, E.; et al. A 14-Item Mediterranean diet assessment tool and obesity indexes among high-risk subjects: The PREDIMED trial. *PLoS ONE* **2012**, *7*, e43134. [CrossRef] [PubMed]
30. Trichopoulou, A.; Costacou, T.; Bamia, C.; Trichopoulos, D. Adherence to a Mediterranean diet and survival in a Greek population *N. Engl. J. Med.* **2003**, *348*, 2599–2608. [CrossRef] [PubMed]
31. Martin-Moreno, J.M.; Boyle, P.; Gorgojo, L.; Maisonneuve, P.; Fernandez-Rodriguez, J.C.; Salvini, S.; Willett, W.C. Development and validation of a food frequency questionnaire in Spain. *Int. J. Epidemiol.* **1993**, *22*, 512–519. [CrossRef] [PubMed]
32. European Food Safety Authority. General principles for the collection of national food consumption data in the view of a Pan-European dietary survey. *EFSA J.* **2009**, *7*, 1435. [CrossRef]
33. Brussaard, J.H.; Löwik, M.R.; Steingrímsdóttir, L.; Møller, A.; Kearney, J.; De Henauw, S. A European food consumption survey method—Conclusions and recommendations. *Eur. J. Clin. Nutr.* **2002**, *56*, S89–S94. [CrossRef]
34. Ortega, R.M.; Pérez-Rodrigo, C.; López-Sobaler, A.M. Dietary assessment methods: Dietary records. *Nutr. Hosp.* **2015**, *31* (Suppl. S3), 38–45. [CrossRef]
35. Trumbo, P.; Schlicker, S.; Yates, A.A.; Poos, M. Dietary reference intakes for energy, carbohydrate, fiber, fat, fatty acids, cholesterol, protein, and amino acids. *J. Am. Diet Assoc.* **2002**, *102*, 1621–1630. [CrossRef]
36. Huang, P.L. A comprehensive definition for metabolic syndrome. *Dis. Model. Mech.* **2009**, *2*, 231–237. [CrossRef]
37. Ascaso, J.F.; Romero, P.; Real, J.T.; Priego, A.; Valdecabres, C.; Carmena, R. Cuantificación de insulinorresistencia con los valores de insulina basal e índice HOMA en una población no diabética [Insulin resistance quantification by fasting insulin plasma values and HOMA index in a non-diabetic population]. *Med. Clin.* **2001**, *117*, 530–533. [CrossRef]
38. Brewer, G.J.; Blue, M.N.M.; Hirsch, K.R.; Saylor, H.E.; Gould, L.M.; Nelson, A.G.; Smith-Ryan, A.E. Validation of InBody 770 bioelectrical impedance analysis compared to a four-compartment model criterion in young adults. *Clin. Physiol. Funct. Imaging* **2021**, *41*, 317–325. [CrossRef]

39. Autier, B.; Gangneux, J.; Robert-Gangneux, F. Evaluation of the AllplexTM gastrointestinal panel-parasite assay for protozoa detection in stool samples: A retrospective and prospective study. *Microorganisms* **2020**, *8*, 569. [CrossRef]
40. Kim, B.; Kim, H.S.; Kim, J.J.; Park, Y.J.; Kim, D.; Yong, D. Detection of intestinal protozoa in Korean patients using BD Max enteric parasite panel and Seegene Allplex gastrointestinal parasite assay. *Lab. Med.* **2020**, *10*, 221–226. [CrossRef]
41. Galán-Puchades, M.T.; Trelis, M.; Sáez-Durán, S.; Cifre, S.; Gosálvez, C.; Sanxis-Furió, J.; Pascual, J.; Bueno-Marí, R.; Franco, S.; Peracho, V.; et al. One Health approach to zoonotic parasites: Molecular detection of intestinal protozoans in an urban population of Norway rats, Rattus norvegicus, in Barcelona, Spain. *Pathogens* **2021**, *10*, 311. [CrossRef]
42. Klindworth, A.; Pruesse, E.; Schweer, T.; Peplies, J.; Quast, C.; Horn, M.; Glöckner, F.O. Evaluation of general 16S ribosomal RNA gene PCR primers for classical and next-generation sequencing-based diversity studies. *Nucleic Acids Res.* **2013**, *41*, e1. [CrossRef]
43. Schmieder, R.; Edwards, R. Quality control and preprocessing of metagenomic datasets. *Bioinformatics* **2011**, *27*, 863–864. [CrossRef]
44. Callahan, B.J.; McMurdie, P.J.; Rosen, M.J.; Han, A.W.; Johnson, A.J.; Holmes, S.P. DADA2: High-resolution sample inference from Illumina amplicon data. *Nat. Methods* **2016**, *13*, 581–583. [CrossRef]
45. Quast, C.; Pruesse, E.; Yilmaz, P.; Gerken, J.; Schweer, T.; Yarza, P.; Peplies, J.; Glöckner, F.O. The SILVA ribosomal RNA gene database project: Improved data processing and web-based tools. *Nucleic Acids Res.* **2013**, *41*, D590–D596. [CrossRef]
46. Caporaso, J.G.; Kuczynski, J.; Stombaugh, J.; Bittinger, K.; Bushman, F.D.; Costello, E.K.; Fierer, N.; Peña, A.G.; Goodrich, J.K.; Gordon, J.I.; et al. QIIME allows analysis of high-throughput community sequencing data. *Nat. Methods* **2010**, *7*, 335–336. [CrossRef]
47. Dao, M.C.; Everard, A.; Aron-Wisnewsky, J.; Sokolovska, N.; Prifti, E.; Verger, E.O.; Kayser, B.D.; Levenez, F.; Chilloux, J.; Hoyles, L.; et al. Akkermansia muciniphila and improved metabolic health during a dietary intervention in obesity: Relationship with gut microbiome richness and ecology. *Gut* **2016**, *65*, 426–436. [CrossRef]
48. Sokol, H.; Pigneur, B.; Watterlot, L.; Lakhdari, O.; Bermúdez-Humarán, L.G.; Gratadoux, J.J.; Blugeon, S.; Bridonneau, C.; Furet, J.P.; Corthier, G.; et al. Faecalibacterium prausnitzii is an anti-inflammatory commensal bacterium identified by gut microbiota analysis of Crohn disease patients. *Proc. Natl. Acad. Sci. USA* **2008**, *105*, 16731–16736. [CrossRef]
49. Tamanai-Shacoori, Z.; Smida, I.; Bousarghin, L.; Loreal, O.; Meuric, V.; Fong, S.B.; Bonnaure-Mallet, M.; Jolivet-Gougeon, A. Roseburia spp.: A marker of health? *Future Microbiol* **2017**, *12*, 157–170. [CrossRef]
50. Russell, D.A.; Ross, R.P.; Fitzgerald, G.F.; Stanton, C. Metabolic activities and probiotic potential of bifidobacteria. *Int. J. Food Microbiol.* **2011**, *149*, 88–105. [CrossRef]
51. Crovesy, L.; Ostrowski, M.; Ferreira, D.; Rosado, E.L.; Soares-Mota, M. Effect of Lactobacillus on body weight and body fat in overweight subjects: A systematic review of randomized controlled clinical trials. *Int. J. Obes.* **2017**, *41*, 1607–1614. [CrossRef] [PubMed]
52. Ley, R.E. Gut microbiota in 2015: Prevotella in the gut: Choose carefully. *Nat. Rev. Gastroenterol. Hepatol.* **2016**, *13*, 69–70. [CrossRef] [PubMed]
53. Christensen, L.; Roager, H.M.; Astrup, A.; Hjorth, M.F. Microbial enterotypes in personalized nutrition and obesity management. *Am. J. Clin. Nutr.* **2018**, *108*, 645–651. [CrossRef] [PubMed]
54. RC Team. *R: A Language and Environment for Statistical Computing*; R Foundation for Statistical Computing: Vienna, Austria, 2013.
55. National Heart, Lung, and Blood Institute; The National Institute of Diabetes and Digestive and Kidney Diseases. *Clinical Guidelines on the Identification, Evaluation, and Treatment of Overweight and Obesity in Adults: The Evidence Report*; National Institutes of Health: Bethesda, MD, USA, 1998.
56. Caudet, J.; Trelis, M.; Cifre, S.; Soriano, J.M.; Merino-Torres, J.F. Presence and significance of intestinal unicellular parasites in a morbidly obese population. *Int. J. Obes.* **2022**, *46*, 220–227. [CrossRef]
57. Lim, M.Y.; You, H.J.; Yoon, H.S.; Kwon, B.; Lee, J.Y.; Lee, S.; Song, Y.M.; Lee, K.; Sung, J.; Ko, G. The effect of heritability and host genetics on the gut microbiota and metabolic syndrome. *Gut* **2017**, *66*, 1031–1038. [CrossRef]
58. Kodio, A.; Menu, E.; Ranque, S. Eukaryotic and prokaryotic microbiota interactions. *Microorganisms* **2020**, *8*, 2018. [CrossRef]
59. Kodio, A.; Coulibaly, D.; Koné, A.K.; Konaté, S.; Doumbo, S.; Guindo, A.; Bittar, F.; Gouriet, F.; Raoult, D.; Thera, M.A.; et al. Blastocystis colonization is associated with increased diversity and altered gut bacterial communities in healthy Malian children. *Microorganisms* **2019**, *7*, 649. [CrossRef]
60. O'Brien Andersen, L.; Karim, A.B.; Roager, H.M.; Vigsnæs, L.K.; Krogfelt, K.A.; Licht, T.R.; Stensvold, C.R. Associations between common intestinal parasites bacteria in humans as revealed by qPCR. *Eur. J. Clin. Microbiol. Infect Dis.* **2016**, *35*, 1427–1431. [CrossRef]
61. Forsell, J.; Bengtsson-Palme, J.; Angelin, M.; Johansson, A.; Evengård, B.; Granlund, M. The relation between Blastocystis and the intestinal microbiota in Swedish travellers. *BMC Microbiol.* **2017**, *17*, 231. [CrossRef]
62. Krogsgaard, L.R.; Andersen La Johannesen, T.B.; Engsbro, A.L.; Stensvold, C.R.; Nielsen, H.V.; Bytzer, P. Characteristics of the bacterial microbiome in association with common intestinal parasites in irritable bowel syndrome. *Clin. Transl. Gastroenterol.* **2018**, *9*, 161. [CrossRef]
63. Mejia, R.; Damania, A.; Jeun, R.; Bryan, P.E.; Vargas, P.; Juarez, M.; Cajal, P.S.; Nasser, J.; Krolewiecki, A.; Lefoulon, E.; et al. Impact of intestinal parasites on microbiota and cobalamin gene sequences: A pilot study. *Parasites Vectors* **2020**, *13*, 200. [CrossRef]
64. Chen, T.L.; Chen, S.; Wu, H.W.; Lee, T.C.; Lu, Y.Z.; Wu, L.L.; Ni, Y.H.; Sun, C.H.; Yu, W.H.; Buret, A.G.; et al. Persistent gut barrier damage and commensal bacterial influx following eradication of Giardia infection in mice. *Gut Pathog.* **2013**, *5*, 26. [CrossRef]

65. Billy, V.; Lhotská, Z.; Jirků, M.; Kadlecová, O.; Frgelecová, L.; Parfrey, L.W.; Pomajbíková, K.J. Blastocystis colonization alters the gut microbiome and, in some cases, promotes faster recovery from induced colitis. *Front. Microbiol.* **2021**, *12*, 641483. [CrossRef]
66. Barash, N.R.; Maloney, J.G.; Singer, S.M.; Dawson, S.C. Giardia alters commensal microbial diversity throughout the murine gut. *Infect. Immun.* **2017**, *85*, e00948-e16. [CrossRef]
67. Calderón de la Barca, A.M.; Castillo-Fimbres, R.S.; Mejía-León, M.E.; Quihui-Cota, L.; Ochoa-Leyva, A.; Aguayo-Patrón, S.V. Enteric parasitic infection disturbs bacterial structure in Mexican children with autoantibodies for type 1 diabetes and/or celiac disease. *Gut Pathog.* **2020**, *12*, 37. [CrossRef]
68. Santacruz, A.; Collado, M.C.; Garcia-Valdes, L.; Segura, M.T.; Martin-Lagos, J.A.; Anjos, T.; Martí-Romero, M.; Lopez, R.M.; Florido, J.; Campoy, C.; et al. Gut microbiota composition is associated with body weight, weight gain and biochemical parameters in pregnant women. *Br. J. Nutr.* **2010**, *104*, 83–92. [CrossRef]
69. Karlsson, C.L.; Önnerfält, J.; Xu, J.; Molin, G.; Ahrné, S.; Thorngren-Jerneck, K. The microbiota of the gut in preschool children with normal and excessive body weight. *Obesity* **2012**, *20*, 2257–2261. [CrossRef]
70. Everard, A.; Belzer, C.; Geurts, L.; Ouwerkerk, J.P.; Druart, C.; Bindels, L.B.; Guiot, Y.; Derrien, M.; Muccioli, G.G.; Delzenne, N.M.; et al. Cross-talk between Akkermansia muciniphila and intestinal epithelium controls diet-induced obesity. *Proc. Natl. Acad. Sci. USA* **2013**, *110*, 9066–9071. [CrossRef]
71. Anhê, F.F.; Roy, D.; Pilon, G.; Dudonné, S.; Matamoros, S.; Varin, T.V.; Garofalo, C.; Moine, Q.; Desjardins, Y.; Levy, E.; et al. A polyphenol-rich cranberry extract protects from diet-induced obesity, insulin resistance and intestinal inflammation in association with increased Akkermansia spp. population in the gut microbiota of mice. *Gut* **2015**, *64*, 872–883. [CrossRef]
72. Depommier, C.; Everard, A.; Druart, C.; Plovier, H.; Van Hul, M.; Vieira-Silva, S.; Falony, G.; Raes, J.; Maiter, D.; Delzenne, N.M.; et al. Supplementation with Akkermansia muciniphila in overweight and obese human volunteers: A proof-of-concept exploratory study. *Nat. Med.* **2019**, *25*, 1096–1103. [CrossRef] [PubMed]
73. Machado, M.V.; Cortez-Pinto, H. Diet, microbiota, obesity, and NAFLD: A dangerous quartet. *Int. J. Mol. Sci.* **2016**, *17*, 481. [CrossRef] [PubMed]
74. Mouzaki, M.; Comelli, E.M.; Arendt, B.M.; Bonengel, J.; Fung, S.K.; Fischer, S.E.; McGilvray, I.D.; Allard, J.P. Intestinal microbiota in patients with nonalcoholic fatty liver disease. *Hepatology* **2013**, *58*, 120–127. [CrossRef] [PubMed]
75. Wong, V.W.S.; Tse, C.H.; Lam, T.T.Y.; Wong, G.L.H.; Chim, A.M.L.; Chu, W.C.W.; Yeung, D.K.W.; Law, P.T.W.; Kwan, H.S.; Yu, J.; et al. Molecular characterization of the fecal microbiota in patients with nonalcoholic steatohepatitis—A longitudinal study. *PLoS ONE* **2013**, *8*, e62885. [CrossRef]
76. Boursier, J.; Mueller, O.; Barret, M.; Machado, M.; Fizanne, L.; Araujo-Perez, F.; Guy, C.D.; Seed, P.C.; Rawls, J.F.; David, L.A.; et al. The severity of nonalcoholic fatty liver disease is associated with gut dysbiosis and shift in the metabolic function of the gut microbiota. *Hepatology* **2016**, *63*, 764–775. [CrossRef]
77. Yoon, W.J.; Kim, H.; Park, E.; Ryu, S.; Chang, Y.; Shin, H.; Kim, H.L.; Yi, S.Y. The impact of cholecystectomy on the gut microbiota: A case-control study. *J. Clin. Med.* **2019**, *8*, 79. [CrossRef]

nutrients

MDPI

Review

5-HT_{2C} Receptor Stimulation in Obesity Treatment: Orthosteric Agonists vs. Allosteric Modulators

Edmund Przegaliński [1,*], Kacper Witek [1], Karolina Wydra [1], Jolanta H. Kotlińska [2] and Małgorzata Filip [1]

[1] Department of Drug Addiction Pharmacology, Maj Institute of Pharmacology Polish Academy of Sciences, Smętna Street 12, 31-343 Krakow, Poland; witek@if-pan.krakow.pl (K.W.); wydra@if-pan.krakow.pl (K.W.); mal.fil@if-pan.krakow.pl (M.F.)
[2] Department of Pharmacology and Pharmacodynamics, Medical University of Lublin, Chodźki Street 4a, 20-093 Lublin, Poland; jolanta.kotlinska@umlub.pl
* Correspondence: przegal@if-pan.krakow.pl

Abstract: Obesity is a substantial health and economic issue, and serotonin (5-hydroxytryptamine, 5-HT) is an important neurotransmitter system involved in the regulation of body weight. The 5-HT_{2C} receptors (5-HT_{2C}Rs), one of 16 of the 5-HT receptor (5-HTRs) subtypes, play a significant role in food intake and body weight control. In this review, we focused on the 5-HTR agonists, such as fenfluramines, sibutramine, and lorcaserin, which act directly or indirectly at 5-HT_{2C}Rs and have been introduced into the clinic as antiobesity medications. Due to their unwanted effects, they were withdrawn from the market. The 5-HT_{2C}R positive allosteric modulators (PAMs) can be potentially safer active drugs than 5-HT_{2C}R agonists. However, more in vivo validation of PAMs is required to fully determine if these drugs will be effective in obesity prevention and antiobesity pharmacology treatment. Methodology strategy: This review focuses on the role of 5-HT_{2C}R agonism in obesity treatment, such as food intake regulation and weight gain. The literature was reviewed according to the review topic. We searched the PubMed and Scopus databases and Multidisciplinary Digital Publishing Institute open-access scientific journals using the following keyword search strategy depending on the chapter phrases: (1) "5-HT_{2C} receptor" AND "food intake", and (2) "5-HT_{2C} receptor" AND "obesity" AND "respective agonists", and (3) "5-HT_{2C} receptor" AND "PAM". We included preclinical studies (only present the weight loss effects) and double-blind, placebo-controlled, randomized clinical trials published since the 1975s (mostly related to antiobesity treatment), and excluded the pay-walled articles. After the search process, the authors selected, carefully screened, and reviewed appropriate papers. In total, 136 articles were included in this review.

Keywords: antiobesity drugs; obesity; PAMs; 5-HT_{2C} receptor agonists

1. Introduction

Overweight and obesity are global epidemics affecting more than 2.5 billion people worldwide. Overweight and obesity are related to a body mass index (BMI) >25 kg/m^2 and >30 kg/m^2, respectively, and result in substantial health and economic problems. Importantly, obesity is associated with several comorbidities, including chronic diseases, such as diabetes (type 2), cardiovascular pathologies (atherosclerosis, hypertension, and myocardial infarction), stroke, and different kinds of cancers. Thus, obesity is responsible for approximately 15% of human mortality [1]. Therefore, respective medications for obesity are important and are still being investigated in several laboratories.

Serotonin (5-hydroxytryptamine, 5-HT) is a key monoaminergic neurotransmitter in the central nervous system. Mammalian 5-HT is synthesized from the amino acid L-tryptophan by tryptophan hydroxylase to 5-hydroxy-L-tryptophan, and finally by aromatic amino acid decarboxylase enzymes. The 5-HT controls numerous physiological functions, such as thermoregulation, motor activity, wakefulness, cognitive function, and mood [2]. The 5-HT plays a crucial role in food intake modulation and body weight control. In fact, manipulations at a presynaptic level to reduce 5-HT function (e.g., after central administration of 5,7-dihydroxytryptamine, which is a 5-HT neurotoxin) or to enhance 5-HT tone (after 5-hydroxytryptophan, which is the precursor of 5-HT or fenfluramine that releases and inhibits the uptake of 5-HT) provoke an increase or decrease in food intake, respectively [3–5].

The multiplicity of 5-HT effects is controlled by a family of 5-HT receptor (5-HTRs) classes, 5-$HT_{1\text{-}7}$R [6]. Preclinical studies using 5-HT_{2C}R knockout demonstrated significantly higher food intake and body weight gain [7,8], while several selective or non-selective 5-HT_{2C}R agonists caused anorectic effects [9]. In addition, the 5-HT_{2C}R antagonist can increase weight gain and food intake [10,11]. This suggests that the 5-HT_{2C}R may be considered the principal therapeutic target of antiobesity drugs among 5-HT signaling.

The 5-HT_{2C}Rs are seven transmembrane spanning helices G protein-coupled receptors (GPCRs) with three extracellular, three intracellular loops, and an extracellular amino-terminus. The 5-HT_{2C}Rs primarily are distributed postsynaptically in the central nervous system and are especially present in the epithelial cells of the choroid plexus, limbic areas, hippocampal regions, the amygdala, and basal ganglia [12]. The latter receptors are located on neuronal cell types expressed acetylcholine, dopamine, and gamma-aminobutyric acid neurotransmitters. The 5-HT_{2C}Rs activate the phospholipase Cβ via $G\alpha^{q/11}$ protein and are coupled to phospholipase C in neurons and choroid plexus, and their activation leads to a cellular accumulation of inositol 1,4,5-triphosphate and diglyceride. In addition, 5-HT_{2C}Rs have also been shown to regulate ion channels and transport processes as well as activate other downstream effectors [6].

Nowadays, when obesity and overweight are epidemics, the effectiveness of medications is necessary and must be investigated. Whereas the 5-HT system plays a crucial role in food intake and body weight control, 5-HT_{2C}Rs are one of the therapeutic targets of antiobesity drugs. Our study aimed to show preclinical research and systematize the obesity treatment efficacy of 5-HT_{2C}R agonists in double-blind, placebo-controlled, and randomized clinical trials. Besides, we focused on the future perspective of newly synthesized pharmaceutical molecules, with 5-HT_{2C}R activity modulation, as a potential antiobesity treatment.

2. 5-HT_{2C} Receptor Action in Food Intake Regulation

The hypothalamus is the most important brain region involved in the central control of feeding and energy expenditure. Within the hypothalamus, the arcuate nucleus controls food intake and metabolism [13]. Functionally, the arcuate nucleus neurons are divided into two antagonistic groups that express specific neuropeptides and elicit disparate physiological actions. The first group consists of orexigenic neurons that express neuropeptide Y and agouti-related peptide to stimulate appetite. The second, anorexigenic group of neurons suppresses appetite with pro-opiomelanocortin (POMC) [14,15]. The modulation of feeding behavior via local 5-HT signaling acts mainly by an anorexigenic effect on POMC neurons. They are controlled by excitatory projections from the raphe nuclei 5-HT-reactive neurons stimulate the POMC-expressing arcuate nucleus neurons [16].

Approximately 25% of adult mouse POMC neurons express the 5-HT_{2C}Rs, but activation of POMC neurons via their receptor has been shown to account for the anorexigenic effects of several 5-HT drugs [17]. It has been demonstrated that 5-HT_{2C}Rs expressed in hypothalamic POMC/cocaine amphetamine-regulated transcript neurons are required to control energy and glucose homeostasis, implicating POMC neurons as the target for the effect of 5-HT_{2C}R agonists on weight-loss induction and improved glycemic control [6,18]. Moreover, 5-HT_{2C}R activation in POMC neurons both induces the *Pomc* mRNA expression and increases POMC neuronal activity [19]. Notably, the 5-HT_{2C}R knockout phenotype in POMC neurons provokes hyperphagia, sensitizes mice to diet-induced obesity, and directly dysregulates glucose homeostasis [18]. Moreover, selectively reintroducing the 5-

$HT_{2C}R$ to POMC neurons in whole-body 5-$HT_{2C}R$ knockout mice is sufficient to completely negate the knockout phenotype [20]. Finally, 5-$HT_{2C}Rs$ re-expression solely in POMC mice neurons is sufficient to mediate the effects of 5-HT drugs on food intake [21].

Food intake is also regulated by the reward brain system (the mesocorticolimbic pathway) structures, such as the ventral tegmental area, nucleus accumbens, prefrontal cortex, hippocampus, and amygdala [22,23]. Changes in reward processing are hypothesized to play a crucial role in the onset and maintenance of binge eating. Binge eating disorder is related to recurrent episodes of frequently consuming unusually large amounts of food and feeling unable to stop eating. Binge eating disorder is also related to its frequent comorbidity, obesity, as well as complications of being overweight [24]. Similar to addictive substances, such as cocaine, food activates the ventral tegmental area–nucleus accumbens pathways and stimulates pleasure by increasing the release of dopamine [25,26]. Moreover, a subset of dopamine neurons of the ventral tegmental area has recently been demonstrated as a key stimulator of binge-like eating behavior in mice [27]. At the same time, 5-HT cell bodies, projecting from the dorsal raphe nuclei to the ventral tegmental area and the nucleus accumbens, and a subset of dopamine and gamma-aminobutyric acid neurons in the ventral tegmental area express the 5-$HT_{2C}Rs$ [28,29]. Generally, the activation of 5-$HT_{2C}Rs$ plays an inhibitory role in the regulation of reward-related behavior by inhibiting release in certain areas of the brain [30,31]. Activation of ventral tegmental area 5-$HT_{2C}R$-expressing neurons significantly reduces homeostatic feeding in mice [32].

3. 5-HT_{2C} Receptor Agonists in Control over Food Intake Preclinical Research

Functionally, the 5-HTR agonists are drugs that orthosterically bind to one (=selective agonist) or more (=nonselective agonist) subtypes of 5-HTR. Direct or indirect (through additional mechanisms) 5-HTR activation by agonists provides a similar response to the intended activation by endogenous 5-HT (Table 1). In rodents, the 5-$HT_{2C}R$ agonist drugs reduce food intake in a manner consistent with an enhancement of satiety by action in the 5-$HT_{2C}R$ binding site in the brain hypothalamus.

Table 1. Description of antiobesity drugs affinity to 5-$HT_{1\text{-}2}$ receptor (5-$HT_{1\text{-}2}R$) subtypes, type of binding and mechanisms of 5-HT_{2C} receptor (5-$HT_{2C}R$) activation.

Drug	Affinity to 5-$HT_{1\text{-}2}R$ Subtypes *	Selectivity to 5-$HT_{2C}R$	Mechanism of 5-$HT_{2C}R$ Activation
piperazine derivatives (e.g., m-chlorophenyl piperazine)	5-$HT_{2B} \geq$ 5-HT_{2C} > 5-HT_{2A} > 5-$HT_{1A} \geq$ 5-HT_{1B} [33]	nonselective ligand	indirect agonism (affinity to 5-HT transporter and followed by 5-HT reuptake inhibition or 5-HT release enhancement)
fenfluramines	5-$HT_{2B} \geq$ 5-HT_{2C} > 5-HT_{2A} [34]	nonselective ligand	indirect agonism (affinity to 5-HT transporter and followed by 5-HT reuptake inhibition)
sibutramine	5-HT_{1A} = 5-HT_{1B} = 5-HT_{2A} = 5-HT_{2C} [35]	nonselective ligand	indirect agonism (affinity to 5-HT transporter and followed by 5-HT reuptake inhibition)
lorcaserin	5-HT_{2C} > 5-HT_{2A} > 5-HT_{2B} [36]	selective ligand	direct agonism

* mostly important for food intake and unwanted effects.

3.1. *Piperazine Derivatives*

The first reports showing that the stimulation of 5-$HT_{2C}Rs$ is responsible for the reduction of food intake were based on experiments performed with piperazine derivatives (m-chlorophenyl piperazine; m-CPP and tri-fluoromethylphenylpiperazine; TFMPP), which are nonselective 5-HT receptor agonists (Table 1). These compounds reduced food intake in rodents, and such an effect did not appear in mice lacking 5-HT_{2C}Rs [7] or in rats pretreated with 5-HT_{2C}R antagonists [37]. It has also been shown that piperazine 5-HT receptor agonists (especially m-CPP) reduce hepatic glucose production and insulin tolerance, and both effects are independent of the reduction in food intake [38]. Other authors presented evidence that the effect of m-CPP and other compounds acting via 5-HT_{2C}Rs increases satiety, reduces food intake, does not affect energy expenditure, and decreases body weight [39]. It should also be emphasized that hypophagia, an effect depending on the activation of 5-HT_{2C}Rs, is also related to an increase in POMC release in the nucleus arcuatus of the hypothalamus and stimulation of melanocortin receptors in the paraventricular nucleus (PVH) [38,40]. In contrast to the above-mentioned piperazine derivatives, several compounds with different chemical structures that have been previously described are selective 5-HT_{2C}R agonists that reduce food intake in rodents. In fact, Org 37684, Ro 60-175, PNU 22394, VER 3323, YM 348, and WAY 163909 have been found to induce hypophagia, which is reduced or blocked by 5-HT_{2C}R antagonists [37,41–44]. Interestingly, the hypophagia induced by 5-HT_{2C}R agonists seems to be selective. There is a lack of effect on water intake, and tolerance is not induced after chronic administration. Furthermore, some of these compounds (e.g., PNU 22394) appeared to be clinically active [37].

3.2. Fenfluramines

Acting at the presynaptic level, fenfluramine and d-fenfluramine are indirect agonists of 5-HT receptors (Table 1), among which the 5-HT_{2C}R are mostly required for the antiobesity effect. Accordingly, it has been demonstrated that, in 5-HT_{2C}R knockout mice, the anorexic effect of d-fenfluramine was not induced [21,45]. Furthermore, the hypophagic effect of d-fenfluramine was blocked by 5-HT_{2C}R antagonists [39,46]. Preclinical studies show that low (2.5 or 3 mg/kg) and high (10 mg/kg) doses of fenfluramine or d-fenfluramine reduced food intake and decreased body weight in rat models [47–49]. Moreover, in the case of cue-induced relapse, d-fenfluramine (3 mg/kg) blocked the reinstatement of lever pressing to food-seeking behavior in male rats [50].

3.3. Sibutramine

Similar to the antiobesity effect of fenfluramines, another selective inhibitor of presynaptic reuptake of the 5-HT and noradrenaline (NA) is β-phenethylamine—sibutramine (Table 1). Sibutramine action has also been suggested to be connected to the activation of 5-HT_{2C}R and enhancement of POMC [51,52]. Sibutramine (3–10 mg/kg) treatment rats showed reduced food intake and decreased body weight [53–58]. Interestingly, intraperitoneal injections of sibutramine (0.5–3.0 mg/kg) reduced feeding on a high fat/high sucrose diet across 2-h feeding sessions, but bilateral injections of sibutramine (2.0–10.0 μg) into either the PVN or the medial nucleus accumbens shell increased the food intake of the sweetened fat diet [59].

3.4. Lorcaserin

A series of new 5-HT_{2C}R agonists, as derivatives of 3-benzazepine, were synthesized by Smith et al. [60]. The most potent and selective compound was (1R)-8-chloro-2,3,4,5-tetrahydro-1-methyl-1H-3-benzazepine (APD 356, lorcaserin) (Table 1). The authors performed in vitro (effect on turnover of [3H]phosphoinositol) and in vivo (effect on food intake and body weight after acute or chronic *per os* administration of lorcaserin) experiments. The results demonstrated its 5-HT_{2C}R selectivity (versus 5-HT_{2A} and 5-HT_{2B} sharing sequence homology) as well as a reduction in food intake after acute administration and reductions in both food intake and body weight after 28 days of treatment. The effect of lorcaserin on food intake has been examined in different animal models of obesity. Some authors used a regular diet [60,61], and other investigators evaluated lorcaserin in rats maintained on a high-fat diet [36,62,63]. Lorcaserin treatment rats (1–2 mg/kg) reduced the percentage of body weight by selective reduction of body fat mass [36,60]. Moreover,

Xu et al. performed their experiments using binge-like eating and hunger-driven feeding in mice, where lorcaserin reduced food intake [27]. Lorcaserin also reversed the binge-like feeding observed following stimulation of the nucleus accumbens μ-opioid receptors and blocked nucleus accumbens μ-opioid enhancement of fat intake [64]. The simple antiobesity effect of lorcaserin may be related to the 5-HT_{2C}Rs location in brain structures associated with food intake control. It has been shown that the stimulation of such receptors expressed in POMC neurons induces anorexia [20,65], and the stimulation of 5-HT_{2C}Rs located on the brain patterning transcription factor single-minded 1 expressing neurons in the PVH increases food intake in mice [66,67].

Other studies showed a reduction in glucose consumption [61] and decreased binge food intake in rats [63] after lorcaserin (1 or 3 mg/kg) treatment. In addition, the above-mentioned antiobesity activity of 5-HT_{2C}R agonists is related to increased satiety and decreased food intake. Such effects of lorcaserin can also be connected with its inhibitory effect on motivation and impulsivity [68]. In some experiments, the effect of lorcaserin on glycemic control has been shown. It reduced the production of glucose and increased the sensitivity to insulin. However, it did not affect the secretion of insulin. The above effects were independent of weight loss [69]. Importantly, single-dose pharmacokinetic studies have shown rapid absorption, high oral bioavailability, and a moderate half-life of lorcaserin [60].

4. Clinical Effects of 5-HT_{2C} Receptor Agonist Drugs

4.1. Fenfluramines

At the beginning of 1970, fenfluramine and d-fenfluramine (an active dextro-rotatory stereoisomer of fenfluramine) were the first antiobesity drugs acting via the 5-HT system to be introduced on the market. In clinical trials, d-fenfluramine showed dose- and time-dependent weight loss (Table 2). In short-term treatment (3–6 months), a higher dose (30–60 mg) of d-fenfluramine led to greater weight loss than low doses (10–15 mg), compared to placebo patients. Long-term treatment (12 months or more) showed greater weight loss in d-fenfluramine patients compared to short-term treatment. Despite the efficacy of fenfluramine or d-fenfluramine in anorexic action, undesirable effects have been observed in obese patients.

Table 2. Efficacy of 5-HT_{2C} receptor agonist properties in double-blind, placebo-controlled, randomized clinical obesity trials. The patient's inclusion criteria are increased body mass index (BMI; >25 kg/m^2) or ideal body weight (IBW; 120–180%). The mean weight loss (kg or %) of the drug group (D) is compared to the placebo group (P). Multicenter studies were marked by an asterisk (*). QD—once-a-day treatment; BID—two times-a-day treatment.

Drug	Dosage (mg)	Duration (Months)	Patients Completed Study D I P	Key Inclusion Criteria (BMI > 25 kg/m² or IBW 120–180%)	Mean Weight Loss D vs. P (kg or %)	Ref.
d-fenfluramine	10 BID	3	85 I 85 *	120–180%	2.79 vs. 2.83 kg	[70]
	15 BID		168 I 169	120–180%	5.84 vs. 1.85 kg	[71]
			12 I 12	28–35 kg/m²	3.1 ± 2.3 vs. 0.1 ± 1.2 kg	[72]
		12	404 I 418 *	≥120%	9.82 vs. 7.15 kg	[73]
	30 QD or BID	3	82 I 85 *	120–180%	5.63 vs. 2.83 kg	[70]
			30 I 30	120–180%	4.6 ± 1.6 kg vs. no changed	[74]
		12	36 I 39	≥135%	12.8 vs. 8.6 kg	[75]
	60 BID	3	87 I 85 *	120–180%	7.23 vs. 2.83 kg	[70]
Sibutramine	5 QD	2	19 I 20	130–180%	2.9 ± 2.3 vs. 1.4 ± 2.1 kg	[76]
		3	56 I 59 *	27–40 kg/m²	2.4 ± 0.5 vs. 1.4 ± 0.5 kg	[77]
		6	107 I 87 *	30–40 kg/m²	3.7 vs. 1.3 kg	[78]

Table 2. *Cont.*

Drug	Dosage (mg)	Duration (Months)	Patients Completed Study D I P	Key Inclusion Criteria (BMI > 25 kg/m^2 or IBW 120–180%)	Mean Weight Loss D vs. P (kg or %)	Ref.
Sibutramine	10 QD	3	59 I 59 *	27–40 kg/m^2	5.1 ± 0.5 vs. 1.4 ± 0.5 kg	[77]
		6	99 I 87 *	30–40 kg/m^2	5.7 vs. 1.3 kg	[78]
			104 I 94 *	≥30 and ≤40 kg/m^2	8.2 vs. 3.9 kg	[79]
		40	2933 I 2825 *	25–45 kg/m^2	1.7 vs. +0.7 kg	[80]
	15 QD	3	62 I 59 *	27–40 kg/m^2	2 4.9 ± 0.5 vs. 1.4 ± 0.5 kg	[77]
		6	98 I 87 *	30–40 kg/m^2	7.0 vs. 1.3 kg	[78]
		12	281 I 80	±44 kg/m^2	6.5 ± 0.31 vs. 1.9 ± 0.56 kg	[81]
			68 I 64 *	>27 kg/m^2	5.5 ± 0.6 vs. 0.2 ± 0.5 kg	[82]
		~14	114 I 103 *	≥30 and <40 kg/m^2	8.1 ± 8.2 vs. 5.1 ± 6.5 kg	[83]
	20 QD	2	21 I 20	130–180%	5.0 ± 2.7 vs. 1.4 ± 2.1	[76]
		6	96 I 87 *	30–40 kg/m^2	8.2 vs. 1.3 kg	[78]
			151 I 152 *	≥27 kg/m^2	4.9 vs. 0.6 kg	[84]
		12	62 I 64 *	>27 kg/m^2	8.0 ± 0.9 vs. 0.2 ± 0.5 kg	[82]
	30 QD	6	101 I 87 *	30–40 kg/m^2	9.0 vs. 1.3 kg	[78]
Lorcaserin	10 QD or 10 BID	~2	29 I 28	27–45 kg/m^2	3.8 ± 0.4 vs. 2.2 ± 0.5 kg	[85]
		3	86 or 77 I 88 *	30–45 kg/m^2	1.8 or 3.6 vs. 0.3 kg	[86]
		6	59 I 53 *	≥33 and ≤55 kg/m^2	2.4 ± 0.8 vs. +0.6 ± 0.8 kg	[87]
		12	748 I 243 *	≥27 kg/m^2	4.2 vs. 1.4 kg	[88]
		12	75 or 169 I 157 *	27–45 kg/m^2	44.7 or 37.5 vs. 16.1%	[89]
			275 I 684 *	27–45 kg/m^2	5.81 ± 0.16 vs. 2.16 ± 0.14%	[90]
		13	1800 I 1550	30–45 kg/m^2	47.1 vs. 22.6%	[91]
		24	564 I 684 *	27–45 kg/m^2	7.0 ± 0.2 vs. 3.0 ± 0.2%	[90]
		40	748 I 243 *	≥27 kg/m^2	4.0 kg vs. 2.1 kg	[88]
	15 QD	3	82 I 88 *	30–45 kg/m^2	2.6 vs. 0.3 kg	[86]

In several clinical trials, cardiovascular and heart valve disorders were observed. Echocardiography performed 12 months after the initiation of fenfluramine-phentermine therapy in twenty-four women demonstrated unusual heart valvular morphology and regurgitation in all patients. Moreover, 30% of them also had newly documented pulmonary hypertension [92]. Another study reported that, of 233 obese patients who took appetite suppressants containing d-fenfluramine, 12.7% of them had a prevalence of cardiac valvular insufficiency [93]. Moreover, after the echocardiography of 200 patients with a history of exposure to anorectic medications, significant aortic valve regurgitation was observed in 14% of patients exposed to d-fenfluramine [94].

Other authors showed occurrences of multivalvular disease and pulmonary hypertension after fenfluramine treatment [95–98]. Nine controlled studies of fenfluramine showed mild or greater aortic valve regurgitation in 9.6% of treated almost 3300 patients compared with 3.9% of 2000 control subjects [99]. Besides the cardiovascular problems, the most common events reported during d-fenfluramine (15 mg twice daily) treatment were diarrhea, asthenia, dry mouth, headache, and tiredness. Side effects were reported significantly more frequently in patients receiving dexfenfluramine 30 mg twice daily than in those receiving 15 mg twice daily [100].

In 1997, fenfluramines were withdrawn from clinical use due to adverse side effects, such as cardiac valvulopathy and pulmonary hypertension. The most likely explanation for fenfluramine-associated valvulopathy is the activation of 5-HT_{2B}Rs by norfenfluramine, being a fenfluramine metabolite. Fenfluramines bind weakly to 5-HT_{2A}Rs, 5-HT_{2B}Rs, and 5-HT_{2C}Rs. Norfenfluramine exhibited a high affinity for 5-HT_{2B}Rs, and 5-HT_{2C}Rs, and a more moderate affinity for 5-HT_{2A}Rs [33]. In cells expressing recombinant 5-HT_{2B}Rs, norfenfluramine potently stimulated the hydrolysis of inositol phosphates, increased intracellular Ca^{2+}, and activated the mitogen-activated protein kinase cascade, the latter of which has been linked to mitogenic actions of the 5-HT_{2B}Rs. This 5-HT_{2B}Rs action is important for heart valvulopathy occurrence. Moreover, the level of 5-HT_{2B}Rs and 5-HT_{2A}Rs transcripts in heart valves was at least 300-fold higher than the levels of the 5-HT_{2C}R transcript, which were barely detectable [101].

4.2. *Sibutramine*

Sibutramine was approved by the U.S. Food and Drug Administration (FDA) in 1997 for weight loss in the short- and long-term treatment of obesity. Sibutramine has dose- and time- dependent antiobesity effectiveness, as evidenced in clinical studies (Table 2). Compared to placebo-treated patients, higher doses (15–30 mg) of sibutramine result in greater weight loss than low doses (10 mg). Moreover, sibutramine efficacy in reducing body weight in a long-term period (over one year) was greater than in short-term treatment (six months). However, the Sibutramine Cardiovascular Outcomes (SCOUT) trial showed that, at 12 months but not six months of sibutramine treatment, patients with marked lower baseline blood pressure had the tendency to increase [102]. In some other clinical studies, sibutramine did not increase blood pressure in obese patients [103,104]. Besides, patients taking sibutramine experienced a significant increase in heart rate [83,105–109], but without difference in the overall status of the cardiac valves compared to placebo subjects [105,110–112]. Otherwise, sibutramine's most frequently encountered adverse effects were constipation, dry mouth, headache, insomnia, and nausea.

In 2010, the FDA decided to withdraw sibutramine from the market as a consequence of increased primary outcome events (POEs), such as nonfatal myocardial infarction, nonfatal stroke, resuscitation after cardiac arrest, or cardiovascular death. Indeed, the risk of POEs was increased by 16% in the sibutramine treatment group as compared with the placebo [80]. Nevertheless, other results from SCOUTs did not show an overall deleterious effect of treatment but an increase in POEs in subjects with a history of cardiovascular disease and type 2 diabetes [113,114]. Unexpectedly, sibutramine therapy in obese or overweight high-risk patients induced significant mean reductions for all blood lipids [115]. Although sibutramine and its metabolites exhibit low affinity for 5-$HT_{1A\text{-}B}$Rs and 5-HT_{2A}Rs, these receptors are reported as a possible target for the causation of unwanted cardiovascular effects [116].

4.3. *Lorcaserin*

In 2012, the FDA approved lorcaserin on the market as a weight loss medication. The results of several clinical studies have shown its antiobesity effect (Table 2). Despite the time of treatment, lorcaserin (10 mg once and twice daily) caused greater weight loss than with a placebo. The most commonly reported adverse effects were headache, nausea, dizziness, and fatigue, but generally, lorcaserin was well-tolerated. In contrast, the unwanted effects of fenfluramines and sibutramine, in randomized, double-blind, placebo-controlled, multinational clinical trials of lorcaserin treatment, were not associated with any increase in cardiovascular events among patients with high cardiovascular risk [88]. Interestingly, lorcaserin treatment for 6–13 months showed an improvement in metabolic and cardiovascular parameters in obese patients [91,117,118]. It has also been reported that this drug decreases the risk of developing diabetes [119]. At the same time, compared to a placebo, lorcaserin did not affect blood pressure, heart rate, or heart valves [120–122].

However, the US Food and Drug Administration Adverse Event Reporting System (FAERS) database scrutinization identified that lorcaserin medication was associated with a significantly greater valvular disorder [123]. Only in overweight and obese patients with renal dysfunction, lorcaserin treatment barely increased cardiovascular disease risk [124]. At the same time, the results of several clinical studies have shown its modest antiobesity effects, and lorcaserin's position on the market slowly declined. Moreover, patients treated with lorcaserin were diagnosed with more frequent occurrences of cancer. Indeed, incidences of malignancies during lorcaserin pharmacotherapy (though not different from the respective placebo groups) were the reason that it was withdrawn as an antiobesity medication in 2020 [125–127].

5. Positive-Allosteric Modulators of the 5-HT$_{2C}$R

The 5-HT$_{2C}$R is not only an antiobesity drug target, but also a binding site for positive-allosteric modulators (PAMs). PAMs are groups of substances that increase the affinity and/or efficacy of respective receptor ligands (Figure 1). A potential PAM therapeutic role is the ability to potentiate the effect of an endogenous cognate ligand or other probes interacting orthosterically by binding at a distinct, allosteric, receptor recognition site [128]. Thereafter, several new molecules related to 5-HT$_{2C}$R PAMs were pharmacologically evaluated. Recently, there have been a few papers showing 5-HT$_{2C}$R PAM to be potentially safer antiobesity drugs. Garcia-Carceles et al. [129] screened a chemical library from Vivia Biotech using the ExviTech platform and validated and synthesized analogues of Compound 5 (VA240). Among 35 synthesized akins, the most interesting was Compound 11 (PAM 11: (N-[(1-benzyl-1H-indol-3-yl)methyl]pyridin-3-amine, VA012). This compound dose-dependently enhanced 5-HT efficacy (highest potentiation—by 35% at 10 μM—of 5-HT-induced inositol monophosphate release in 5-HT$_{2C}$R HeLa cells), displayed low binding competition with 5-HT or other orthosteric ligands, and did not exhibit significant off-target activities. Importantly, PAM 11 and WAY 161503 (an agonist of 5-HT$_{2C}$Rs used as a reference drug) were administered acutely to reduce food intake in rats, and PAM 11 acted with higher efficacy and with more prolonged action. Moreover, PAM 11-evoked food intake inhibition was not eliminated after pretreatment with the 5-HT$_{2A}$R antagonist ketanserin. These findings indicate that the effect of PAM 11 was not related to the activation of 5-HT$_{2A}$Rs and suggest that it has no direct action at the orthosteric site of the 5-HT$_{2C}$R. Furthermore, PAM 11 administered subchronically (seven days) in a restricted food access model also reduced both food intake and body weight gain in rats. Finally, after combined treatment with PAM 11 and sertraline (a 5-HT reuptake inhibitor) administered in a dose-induced mild feeding suppression, potentiation of feeding reduction was demonstrated. This is clear evidence for the allosteric potentiation of 5-HT-induced anorexia, especially 5-HT$_{2C}$R-induced anorexia [129]. Another study synthesized a series of N-heterocycle imidazole-linked phenyl cyclopropyl methanone molecules. One of three active 5-HT$_{2C}$R allosteric modulator molecules, Compound 58, showed unique and beneficial dual characteristics. Compound 58 selectively exhibited PAM response at 5-HT$_{2C}$Rs and negative-allosteric modulator at 5-HT$_{2B}$Rs, which is rarely reported for allosteric modulators. From the point of view of 5-HT$_{2C}$R agonist's unwanted cardiovascular effects (depending on 5-HT$_{2B}$Rs activation), the negative 5-HT$_{2B}$Rs modulation is a unique property. Besides, at the same dose, both Compound 58 and lorcaserin reduced food intake in rats [130].

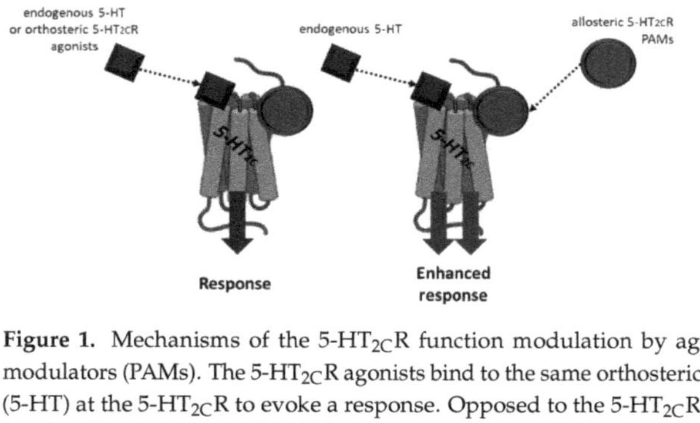

Figure 1. Mechanisms of the 5-HT$_{2C}$R function modulation by agonists and positive-allosteric modulators (PAMs). The 5-HT$_{2C}$R agonists bind to the same orthosteric sites as endogenous serotonin (5-HT) at the 5-HT$_{2C}$R to evoke a response. Opposed to the 5-HT$_{2C}$R agonists, the 5-HT$_{2C}$R PAMs bind to allosteric sites at the 5-HT$_{2C}$R, enhancing the affinity and efficacy of the 5-HT$_{2C}$R response by 5-HT.

6. Conclusions and Perspectives

This paper reviews the preclinical and clinical efficacy of 5-HT_{2C}R agonists in obesity treatment. Moreover, we showed evidence of new therapeutic molecules, based on 5-HT_{2C}R targets, as potential antiobesity drugs.

In preclinical studies, nonselective or more selective 5-HT_{2C}R agonists showed effectiveness in decreasing body weight, reducing food intake, and inhibiting food seeking-behavior. Consequently, 5-HT_{2C}R drugs, such as fenfluramines, sibutramine, and lorcaserin, were approved in the trade as obesity pharmacology medications. Clinical trials confirmed 5-HT_{2C}R agonist's action in reduced food intake and decreased body weight in patients with BMI >25 kg/m^2 or an ideal body weight of 120–180%. However, after a few years, the 5-HT_{2C}R agonist's position on the market slowly declined, until being withdrawn from the market due to unwanted effects (higher risk of cardiac valvular abnormalities) occurrence. Nonetheless, the above-mentioned drugs have contributed to understanding the mechanisms of 5-HTR action that permitted the design of new selective molecules. Herein, we showed that 5-HT_{2C}R PAM intensifies 5-HT action for reduced food intake and decreased weight loss in a few in vivo studies. Moreover, we presented selective 5-HT_{2C}R PAM without 5-HT_{2B}R-linked cardiac valve affinity that offers a new angle into the pharmacological potential safer in obesity treatment.

Nowadays, more attention is being paid to precision medicine that offers new grounds for obesity prevention and targeting correct treatment based on genetic, pharmacogenomic, and environmental factors [131–133]. Recent human studies underline the connectivity between 5-HT availability and BMI as a predictor of obesity treatment success [134]. Furthermore, the loss of 5-HT_{2C}R function due to mutation can predispose humans to obesity. Thus, sequencing genes encoding the 5-HT_{2C}R should be included in diagnostic panels for obesity [135]. Currently, a series of highly specific 5-HT_{2C}R PAM selectively increase in vitro 5-HT efficacy [136]. This elevates the possibility of 5-HT_{2C}R PAM being used in a more directed way as precision medicine.

In conclusion, we underline the role of 5-HT_{2C}R as a crucial therapeutic target in obesity treatment. Further, 5-HT_{2C}R PAM discovery and syntheses are recommended. Furthermore, 5-HT_{2C}R PAM optimization and clinical weight loss validation are necessary for successful antiobesity treatment and to reveal the full therapeutic potential of PAM.

Author Contributions: Conceptualization and supervision, E.P. and M.F.; methodology, K.W. (Kacper Witek); writing—original draft preparation, E.P., K.W. (Kacper Witek), K.W. (Karolina Wydra), J.H.K. and M.F.; writing—review and editing, E.P. and K.W. (Kacper Witek). All authors have read and agreed to the published version of the manuscript.

Funding: This research was supported by the statutory fund of the Department of Drug Addiction Pharmacology, Maj Institute of Pharmacology Polish Academy of Sciences.

Institutional Review Board Statement: Not applicable.

Informed Consent Statement: Not applicable.

Data Availability Statement: Not applicable.

Conflicts of Interest: The authors declare no conflict of interest.

References

. Hurt, R.T.; Mundi, M.S.; Ebbert, J.O. Challenging Obesity, Diabetes, and Addiction: The Potential of Lorcaserin Extended Release. *Diabetes Metab. Syndr. Obes.* **2018**, *11*, 469–478. [CrossRef] [PubMed]
. Dutton, A.C.; Barnes, N.M. Anti-Obesity Pharmacotherapy: Future Perspectives Utilising 5-HT_{2C} Receptor Agonists. *Drug Discov. Today Ther. Strat.* **2006**, *3*, 577–583. [CrossRef]
. Saller, C.F.; Stricker, E.M. Hyperphagia and Increased Growth in Rats After Intraventricular Injection of 5,7-Dihydroxytryptamine. *Science* **1976**, *191*, 385–387. [CrossRef] [PubMed]
. Blundell, J.E.; Leshem, M.B. The Effect of 5-Hydroxytryptophan on Food Intake and on the Anorexic Action of Amphetamine and Fenfluramine. *J Pharm. Pharmacol.* **1975**, *27*, 31–37. [CrossRef] [PubMed]

5. Duhault, J.; Malen, C.; Boulanger, M.; Voisin, C.; Beregi, L.; Schmitt, H. Fenfluramine and 5 Hydroxytryptamine. I: Is Fenfluramine or Norfenfluramine Involved in the Decrease of Brain 5 Hydroxytryptamine? *Arzneim.-Forsch./Drug Res.* **1975**, *25*, 1755–1758.
6. Masson, J.; Emerit, M.B.; Hamon, M.; Darmon, M. Serotonergic Signaling: Multiple Effectors and Pleiotropic Effects. *Wiley Interdiscip. Rev. Membr. Transp. Signal.* **2012**, *1*, 685–713. [CrossRef]
7. Tecott, L.H.; Sun, L.M.; Akana, S.F.; Strack, A.M.; Lowenstein, D.H.; Dallman, M.F.; Julius, D. Eating Disorder and Epilepsy in Mice Lacking 5-HT^{2C} Serotonin Receptors. *Nature* **1995**, *374*, 542–546. [CrossRef]
8. Nonogaki, K.; Nozue, K.; Oka, Y. Hyperphagia Alters Expression of Hypothalamic 5-HT_{2C} and 5-HT_{1B} Receptor Genes and Plasma Des-Acyl Ghrelin Levels in Ay Mice. *Endocrinology* **2006**, *147*, 5893–5900. [CrossRef]
9. Bello, N.T.; Liang, N.C. The Use of Serotonergic Drugs to Treat Obesity—Is There Any Hope? *Drug Des. Dev. Ther.* **2011**, *5*, 95–109. [CrossRef]
10. Schuhler, S.; Clark, A.; Joseph, W.; Patel, A.; Lehnen, K.; Stratford, E.; Horan, T.L.; Fone, K.C.F.; Ebling, F.J.P.; Schuhler, A. Involvement of 5-HT Receptors in the Regulation of Food Intake in Siberian Hamsters. *J. Neuroendocrinol.* **2005**, *17*, 276–285. [CrossRef]
11. Bonhaus, D.W.; Weinhardt, K.K.; Taylor, M.; Desouza, A.; Mcneeley, P.M.; Szczepanski, K.; Fontana, D.J.; Trinh, J.; Rocha, C.L.; Dawson, M.W.; et al. RS-102221: A Novel High Affinity and Selective, 5-HT_{2C} Receptor Antagonist. *Neuropharmacology* **1997**, *36*, 621–629. [CrossRef] [PubMed]
12. Wold, E.A.; Wild, C.T.; Cunningham, K.A.; Zhou, J. Targeting the 5-HT_{2C} Receptor in Biological Context and the Current State of 5-HT_{2C} Receptor Ligand Development. *Curr. Top. Med. Chem.* **2019**, *19*, 1381–1398. [CrossRef] [PubMed]
13. Myers, M.G.; Olson, D.P. Central Nervous System Control of Metabolism. *Nature* **2012**, *491*, 357–363. [CrossRef] [PubMed]
14. Gropp, E.; Shanabrough, M.; Borok, E.; Xu, A.W.; Janoschek, R.; Buch, T.; Plum, L.; Balthasar, N.; Hampel, B.; Waisman, A.; et al. Agouti-Related Peptide–Expressing Neurons Are Mandatory for Feeding. *Nat. Neurosci.* **2005**, *8*, 1289–1291. [CrossRef]
15. Balthasar, N.; Dalgaard, L.T.; Lee, C.E.; Yu, J.; Funahashi, H.; Williams, T.; Ferreira, M.; Tang, V.; McGovern, R.A.; Kenny, C.D.; et al. Divergence of Melanocortin Pathways in the Control of Food Intake and Energy Expenditure. *Cell* **2005**, *123*, 493–505. [CrossRef]
16. Van Galen, K.A.; Ter Horst, K.W.; Serlie, M.J. Serotonin, Food Intake, and Obesity. *Obes. Rev.* **2021**, *22*, e13210. [CrossRef]
17. Doslikova, B.; Garfield, A.S.; Shaw, J.; Evans, M.L.; Burdakov, D.; Billups, B.; Heisler, L.K. 5-HT_{2C} Receptor agonist Anorectic Efficacy Potentiated by 5-HT_{1B} Receptor agonist Coapplication: An Effect Mediated via Increased Proportion of Pro-Opiomelanocortin Neurons Activated. *J. Neurosci.* **2013**, *33*, 9800–9804. [CrossRef]
18. Berglund, E.D.; Liu, C.; Sohn, J.W.; Liu, T.; Kim, M.H.; Lee, C.E.; Vianna, C.R.; Williams, K.W.; Xu, Y.; Elmquist, J.K. Serotonin 2C Receptors in Pro-Opiomelanocortin Neurons Regulate Energy and Glucose Homeostasis. *J. Clin. Investig.* **2013**, *123*, 5061–5070. [CrossRef]
19. Wyler, S.C.; Lord, C.C.; Lee, S.; Elmquist, J.K.; Liu, C. Serotonergic Control of Metabolic Homeostasis. *Front. Cell. Neurosci.* **2017**, *11*, 277. [CrossRef]
20. Roepke, T.A.; Smith, A.W.; Rønnekleiv, O.K.; Kelly, M.J. Serotonin 5-HT_{2C} Receptor-Mediated Inhibition of the M-Current in Hypothalamic POMC Neurons. *Am. J. Physiol. Endocrinol. Metab.* **2012**, *302*, E1399–E1406. [CrossRef]
21. Xu, Y.; Jones, J.E.; Kohno, D.; Williams, K.W.; Lee, C.E.; Choi, M.J.; Anderson, J.G.; Heisler, L.K.; Zigman, J.M.; Lowell, B.B.; et al. 5-HT_{2C}Rs Expressed by Pro-Opiomelanocortin Neurons Regulate Energy Homeostasis. *Neuron* **2008**, *60*, 582–589. [CrossRef] [PubMed]
22. Alonso-Alonso, M.; Woods, S.C.; Pelchat, M.; Grigson, P.S.; Stice, E.; Farooqi, S.; Khoo, C.S.; Mattes, R.D.; Beauchamp, G.K. Food Reward System: Current Perspectives and Future Research Needs. *Nutr. Rev.* **2015**, *73*, 296–307. [CrossRef]
23. Leenaerts, N.; Jongen, D.; Ceccarini, J.; van Oudenhove, L.; Vrieze, E. The Neurobiological Reward System and Binge Eating: A Critical Systematic Review of Neuroimaging Studies. *Int. J. Eat. Disord.* **2022**, *55*, 1421–1458. [CrossRef] [PubMed]
24. Amianto, F.; Ottone, L.; Abbate Daga, G.; Fassino, S. Binge-Eating Disorder Diagnosis and Treatment: A Recap in Front of DSM-5. *BMC Psychiatry* **2015**, *15*, 70. [CrossRef] [PubMed]
25. Cunningham, K.A.; Fox, R.G.; Anastasio, N.C.; Bubar, M.J.; Stutz, S.J.; Moeller, F.G.; Gilbertson, S.R.; Rosenzweig-Lipson, S. Selective Serotonin 5-HT(2C) Receptor Activation Suppresses the Reinforcing Efficacy of Cocaine and Sucrose but Differentially Affects the Incentive-Salience Value of Cocaine- vs. Sucrose-Associated Cues. *Neuropharmacology* **2011**, *61*, 513–523. [CrossRef]
26. Price, A.E.; Anastasio, N.C.; Stutz, S.J.; Hommel, J.D.; Cunningham, K.A. Serotonin 5-HT_{2C} Receptor Activation Suppresses Binge Intake and the Reinforcing and Motivational Properties of High-Fat Food. *Front. Pharmacol.* **2018**, *9*, 821. [CrossRef]
27. Xu, P.; He, Y.; Cao, X.; Valencia-Torres, L.; Yan, X.; Saito, K.; Wang, C.; Yang, Y.; Hinton, A.; Zhu, L.; et al. Activation of Serotonin 2C Receptors in Dopamine Neurons Inhibits Binge-like Eating in Mice. *Biol. Psychiatry* **2017**, *81*, 737–747. [CrossRef]
28. Bubar, M.J.; Cunningham, K.A. Distribution of Serotonin 5-HT_{2C} Receptors in the Ventral Tegmental Area. *Neuroscience* **2007**, *146*, 286–297. [CrossRef]
29. Bubar, M.J.; Stutz, S.J.; Cunningham, K.A. 5-HT_{2C} Receptors Localize to Dopamine and GABA Neurons in the Rat Mesoaccumbens Pathway. *PLoS ONE* **2011**, *6*, e20508. [CrossRef]
30. De Deurwaerdère, P.; Navailles, S.; Berg, K.A.; Clarke, W.P.; Spampinato, U. Constitutive Activity of the Serotonin2C Receptor Inhibits In Vivo Dopamine Release in the Rat Striatum and Nucleus Accumbens. *J. Neurosci.* **2004**, *24*, 3235. [CrossRef] [PubMed]
31. Hayes, D.J.; Mosher, T.M.; Greenshaw, A.J. Differential Effects of 5-HT_{2C} Receptor Activation by WAY 161503 on Nicotine-Induced Place Conditioning and Locomotor Activity in Rats. *Behav. Brain Res.* **2009**, *197*, 323–330. [CrossRef] [PubMed]

32. Valencia-Torres, L.; Olarte-Sánchez, C.M.; Lyons, D.J.; Georgescu, T.; Greenwald-Yarnell, M.; Myers, M.G.; Bradshaw, C.M.; Heisler, L.K. Activation of Ventral Tegmental Area 5-HT_{2C} Receptors Reduces Incentive Motivation. *Neuropsychopharmacology* **2017**, *42*, 1511–1521. [CrossRef] [PubMed]
33. Rothman, R.B.; Baumann, M.H.; Savage, J.E.; Rauser, L.; McBride, A.; Hufeisen, S.J.; Roth, B.L. Evidence for Possible Involvement of 5-HT_{2B} Receptors in the Cardiac Valvulopathy Associated With Fenfluramine and Other Serotonergic Medications. *Circulation* **2000**, *102*, 2836–2841. [CrossRef]
34. Setola, V.; Dukat, M.; Glennon, R.A.; Roth, B.L. Molecular Determinants for the Interaction of the Valvulopathic Anorexigen Norfenfluramine with the 5-HT_{2B} Receptor. *Mol. Pharmacol.* **2005**, *68*, 20–33. [CrossRef] [PubMed]
35. Frassetto, S.S.; Delia Santa Rubio, Â.; Lopes, J.J.; Pereira, P.; Brum, C.; Khazzaka, M.; Vinagre, A.S. Locomotor and Peripheral Effects of Sibutramine Modulated by 5-HT_2 Receptors. *Can. J. Physiol. Pharmacol.* **2006**, *84*, 1239–1244. [CrossRef]
36. Thomsen, W.J.; Grottick, A.J.; Menzaghi, F.; Reyes-Saldana, H.; Espitia, S.; Yuskin, D.; Whelan, K.; Martin, M.; Morgan, M.; Chen, W.; et al. Lorcaserin, a Novel Selective Human 5-Hydroxytryptamine2C Agonist: In Vitro and in Vivo Pharmacological Characterization. *J. Pharmacol. Exp. Ther.* **2008**, *325*, 577–587. [CrossRef] [PubMed]
37. Bickerdike, M. 5-HT_{2C} Receptor agonists as Potential Drugs for the Treatment of Obesity. *Curr. Top. Med. Chem.* **2003**, *3*, 885–897. [CrossRef]
38. Georgescu, T.; Lyons, D.; Heisler, L.K. Role of Serotonin in Body Weight, Insulin Secretion and Glycaemic Control. *J. Neuroendocrinol.* **2021**, *33*, e12960. [CrossRef]
39. Hayashi, A.; Suzuki, M.; Sasamata, M.; Miyata, K. Agonist diversity in 5-HT_{2C} receptor-mediated weight control in rats. *Psychopharmacology* **2005**, *178*, 241–249. [CrossRef]
40. Xu, Y.; Jones, J.E.; Lauzon, D.A.; Anderson, J.G.; Balthasar, N.; Heisler, L.K.; Zinn, A.R.; Lowell, B.B.; Elmquist, J.K. A Serotonin and Melanocortin Circuit Mediates D-Fenfluramine Anorexia. *J. Neurosci.* **2010**, *30*, 14630–14634. [CrossRef]
41. Martin, J.R.; Bös, M.; Jenck, F.; Moreau, J.L.; Mutel, V.; Sleight, A.J.; Wichmann, J.; Andrews, J.S.; Berendsen, H.H.G.; Broekkamp, C.L.E.; et al. 5-HT_{2C} Receptor Agonists: Pharmacological Characteristics and Therapeutic Potential. *J. Pharmacol. Exp. Ther.* **1998**, *286*, 913–924. [PubMed]
42. Kimura, Y.; Hatanaka, K.I.; Naitou, Y.; Maeno, K.; Shimada, I.; Koakutsu, A.; Wanibuchi, F.; Yamaguchi, T. Pharmacological Profile of YM348, a Novel, Potent and Orally Active 5-HT_{2C} Receptor Agonist. *Eur. J. Pharmacol.* **2004**, *483*, 37–43. [CrossRef] [PubMed]
43. Vickers, S.P.; Benwell, K.R.; Porter, R.H.; Bickerdike, M.J.; Kennett, G.A.; Dourish, C.T. Comparative Effects of Continuous Infusion of MCPP, Ro 60-0175 and d-Fenfluramine on Food Intake, Water Intake, Body Weight and Locomotor Activity in Rats. *Br. J. Pharmacol.* **2000**, *130*, 1305–1314. [CrossRef] [PubMed]
44. Dunlop, J.; Sabb, A.L.; Mazandarani, H.; Zhang, J.; Kalgaonker, S.; Shukhina, E.; Sukoff, S.; Vogel, R.L.; Stack, G.; Schechter, L.; et al. WAY-163909 [(7bR, 10aR)-1,2,3,4,8,9,10,10a-Octahydro-7bH-Cyclopenta-[b][1,4]Diazepino[6,7,1hi]Indole], a Novel 5-Hydroxytryptamine 2C Receptor-Selective Agonist with Anorectic Activity. *J. Pharmacol. Exp. Ther.* **2005**, *313*, 862–869. [CrossRef]
45. Vickers, S.P.; Clifton, P.G.; Dourish, C.T.; Tecott, L.H. Reduced Satiating Effect of D-Fenfluramine in Serotonin 5-HT(2C) Receptor Mutant Mice. *Psychopharmacology* **1999**, *143*, 309–314. [CrossRef]
46. Vickers, S.P.; Dourish, C.T.; Kennett, G.A. Evidence That Hypophagia Induced by D-Fenfluramine and d-Norfenfluramine in the Rat Is Mediated by 5-HT_{2C} Receptors. *Neuropharmacology* **2001**, *41*, 200–209. [CrossRef]
47. Fisler, J.S.; Underberger, S.J.; York, D.A.; Bray, G.A. D-Fenfluramine in a Rat Model of Dietary Fat-Induced Obesity. *Pharmacol. Biochem. Behav.* **1993**, *45*, 487–493. [CrossRef]
48. Clifton, P.G.; Lee, M.D.; Dourish, C.T. Similarities in the Action of Ro 60-0175, a 5-HT_{2C} Receptor Agonist, and d-Fenfluramine on Feeding Patterns in the Rat. *Psychopharmacology* **2000**, *152*, 256–267. [CrossRef]
49. Brindley, D.N.; Hales, P.; Al-Sieni, A.I.I.; Russell, J.C. Sustained Decreases in Weight and Serum Insulin, Glucose, Triacylglycerol and Cholesterol in JCR:LA-Corpulent Rats Treated with D-Fenfluramine. *Br. J. Pharmacol.* **1992**, *105*, 679–685. [CrossRef]
50. Pratt, W.E.; Ford, R.T. Systemic Treatment with D-Fenfluramine, but Not Sibutramine, Blocks Cue-Induced Reinstatement of Food-Seeking Behavior in the Rat. *Neurosci. Lett.* **2013**, *556*, 232–237. [CrossRef]
51. Burke, L.K.; Doslikova, B.; D'Agostino, G.; Garfield, A.S.; Farooq, G.; Burdakov, D.; Low, M.J.; Rubinstein, M.; Evans, M.L.; Billups, B.; et al. 5-HT Obesity Medication Efficacy via POMC Activation Is Maintained During Aging. *Endocrinology* **2014**, *155*, 3732–3738. [CrossRef] [PubMed]
52. Higgs, S.; Cooper, A.J.; Barnes, N.M. Reversal of Sibutramine-Induced Anorexia with a Selective 5-HT(2C) Receptor Antagonist. *Psychopharmacology* **2011**, *214*, 941–947. [CrossRef] [PubMed]
53. Levin, B.E.; Dunn-Meynell, A.A. Sibutramine Alters the Central Mechanisms Regulating the Defended Body Weight in Diet-Induced Obese Rats. *Am. J. Physiol. Regul. Integr. Comp. Physiol.* **2000**, *279*, R2222–R2228. [CrossRef]
54. Hansen, H.H.; Hansen, G.; Tang-Christensen, M.; Larsen, P.J.; Axel, A.M.D.; Raben, A.; Mikkelsen, J.D. The Novel Triple Monoamine Reuptake Inhibitor Tesofensine Induces Sustained Weight Loss and Improves Glycemic Control in the Diet-Induced Obese Rat: Comparison to Sibutramine and Rimonabant. *Eur. J. Pharmacol.* **2010**, *636*, 88–95. [CrossRef] [PubMed]
55. Madsen, A.N.; Hansen, G.; Paulsen, S.J.; Lykkegaard, K.; Tang-Christensen, M.; Hansen, H.S.; Levin, B.E.; Larsen, P.J.; Knudsen, L.B.; Fosgerau, K.; et al. Long-Term Characterization of the Diet-Induced Obese and Diet-Resistant Rat Model: A Polygenetic Rat Model Mimicking the Human Obesity Syndrome. *J. Endocrinol.* **2010**, *206*, 287–296. [CrossRef]

56. Hansen, G.; Jelsing, J.; Vrang, N. Effects of Liraglutide and Sibutramine on Food Intake, Palatability, Body Weight and Glucose Tolerance in the Gubra DIO-Rats. *Acta Pharmacol. Sin.* **2012**, *33*, 194–200. [CrossRef]
57. Casado, A.; Rodríguez, V.M.; Portillo, M.P.; Macarulla, M.T.; Abecia, L.C.; Echevarría, E.; Casis, L. Sibutramine Decreases Body Weight Gain and Increases Energy Expenditure in Obese Zucker Rats without Changes in NPY and Orexins. *Nutr. Neurosci.* **2003**, *6*, 102–111. [CrossRef]
58. Jackson, H.C.; Needham, A.M.; Hutchins, L.J.; Mazurkiewicz, S.E.; Heal, D.J. Comparison of the Effects of Sibutramine and Other Monoamine Reuptake Inhibitors on Food Intake in the Rat. *Br. J. Pharmacol.* **1997**, *121*, 1758–1762. [CrossRef]
59. Pratt, W.E.; Connolly, M.E. Contrasting Effects of Systemic and Central Sibutramine Administration on the Intake of a Palatable Diet in the Rat. *Neurosci. Lett.* **2010**, *484*, 30–34. [CrossRef]
60. Smith, B.M.; Smith, J.M.; Tsai, J.H.; Schultz, J.A.; Gilson, C.A.; Estrada, S.A.; Chen, R.R.; Park, D.M.; Prieto, E.B.; Gallardo, C.S.; et al. Discovery and Structure-Activity Relationship of (1R)-8-Chloro-2,3,4,5-Tetrahydro-1-Methyl-1H-3-Benzazepine (Lorcaserin), a Selective Serotonin 5-HT_{2C} Receptor Agonist for the Treatment of Obesity. *J. Med. Chem.* **2008**, *51*, 305–313. [CrossRef]
61. Higgs, S.; Cooper, A.J.; Barnes, N.M. The 5-HT_{2C} Receptor Agonist, Lorcaserin, and the 5-HT6 Receptor Antagonist, SB-742457, Promote Satiety; A Microstructural Analysis of Feeding Behaviour. *Psychopharmacology* **2016**, *233*, 417–424. [CrossRef] [PubMed]
62. Higgins, G.A.; Desnoyer, J.; van Niekerk, A.; Silenieks, L.B.; Lau, W.; Thevarkunnel, S.; Izhakova, J.; Delannoy, I.A.M.; Fletcher, P.J.; Delay, J.; et al. Characterization of the 5-HT_{2C} Receptor Agonist Lorcaserin on Efficacy and Safety Measures in a Rat Model of Diet-Induced Obesity. *Pharmacol. Res. Perspect.* **2015**, *3*, e00084. [CrossRef] [PubMed]
63. Price, A.E.; Brehm, V.D.; Hommel, J.D.; Anastasio, N.C.; Cunningham, K.A. Pimavanserin and Lorcaserin Attenuate Measures of Binge Eating in Male Sprague-Dawley Rats. *Front. Pharmacol.* **2018**, *9*, 1424. [CrossRef] [PubMed]
64. Blumenthal, S.A.; Pratt, W.E. D-Fenfluramine and Lorcaserin Inhibit the Binge-like Feeding Induced by μ-Opioid Receptor Stimulation of the Nucleus Accumbens in the Rat. *Neurosci. Lett.* **2018**, *687*, 43–48. [CrossRef] [PubMed]
65. D'Agostino, G.; Lyons, D.; Cristiano, C.; Lettieri, M.; Olarte-Sanchez, C.; Burke, L.K.; Greenwald-Yarnell, M.; Cansell, C.; Doslikova, B.; Georgescu, T.; et al. Nucleus of the Solitary Tract Serotonin 5-HT_{2C} Receptors Modulate Food Intake. *Cell Metab.* **2018**, *28*, 619. [CrossRef] [PubMed]
66. Zhan, C.; Zhou, J.; Feng, Q.; Zhang, J.E.; Lin, S.; Bao, J.; Wu, P.; Luo, M. Acute and Long-Term Suppression of Feeding Behavior by POMC Neurons in the Brainstem and Hypothalamus, Respectively. *J. Neurosci.* **2013**, *33*, 3624. [CrossRef]
67. Kwon, E.; Jo, Y.H. Activation of the ARCPOMC→MeA Projection Reduces Food Intake. *Front. Neural Circuits* **2020**, *14*, 595783. [CrossRef]
68. Higgins, G.A.; Zeeb, F.D.; Fletcher, P.J. Role of Impulsivity and Reward in the Anti-Obesity Actions of 5-HT 2C Receptor Agonists. *J. Psychopharmacol.* **2017**, *31*, 1403–1418. [CrossRef]
69. Burke, L.K.; Ogunnowo-Bada, E.; Georgescu, T.; Cristiano, C.; de Morentin, P.B.M.; Valencia Torres, L.; D'Agostino, G.; Riches, C.; Heeley, N.; Ruan, Y.; et al. Lorcaserin Improves Glycemic Control via a Melanocortin Neurocircuit. *Mol. Metab.* **2017**, *6*, 1092–1102. [CrossRef]
70. Marbury, T.C.; Angelo, J.E.; Michael Gulley, R.; Krosnick, A.; Sugimoto, D.H.; Zellner, S.R. A Placebo-Controlled, Dose-Response Study of Dexfenfluramine in the Treatment of Obese Patients. *Curr. Ther. Res.* **1996**, *57*, 663–674. [CrossRef]
71. Lucas, C.P.; Sandage, B.W. Treatment of Obese Patients with Dexfenfluramine: A Multicenter, Placebo-Controlled Study. *Am. J. Ther.* **1995**, *2*, 962–967. [CrossRef] [PubMed]
72. Drent, M.L.; Adèr, H.J.; van der Veen, E.A. The Influence of Chronic Administration of the Serotonin Agonist Dexfenfluramine on Responsiveness to Corticotropin Releasing Hormone and Growth Hormone-Releasing Hormone in Moderately Obese People. *J. Endocrinol. Investig.* **1995**, *18*, 780–788. [CrossRef] [PubMed]
73. Guy-Grand, B.; Crepaldi, G.; Vre, P.L.; Apfelbaum, M.; Gries, A.; Turner, P. International Trial of Long-Term Dexfenfluramine in Obesity. *Lancet* **1989**, *2*, 1142–1145. [CrossRef] [PubMed]
74. Lafreniere, F.; Lambert, L.J.; Rasio, E.; Serri, O. Effects of Dexfenfluramine Treatment on Body Weight and Postprandial Thermogenesis in Obese Subjects. A Double-Blind Placebo-Controlled Study. *Int. J. Obes. Relat. Metab. Disord.* **1993**, *17*, 25–30. [PubMed]
75. Mathus-Vliegen, E.M.H.; van de Voorde, K.; Kok, A.M.E.; Res, A.M.A. Dexfenfluramine in the Treatment of Severe Obesity: A Placebo-Controlled Investigation of the Effects on Weight Loss, Cardiovascular Risk Factors, Food Intake and Eating Behaviour. *J. Intern. Med.* **1992**, *232*, 119–127. [CrossRef]
76. Weintraub, M.; Rubio, A.; Golik, A.; Byrne, L.; Scheinbaum, M.L. Sibutramine in Weight Control: A Dose-Ranging, Efficacy Study. *Clin. Pharmacol. Ther.* **1991**, *50*, 330–337. [CrossRef]
77. Hanotin, C.; Thomas, F.; Jones, S.P.; Leutenegger, E.; Drouin, P. Efficacy and Tolerability of Sibutramine in Obese Patients: A Dose-Ranging Study. *Int. J. Obes.* **1997**, *22*, 32–38. [CrossRef]
78. Bray, G.A.; Blackburn, G.L.; Ferguson, J.M.; Greenway, F.L.; Jain, A.K.; Mendel, C.M.; Mendels, J.; Ryan, D.H.; Schwartz, S.L.; Scheinbaum, M.L.; et al. Sibutramine Produces Dose-Related Weight Loss. *Obes. Res.* **1999**, *7*, 189–198. [CrossRef]
79. Di Francesco, V.; Sacco, T.; Zamboni, M.; Bissoli, L.; Zoico, E.; Mazzali, G.; Minniti, A.; Salanitri, T.; Cancelli, F.; Bosello, O. Weight Loss and Quality of Life Improvement in Obese Subjects Treated with Sibutramine: A Double-Blind Randomized Multicenter Study. *Ann. Nutr. Metab.* **2007**, *51*, 75–81. [CrossRef]

80. James, W.P.T.; Caterson, I.D.; Coutinho, W.; Finer, N.; van Gaal, L.F.; Maggioni, A.P.; Torp-Pedersen, C.; Sharma, A.M.; Shepherd, G.M.; Rode, R.A.; et al. Effect of Sibutramine on Cardiovascular Outcomes in Overweight and Obese Subjects. *N. Engl. J. Med.* **2010**, *363*, 905–917. [CrossRef]
81. Berkowitz, R.I.; Fujioka, K.; Daniels, S.R.; Hoppin, A.G.; Owen, S.; Perry, A.C.; Sothern, M.S.; Renz, C.L.; Pirner, M.A.; Walch, J.K.; et al. Effects of Sibutramine Treatment in Obese Adolescents: A Randomized Trial. *Ann. Intern. Med.* **2006**, *145*, 81–90. [CrossRef] [PubMed]
82. McNulty, S.J.; Ur, E.; Williams, G. A Randomized Trial of Sibutramine in the Management of Obese Type 2 Diabetic Patients Treated With Metformin. *Diabetes Care* **2003**, *26*, 125–131. [CrossRef] [PubMed]
83. Hauner, H.; Meier, M.; Wendland, G.; Kurscheid, T.; Lauterbach, K. Weight Reduction by Sibutramine in Obese Subjects in Primary Care Medicine: The S.A.T. Study. *Exp. Clin. Endocrinol. Diabetes* **2004**, *112*, 201–207. [CrossRef] [PubMed]
84. Dujovne, C.A.; Zavoral, J.H.; Rowe, E.; Mendel, C.M. Effects of Sibutramine on Body Weight and Serum Lipids: A Double-Blind, Randomized, Placebo-Controlled Study in 322 Overweight and Obese Patients with Dyslipidemia. *Am. Heart J.* **2001**, *142*, 489–497. [CrossRef]
85. Martin, C.K.; Redman, L.M.; Zhang, J.; Sanchez, M.; Anderson, C.M.; Smith, S.R.; Ravussin, E. Lorcaserin, a 5-HT(2C) Receptor Agonist, Reduces Body Weight by Decreasing Energy Intake without Influencing Energy Expenditure. *J. Clin. Endocrinol. Metab.* **2011**, *96*, 837–845. [CrossRef] [PubMed]
86. Smith, S.R.; Prosser, W.A.; Donahue, D.J.; Morgan, M.E.; Anderson, C.M.; Shanahan, W.R. Lorcaserin (APD356), a Selective 5-HT_{2C} Agonist, Reduces Body Weight in Obese Men and Women. *Obesity* **2009**, *17*, 494–503. [CrossRef] [PubMed]
87. Shaw Tronieri, J.; Wadden, T.A.; Berkowitz, R.I.; Chao, A.M.; Pearl, R.L.; Alamuddin, N.; Leonard, S.M.; Carvajal, R.; Bakizada, Z.M.; Pinkasavage, E.; et al. A Randomized Trial of Lorcaserin and Lifestyle Counseling for Maintaining Weight Loss Achieved with a Low-Calorie Diet. *Obesity* **2018**, *26*, 299–309. [CrossRef]
88. Bohula, E.A.; Wiviott, S.D.; McGuire, D.K.; Inzucchi, S.E.; Kuder, J.; Im, K.; Fanola, C.L.; Qamar, A.; Brown, C.; Budaj, A.; et al. Cardiovascular Safety of Lorcaserin in Overweight or Obese Patients. *N. Engl. J. Med.* **2018**, *379*, 1107–1117. [CrossRef]
89. O'Neil, P.M.; Smith, S.R.; Weissman, N.J.; Fidler, M.C.; Sanchez, M.; Zhang, J.; Raether, B.; Anderson, C.M.; Shanahan, W.R. Randomized Placebo-Controlled Clinical Trial of Lorcaserin for Weight Loss in Type 2 Diabetes Mellitus: The BLOOM-DM Study. *Obesity* **2012**, *20*, 1426–1436. [CrossRef]
90. Smith, S.R.; Weissman, N.J.; Anderson, C.M.; Sanchez, M.; Chuang, E.; Stubbe, S.; Bays, H.; Shanahan, W.R. Multicenter, Placebo-Controlled Trial of Lorcaserin for Weight Management. *N. Engl. J. Med.* **2010**, *363*, 245–256. [CrossRef]
91. Aronne, L.; Shanahan, W.; Fain, R.; Glicklich, A.; Soliman, W.; Li, Y.; Smith, S. Safety and Efficacy of Lorcaserin: A Combined Analysis of the BLOOM and BLOSSOM Trials. *Postgrad. Med.* **2014**, *126*, 7–18. [CrossRef] [PubMed]
92. Connolly, H.M.; Crary, J.L.; McGoon, M.D.; Hensrud, D.D.; Edwards, B.S.; Edwards, W.D.; Schaff, H.V. Valvular Heart Disease Associated with Fenfluramine-Phentermine. *N. Engl. J. Med.* **1997**, *337*, 141. [CrossRef]
93. Khan, M.A.; Herzog, C.A.; Peter, J.V.S.; Hartley, G.G.; Madlon-Kay, R.; Dick, C.D.; Asinger, R.W.; Vessey, J.T. The Prevalence of Cardiac Valvular Insufficiency Assessed by Transthoracic Echocardiography in Obese Patients Treated with Appetite-Suppressant Drugs. *N. Engl. J. Med.* **1998**, *339*, 713–718. [CrossRef]
94. Kancherla, M.K.; Salti, H.I.; Mulderink, T.A.; Parker, M.; Bonow, R.O.; Mehlman, D.J. Echocardiographic Prevalence of Mitral and/or Aortic Regurgitation in Patients Exposed to Either Fenfluramine-Phentermine Combination or to Dexfenfluramine. *Am. J. Cardiol.* **1999**, *84*, 1335–1338. [CrossRef] [PubMed]
95. Surapaneni, P.; Vinales, K.L.; Najib, M.Q.; Chaliki, H.P. Valvular Heart Disease with the Use of Fenfluramine-Phentermine. *Tex. Heart Inst. J.* **2011**, *38*, 581.
96. McMurray, C.; Bloomfield, P.; Miller, H.C. Irreversible Pulmonary Hypertension after Treatment with Fenfluramine. *Br. Med. J.* **1986**, *292*, 239. [CrossRef] [PubMed]
97. Pouwels, H.; Smeets, J.; Cheriex, E.; Wouters, E. Pulmonary Hypertension and Fenfluramine. *Eur. Respir. J.* **1990**, *3*, 606–607. [CrossRef] [PubMed]
98. Bang, W.D.; Kim, J.Y.; Yu, H.T.; Cho, S.S.; Jang, J.Y.; Oh, C.M.; Joung, B.; Chang, H.J. Pulmonary Hypertension Associated with Use of Phentermine. *Yonsei Med. J.* **2010**, *51*, 971–973. [CrossRef]
99. Schoonjans, A.S.; Marchau, F.; Paelinck, B.P.; Lagae, L.; Gammaitoni, A.; Pringsheim, M.; Keane, M.G.; Ceulemans, B. Cardiovascular Safety of Low-Dose Fenfluramine in Dravet Syndrome: A Review of Its Benefit-Risk Profile in a New Patient Population. *Curr. Med. Res. Opin.* **2017**, *33*, 1773–1781. [CrossRef]
100. Davis, R.; Faulds, D. Dexfenfluramine. An Updated Review of Its Therapeutic Use in the Management of Obesity. *Drugs* **1996**, *52*, 696–724. [CrossRef]
101. Fitzgerald, L.W.; Burn, T.C.; Brown, B.S.; Patterson, J.P.; Corjay, M.H.; Valentine, P.A.; Sun, J.H.; Link, J.R.; Abbaszade, I.; Hollis, J.M.; et al. Possible Role of Valvular Serotonin 5-HT(2B) Receptors in the Cardiopathy Associated with Fenfluramine. *Mol. Pharmacol.* **2000**, *57*, 75–81. [PubMed]
102. Seimon, R.V.; Espinoza, D.; Ivers, L.; Gebski, V.; Finer, N.; Legler, U.F.; Sharma, A.M.; James, W.P.T.; Coutinho, W.; Caterson, I.D. Changes in Body Weight and Blood Pressure: Paradoxical Outcome Events in Overweight and Obese Subjects with Cardiovascular Disease. *Int. J. Obes.* **2014**, *38*, 1165–1171. [CrossRef] [PubMed]

103. Daniels, S.R.; Long, B.; Crow, S.; Styne, D.; Sothern, M.; Vargas-Rodriguez, I.; Harris, L.; Walch, J.; Jasinsky, O.; Cwik, K.; et al. Cardiovascular Effects of Sibutramine in the Treatment of Obese Adolescents: Results of a Randomized, Double-Blind, Placebo-Controlled Study. *Pediatrics* **2007**, *120*, e147–e157. [CrossRef] [PubMed]
104. Torp-Pedersen, C.; Caterson, I.; Coutinho, W.; Finer, N.; van Gaal, L.; Maggioni, A.; Sharma, A.; Brisco, W.; Deaton, R.; Shepherd, G.; et al. Cardiovascular Responses to Weight Management and Sibutramine in High-Risk Subjects: An Analysis from the SCOUT Trial. *Eur. Heart J.* **2007**, *28*, 2915–2923. [CrossRef] [PubMed]
105. Zannad, F.; Gille, B.; Grentzinger, A.; Bruntz, J.F.; Hammadi, M.; Boivin, J.M.; Hanotin, C.; Igau, B.; Drouin, P. Effects of Sibutramine on Ventricular Dimensions and Heart Valves in Obese Patients during Weight Reduction. *Am. Heart J.* **2002**, *144*, 508–515. [CrossRef]
106. Gürsoy, A.; Erdoğan, M.F.; Cin, M.Ö.; Cesur, M.; Başkal, N. Effect of Sibutramine on Blood Pressure in Patients with Obesity and Well-Controlled Hypertension or Normotension. *Endocr. Pract.* **2005**, *11*, 308–312. [CrossRef]
107. De Simone, G.; Romano, C.; de Caprio, C.; Contaldo, F.; Salanitri, T.; di Luzio Paparatti, U.; Pasanisi, F. Effects of Sibutramine-Induced Weight Loss on Cardiovascular System in Obese Subjects. *Nutr. Metab. Cardiovasc. Dis.* **2005**, *15*, 24–30. [CrossRef]
108. Heusser, K.; Engeli, S.; Tank, J.; Diedrich, A.; Wiesner, S.; Janke, J.; Luft, F.C.; Jordan, J. Sympathetic Vasomotor Tone Determines Blood Pressure Response to Long-Term Sibutramine Treatment. *J. Clin. Endocrinol. Metab.* **2007**, *92*, 1560–1563. [CrossRef]
109. Merenich, J.A. The Long-Term Outcomes of Sibutramine Effectiveness on Weight (LOSE Weight) Study: Evaluating the Role of Drug Therapy Within a Weight Management Program in a Group-Model Health Maintenance Organizati. *Am. J. Manag. Care* **2004**, *10*, 369–376. [CrossRef]
110. Fanghänel, G.; Cortinas, L.; Sánchez-Reyes, L.; Berber, A. A Clinical Trial of the Use of Sibutramine for the Treatment of Patients Suffering Essential Obesity. *Int. J. Obes. Relat. Metab. Disord.* **2000**, *24*, 144–150. [CrossRef]
111. Guven, A.; Koksal, N.; Cetinkaya, A.; Sokmen, G.; Ozdemir, R. Effects of the Sibutramine Therapy on Pulmonary Artery Pressure in Obese Patients. *Diabetes Obes. Metab.* **2004**, *6*, 50–55. [CrossRef] [PubMed]
112. Saraç, S.; Saraç, F. Cardiac Valve Evaluation and Adipokine Levels in Obese Women Treated with Sibutramine. *Anadolu Kardiyol. Derg.* **2010**, *10*, 226–232. [CrossRef] [PubMed]
113. Caterson, I.D.; Finer, N.; Coutinho, W.; van Gaal, L.F.; Maggioni, A.P.; Torp-Pedersen, C.; Sharma, A.M.; Legler, U.F.; Shepherd, G.M.; Rode, R.A.; et al. Maintained Intentional Weight Loss Reduces Cardiovascular Outcomes: Results from the Sibutramine Cardiovascular OUTcomes (SCOUT) Trial. *Diabetes Obes. Metab.* **2012**, *14*, 523–530. [CrossRef] [PubMed]
114. Maggioni, A.P.; Caterson, I.; Coutinho, W.; Finer, N.; van Gaal, L.; Sharma, A.M.; Torp-Pedersen, C.; Bacher, P.; Shepherd, G.; Sun, R.; et al. Tolerability of Sibutramine during a 6-Week Treatment Period in High-Risk Patients with Cardiovascular Disease and/or Diabetes: A Preliminary Analysis of the Sibutramine Cardiovascular Outcomes (SCOUT) Trial. *J. Cardiovasc. Pharmacol.* **2008**, *52*, 393–402. [CrossRef]
115. Weeke, P.; Andersson, C.; Fosbøl, E.L.; Brendorp, B.; Køber, L.; Sharma, A.M.; Finer, N.; James, P.T.; Caterson, I.D.; Rode, R.A.; et al. The Weight Lowering Effect of Sibutramine and Its Impact on Serum Lipids in Cardiovascular High Risk Patients with and without Type 2 Diabetes Mellitus—An Analysis from the SCOUT Lead-in Period. *BMC Endocr. Disord.* **2010**, *10*, 3. [CrossRef]
116. Nisoli, E.; Carruba, M.O. An Assessment of the Safety and Efficacy of Sibutramine, an Anti-Obesity Drug with a Novel Mechanism of Action. *Obes. Rev.* **2000**, *1*, 127–139. [CrossRef]
117. Tuccinardi, D.; Farr, O.M.; Upadhyay, J.; Oussaada, S.M.; Mathew, H.; Paschou, S.A.; Perakakis, N.; Koniaris, A.; Kelesidis, T.; Mantzoros, C.S. Lorcaserin Treatment Decreases Body Weight and Reduces Cardiometabolic Risk Factors in Obese Adults: A Six-Month, Randomized, Placebo-Controlled, Double-Blind Clinical Trial. *Diabetes Obes. Metab.* **2019**, *21*, 1487–1492. [CrossRef]
118. Pi-Sunyer, X.; Shanahan, W.; Fain, R.; Ma, T.; Garvey, W.T. Impact of Lorcaserin on Glycemic Control in Overweight and Obese Patients with Type 2 Diabetes: Analysis of Week 52 Responders and Nonresponders. *Postgrad. Med.* **2016**, *128*, 591–597. [CrossRef]
119. Bohula, E.A.; Scirica, B.M.; Inzucchi, S.E.; McGuire, D.K.; Keech, A.C.; Smith, S.R.; Kanevsky, E.; Murphy, S.A.; Leiter, L.A.; Dwyer, J.P.; et al. Effect of Lorcaserin on Prevention and Remission of Type 2 Diabetes in Overweight and Obese Patients (CAMELLIA-TIMI 61): A Randomised, Placebo-Controlled Trial. *Lancet* **2018**, *392*, 2269–2279. [CrossRef]
120. Fidler, M.C.; Sanchez, M.; Raether, B.; Weissman, N.J.; Smith, S.R.; Shanahan, W.R.; Anderson, C.M. A One-Year Randomized Trial of Lorcaserin for Weight Loss in Obese and Overweight Adults: The BLOSSOM Trial. *J. Clin. Endocrinol. Metab.* **2011**, *96*, 3067–3077. [CrossRef]
121. Weissman, N.J.; Sanchez, M.; Koch, G.G.; Smith, S.R.; Shanahan, W.R.; Anderson, C.M. Echocardiographic Assessment of Cardiac Valvular Regurgitation with Lorcaserin from Analysis of 3 Phase 3 Clinical Trials. *Circ. Cardiovasc. Imaging* **2013**, *6*, 560–567. [CrossRef] [PubMed]
122. Greenway, F.L.; Shanahan, W.; Fain, R.; Ma, T.; Rubino, D. Safety and Tolerability Review of Lorcaserin in Clinical Trials. *Clin. Obes.* **2016**, *6*, 285–295. [CrossRef] [PubMed]
123. Gorelik, E.; Gorelik, B.; Masarwa, R.; Perlman, A.; Hirsh-Raccah, B.; Matok, I. The Cardiovascular Safety of Antiobesity Drugs-Analysis of Signals in the FDA Adverse Event Report System Database. *Int. J. Obes.* **2020**, *44*, 1021–1027. [CrossRef] [PubMed]
124. Scirica, B.M.; Bohula, E.A.; Dwyer, J.P.; Qamar, A.; Inzucchi, S.E.; McGuire, D.K.; Keech, A.C.; Smith, S.R.; Murphy, S.A.; Im, K.; et al Lorcaserin and Renal Outcomes in Obese and Overweight Patients in the CAMELLIA-TIMI 61 Trial. *Circulation* **2019**, *139*, 366–375. [CrossRef] [PubMed]

25. Bray, G.A. Medical Treatment of Obesity: The Past, the Present and the Future. *Best Pract. Res. Clin. Gastroenterol.* **2014**, *28*, 665–684. [CrossRef] [PubMed]
26. De Andrade Mesquita, L.; Fagundes Piccoli, G.; Richter da Natividade, G.; Frison Spiazzi, B.; Colpani, V.; Gerchman, F. Is Lorcaserin Really Associated with Increased Risk of Cancer? A Systematic Review and Meta-Analysis. *Obes. Rev.* **2021**, *22*, e13170. [CrossRef] [PubMed]
27. Sharretts, J.; Galescu, O.; Gomatam, S.; Andraca-Carrera, E.; Hampp, C.; Yanoff, L. Cancer Risk Associated with Lorcaserin—The FDA's Review of the CAMELLIA-TIMI 61 Trial. *N. Engl. J. Med.* **2020**, *383*, 1000–1002. [CrossRef]
28. Jeffrey Conn, P.; Christopoulos, A.; Lindsley, C.W. Allosteric Modulators of GPCRs: A Novel Approach for the Treatment of CNS Disorders. *Nat. Rev. Drug Discov.* **2009**, *8*, 41–54. [CrossRef]
29. García-Cárceles, J.; Decara, J.M.; Vázquez-Villa, H.; Rodríguez, R.; Codesido, E.; Cruces, J.; Brea, J.; Loza, M.I.; Alén, F.; Botta, J.; et al. A Positive Allosteric Modulator of the Serotonin 5-HT 2C Receptor for Obesity. *J. Med. Chem.* **2017**, *60*, 9575–9584. [CrossRef]
30. Singh, K.; Sona, C.; Ojha, V.; Singh, M.; Mishra, A.; Kumar, A.; Siddiqi, M.I.; Tripathi, R.P.; Yadav, P.N. Identification of Dual Role of Piperazine-Linked Phenyl Cyclopropyl Methanone as Positive Allosteric Modulator of 5-HT_{2C} and Negative Allosteric Modulator of 5-HT_{2B} Receptors. *Eur. J. Med. Chem.* **2019**, *164*, 499–516. [CrossRef]
31. Cifuentes, L.; Eckel-Passow, J.; Acosta, A. Precision Medicine for Obesity. *Dig. Dis. Interv.* **2021**, *5*, 239. [CrossRef] [PubMed]
32. Severin, R.; Sabbahi, A.; Mahmoud, A.M.; Arena, R.; Phillips, S.A. Precision Medicine in Weight Loss and Healthy Living. *Prog. Cardiovasc. Dis.* **2019**, *62*, 15. [CrossRef] [PubMed]
33. Hurtado, A.M.D.; Acosta, A. Precision Medicine and Obesity. *Gastroenterol. Clin. N. Am.* **2021**, *50*, 127. [CrossRef] [PubMed]
34. Griebsch, N.I.; Kern, J.; Hansen, J.; Rullmann, M.; Luthardt, J.; Helfmeyer, S.; Dekorsy, F.J.; Soeder, M.; Hankir, M.K.; Zientek, F.; et al. Central Serotonin/Noradrenaline Transporter Availability and Treatment Success in Patients with Obesity. *Brain Sci.* **2022**, *12*, 1437. [CrossRef]
35. He, Y.; Brouwers, B.; Liu, H.; Liu, H.; Lawler, K.; Mendes de Oliveira, E.; Lee, D.K.; Yang, Y.; Cox, A.R.; Keogh, J.M.; et al. Human Loss-of-Function Variants in the Serotonin 2C Receptor Associated with Obesity and Maladaptive Behavior. *Nat. Med.* **2022**, *28*, 2537. [CrossRef]
36. Wold, E.A.; Garcia, E.J.; Wild, C.T.; Miszkiel, J.M.; Soto, C.A.; Chen, J.; Pazdrak, K.; Fox, R.G.; Anastasio, N.C.; Cunningham, K.A.; et al. Discovery of 4-Phenylpiperidine-2-Carboxamide Analogues as Serotonin 5-HT_{2C} Receptor-Positive Allosteric Modulators with Enhanced Drug-like Properties. *J. Med. Chem.* **2020**, *63*, 7529. [CrossRef]

nutrients

MDPI

Review

The Influence of Serious Games in the Promotion of Healthy Diet and Physical Activity Health: A Systematic Review

Susana Lamas [1], Sofia Rebelo [2], Sofia da Costa [2,3], Helena Sousa [1], Nelson Zagalo [4] and Elisabete Pinto [2,3,*]

[1] Centro de Estudos de Comunicação e Sociedade, Instituto de Ciências Sociais, Universidade do Minho, Campos de Gualtar, 4710-057 Braga, Portugal
[2] CBQF—Centro de Biotecnologia e Química Fina, Laboratório Associado, Escola Superior de Biotecnologia, Universidade Católica Portuguesa, 1649-023 Porto, Portugal
[3] EPIUnit—Instituto de Saúde Pública, Universidade do Porto, 4099-002 Porto, Portugal
[4] DigiMedia, Universidade de Aveiro, Campus Universitário de Santiago, 3810-193 Aveiro, Portugal
* Correspondence: ecbpinto@ucp.pt; Tel.: +351-225-580-000

Abstract: (1) Background: serious games seem to show promising strategies to promote treatment compliance and motivate behavior changes, and some studies have proven to contribute to the literature on serious games. (2) Methods: this systematic review aimed to analyze the effect of serious games in promoting healthy eating behaviors, effectively preventing childhood obesity, and improving physical activity in children. Five electronic bibliographic databases—PubMed, ACM Digital Library, Games for Health Journal, and IEEE Xplore were used to conduct a systematic literature search based on fixed inclusion and exclusion criteria. Peer-reviewed journal articles published between 2003 and 2021 were selected for data extraction. (3) Results: a total of 26 studies were identified, representing 17 games. Half of the studies tested interventions for healthy eating and physical education. Most of the intervention's games were designed according to specific behavioral change theories, predominantly the social cognitive theory. (4) Conclusions: studies confirmed the potential of serious games for obesity prevention but considering the restrictions encountered, we exhort for novel designs with different theoretical perspectives.

Keywords: serious games; nutrition; childhood obesity; real foods

1. Introduction

In recent decades, the prevalence of obesity in children has increased significantly, and it is now recognized as a global epidemic [1]. Multiple complex factors are associated with this prevalence [2], namely behavioral factors such as decreased PA and increased consumption of unhealthy food choices [3]. There is growing evidence of the impact that being overweight and obese have on short and long-term health and well-being [4], supports the relevance of their prevention as public health priorities [2,5].

The prevalence of obesity in children has increased dramatically, as evidenced in 2015, when a total of 107.7 million children were classified as obese, corresponding to a worldwide prevalence of childhood overweight and obesity of 23% [6]. Once established, it is difficult to reverse and likely to persist into adult life [7].

Obesity is a multisystem disease characterized by the accumulation of excessive fat in the body [3], already defined by the World Health Organization (WHO) as a condition of abnormality in the content of body fat, or an excess of fatty tissue, which affects or deteriorates the health of an individual [1]. This is associated with the development of chronic non-communicable diseases such as hypertension, type 2 diabetes mellitus, hepatic steatosis, and dyslipidemia in children, which were previously considered to be "adult diseases," favoring the increased risk of early mortality in adulthood [1].

One of the most frequent behavior patterns among children is to spend too much time in front of a screen (television (TV), computers, tablets). They often do this while they are eating, which causes a greater food intake as well as less energy expenditure (sedentary behavior). This has created a link between childhood obesity and food intake [8], combined with a lack of PA. In addition, commercials and other programs on TV are one of the drivers of this problem, due to the favorable publicity they give to unhealthy foods, which has a negative impact on the relationship between children and food [9]. It was also detected that destructive health behaviors generally prevail throughout the family, so that the possibility of a child becoming an obese adult is as high as 80%. Therefore, it is clear that an obese child will more likely become an obese adult [8].

It is imperative to find new methods to combat this epidemic that involves children from an early age and the family, rather than individual component programs [10]. Serious games make up part of this diversity of strategies and tools to intervene in young age groups due to the predisposition of children to learn, coupled with their attraction to video games.

Most 10-year-old children spend more than one hour per day playing digital games in Europe and the United States of America [11]. Videogames appeal to both children and their parents (in the USA, 74% of parents play games with their children on a weekly basis at least) [12].

Serious games are video games designed to achieve a change of some type while entertaining [13]. In health, they are targeted towards the rehabilitation of patients suffering from various disabilities [14], for the treatment of specific diseases [15], and also for the promotion of healthy lifestyles [16]. In 2013, video games for self-healthcare and wellness (which exclude games for patients and professional training) accounted for 41% of all health games [17].

Beyond the revision of serious games for promoting good health-related behaviors [18], some reviews addressed nutrition and obesity prevention. Mack et al. (2017) reviewed video games explicitly targeting nutrition, PA, and obesity for children between 7 and 15 years of age [19]. Baranowski et al. (2019a) made a scoping review of nutrition education and dietary behavior change videogames/or interactive games (as part of human-delivered interventions) [20]. Moreover, Chow et al. (2019) gathered forty-three studies that used video or physical games and gamification (i.e., game-based approaches) to influence children's ($\leq$12 years old) eating behavior [21].

From the above, it is still rather unclear what the contribution of challenging games is to a change in lifestyles, mainly in terms of reducing obesity. However, they do show a clear potential to induce change. Effects are minor [19] and are primarily reported in the short term [21]. Games differ remarkably in their targeted knowledge and behaviors, population, game mechanics, behavioral theories, research designs, and findings [20], hampering the analysis. A more solid research-based game design and evaluation would enable a more in-depth analysis of serious games' characteristics and outcomes [20] to conclude their effectiveness [16] properly.

While authors such as Baranowski and colleagues (2019a) appeal to the embracing of behavior change procedures in games' design, trying to change the player's attitudes, beliefs, risk perceptions, knowledge, or skills in the mediation to better health outcomes [20], others such as Guy, Ratzki-Leewing, and Gwadry-Sridhar (2011) [22] remind us that nutritional expertise and financial resources seem not to be the leading solutions to healthy eating. There is a need for an ecological, multilevel approach to childhood obesity prevention [23].

In this light, games would benefit from acknowledging the kid's food environment in their narratives (e.g., the pressure of publicity/markets on children's food choices and the food available in their environment). Likewise, they would benefit from recognizing social stigmas in girls' sports practices as barriers to PA. This would leverage communication beyond solely depicting information (e.g., the nutritional content of foods, pointing to what is good or bad). Games can propose solutions to barriers or provide extra motivational arguments for behavioral change by acknowledging reality.

Additionally, as far as eating behavior is concerned, there seems to be a distinct lack of games to encourage children's (sensorial) food exploration. In analyzing a diversity of games, Chow et al. (2019) [21] only found one article that developed a digital experience with natural foods [24]. EducaTableware hopes to help kids enjoy eating disliked foods in dietary education, by introducing an element of fun into eating, encouraging them to give audio feedback when consuming foods with different textures.

Serious games (video games or interactive games] could introduce children to diverse foods, guiding them to what is good for them [25]. This could help surpass some neophobia and picky eating [26] in particular contexts. It also adds a performative aspect to behavior change, or an in-game transformation perspective, that is more usual in PA.

In pursuing innovative ways to support obesity prevention and being aware of the allure and promise of challenging games in health, this study took shape. It is a systematic review of the existent literature on the effect of serious games for promoting healthy diet behaviors (as well as PA) in children and adolescents. Data were also collected regarding the theories for change behind the game design, the (possible) acknowledgment of the kid's environment, and performative aspects of the game (motion and tangibility).

2. Materials and Methods

In order to conduct the present systematic review of the literature, a slightly modified PRISMA (Preferred Reporting Items for Systematic reviews and Meta-Analyses) checklist was followed [27].

The identification of papers was conducted through a search on PubMed, ACM Digital Library, Games for Health Journal, and IEEE Xplore with the following expression [("serious game" OR gamification) AND (nutrition OR "health promotion")].

The search was carried out in September 2022, where the filters were applied to exclude systematic reviews and meta-analyses and the inclusion of full papers, short papers, and extended abstracts. In total, publications were collected and analyzed, unless they were written in a language different from English, Portuguese, or Spanish.

After collecting all publications to be analyzed, three authors (SA, SL, and SC) reviewed the abstracts—each of them reads the abstract of the papers individually—to seek agreement between them in deciding which publications would be included. A third element (EP) participated in the discussion of included and excluded papers to solve disagreements in the decisions of the other two authors.

The search retrieved duplicate articles, which were removed. The inclusion criteria were: papers evaluating an intervention in nutrition and/or PA, where there was a change in behaviors (for instance, increase in the intake of healthy foods/decrease in the intake of unhealthy foods or beverages; increase in PA; increase in knowledge about healthy behaviors) after the intervention. The exclusion criteria considered were: papers written in languages other than English, Portuguese, or Spanish (n = 3); narrative reviews (n = 70); studies not focused on nutrition and/or PA (n = 50); studies using patients as target population (n = 37); studies not using games, or where their role is only subsidiary (n = 35); studies which did not contemplate any intervention (n = 37); and studies not targeting children and/or adolescents (n = 57).

The revision of the abstracts excluded 289 studies from the 403 initially retrieved (after the exclusion of repeated abstracts), making a total of 95 articles to read in full. Next, the three authors that conducted the abstracts' assessments and analyzed the full papers in detail opted for the exclusion of 83 of them. These exclusions were motivated by: a paper written in Spanish (n = 1); narrative reviews (n = 3); studies not focused on nutrition and/or PA (n = 7); studies using patients as target population (n = 6); studies not using games, or where their role is only subsidiary (n = 24); studies which did not contemplate any intervention (n = 19); and studies not targeting children and/or adolescents (n = 23).

Only 12 papers met the inclusion criteria. Their reference lists were also reviewed, and another 14 studies were included in the revision. All these steps are represented in a flowchart (Figure 1).

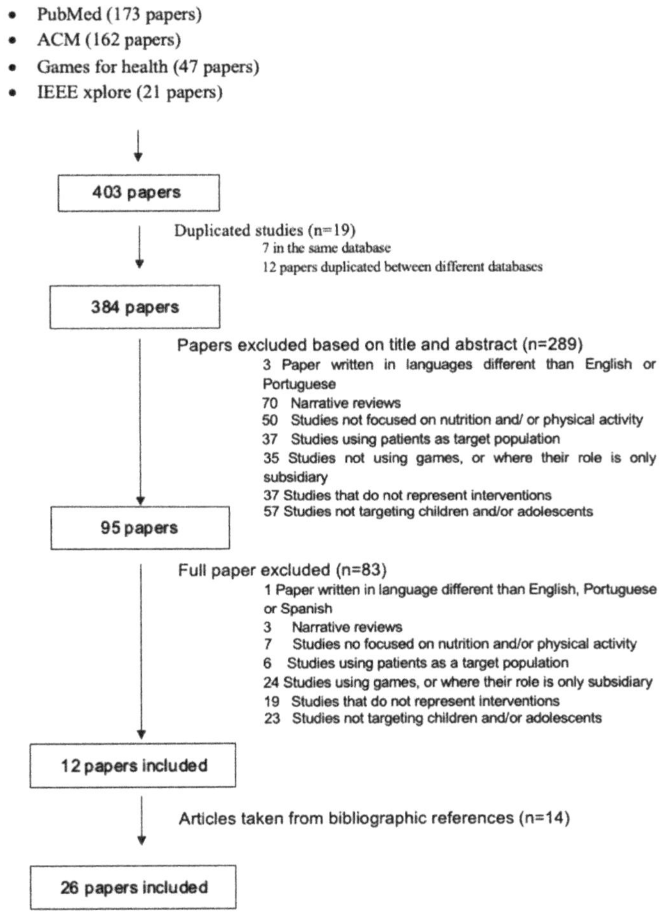

Figure 1. PRISMA diagram showing the screening process.

The study information was systematized in a table including the following characteristics: first author's name, year of publication, country of study, sample's characteristics, area of intervention, type of study, description of the intervention, and finally, the results that each study had. The table is presented in Appendix A.

3. Results

After using the predefined search strategy, 403 results were pulled from the databases. Three hundred and eighty-four remained for screening after duplications were eliminated. Following a review of the titles and abstracts, 95 papers were kept. After reading the studies, 12 papers fulfilled the inclusion criteria and were maintained for data extraction. An additional 14 pertinent papers were found and included in the final analysis by examining the references from the included reviews. The selection of 26 distinct studies for data analysis were totaled. Figure 1 displays the progression of the screening.

The 26 papers included in this revision corresponded to interventions conducted around the world between 2003 and 2022, the majority of them in the USA (n = 15), and the rest in the Netherlands (n = 1), Germany (n = 2), Italy (n = 2), UK (n = 1), Mexico (n = 2), Finland (n = 1), Australia (n = 1), and Canada (n = 1). In total, they represented 17 different games.

Half of the studies (n = 13) tested interventions directed both to healthy eating and PA, six studies focused merely on improving healthy eating, and two focused only on PA. The sample size ranged between 20 and 1578 participants; three of these studies included teams of parents and their offspring. When parents were involved, the primary objective was to receive information about the results of the intervention and to be able to assist with future behavioral change. The age of the participants mostly ranged between eight and fifteen years old, with only one of the studies including participants up to eighteen years old and another three children from three to eight years old.

Fifteen studies were randomized controlled trials, and eleven were quasi-experimental studies, with pre-and post-intervention evaluation. Regarding the period in which the intervention took place, it ranged from one day to three months.

Most of the intervention games (nine out of seventeen) were designed according to specific behavioral change theories, predominantly the social cognitive theory (SCT) [28] and the self-determination theory (SDT) [29], but also the Elaboration Likelihood Model [30]. Other behavioral theories were also used, such as the Transtheoretical Model of Change [31], Behavioral Inoculation Theory [32], Maintenance Theory [33], the Theory of Reasoned Action [34], Transportation Theory [35], and in two cases, Behavior Change procedures from the Michie inventory [36] were applied. Other theories were used from game design and theoretical education areas. Following the concept of serious gaming, one paper [37] reported using the theory of persuasive gaming and the positive gaming concept [38], and another one [39] reported using images from collaborative games in conjunction with parental PA modeling concepts. A third game [40] explored the idea of Situated and Embodied Cognition, including Gestural congruency. No theory was specified in the remaining games [41–47].

Serious games that did not use any particular behavioral theory aimed chiefly at increasing players' nutrition knowledge or PA. Examples of nutrition information are knowledge about healthy/unhealthy foods, energy-dense foods, food quality vs. calorie content, or meal composition. As for the games with embedded behavior change theories, they expected some behavioral change in their players at the postgame (or follow-up), although with diverging goals: increase healthy food intake, fruits, and vegetables (FV) consumption, water intake, or level of PA; positive changes in anthropometric measures or attitudes and intentions; or to decrease consumption of sugary foods, sugar-sweetened beverages (SB), packaged snacks (PS), or non-healthy foods.

Regarding PA, serious games are a potent means to prompt movement and activity during gameplay. Of the ten games that included PA as an interventional area (alone or in conjunction with diet improvement), in five of them, motion control interfaces and movement sensors were used to imbed PA in the game (namely, Microsoft Kinect V2 sensor, SMALLab mixed reality platform, Fitbit activity trackers, or GPS mobile sensor). In the other six, motion does not occur in the game: they are uniquely cognitive-based (e.g., by delivering information on energy expenditure tied to caloric intake and healthy eating concepts).

Games with nutrition as a unique interventional area (n = 7) are solely cognitive-based. As for the others, tangible elements (besides PC keyboards, touchscreens, and touchpads) are almost absent, except for one boardgame (that uses cards, dice, and pawns) and a mixed reality game that uses trackable wands for players to interact with the digital world (e.g., picking digital objects). Thus, natural foods are never present in these games. Nutrition communication is always cognitive-based.

Notwithstanding, in two serious games (Squire's Quest! I and Squire's Quest! II—two versions of the same game) players are elicited to eat FV during the day and to prepare authentic recipes with their parents (or other adults) by establishing specific goals in the game. During gameplay, they are taught how to make simple FV recipes ("Virtual Kitchen") through brief demonstration video clips and then asked to set goals to make an actual recipe at home.

In five games, the children's food environment is somehow acknowledged, ranging from simply referring to a grocer or restaurant and their food availability, to asking children to set solutions for environmental barriers to FV consumption and PA.

Regarding the interventions' impact assessment, this was generally carried out through questionnaires. Some studies, in addition to questionnaires, included anthropometric measurements, the determination of biochemical parameters, and the use of accelerometers to measure PA, as well as data collected during gameplay through in-game log files. One study performed a food-tasting test as a pretext to assess energy-dense food consumption post-intervention. Different measurements were used to assess eating behavior, including the Food Intake Recording Software System (FIRSSt)—a computer-based 24-h dietary recall program for children. Questionnaires were administered in person in most studies. However, five questionnaires were administered by phone to children or parents in cases where they were also the target of the study. One study [48] used the EGameFlow and guessed questionnaires to evaluate children's enjoyment of the game and user experience satisfaction to link these concepts to learning. Besides that, Wengreen et al., 2021, estimated the daily FV consumption of all the children eating a school-prepared lunch using a waste-based measure by weighting and taking photos before/after lunch trays [44].

There was a control group in almost all experimental—sixteen out of seventeen—and four quasi-experimental studies. In some cases, the control group received written information; in others, lectures in a classroom context played generic games (such as web-based games) or participated in incomplete parts of the game. There were cases in which the control group constituted the wait list group and received the intervention sometime after the study.

The vast majority of interventions in nutrition had a positive impact, with changes in knowledge and behavior. Only one of the games [49] did not significantly impact the different variables tested. Several games increased children's nutritional knowledge compared to the control or baseline group. Moreover, most serious games that embedded behavioral change theories registered positive results, despite the diversity of the foreseen goals. Globally, they reported an increase in the consumption of healthy foods or FV and a decrease in sugary or processed foods. Positive changes in intentions and attitudes toward healthy eating and physical exercise were also attained. In one study [48], enjoyment and user experience satisfaction with the game were positively correlated and significant predictors of learning.

Even so, some studies found effectiveness in both interventions (game and control), and others found significant positive results immediately after gameplay (and not in the follow-up). In one study [50], although players decreased the consumption of SB and PS, there were no positive effects in FV and water intake, PA, or screen time (or, generally speaking, a shift to a more balanced diet). The same happened in other studies, especially in variables such as the availability of FV at home or some objective variables (e.g., positive changes in anthropometric measurements—e.g., body mass index or waist measurement—or in fasting insulin (a biological parameter important for preventing diabetes).

None of the selected articles targeted for PA registered an increase in the PA after the game (reported by the kids or measured using an accelerometer); there were only positive changes in attitudes and intentions [39,51]. Solely one game, explicitly designed to increase PA [43], produced positive results during gameplay, with players achieving a speed representative of "moderate to vigorous activity".

Lastly, eight of the seventeen games were designed following formative evaluations, and two included procedures to tailor content to the player's preferences (e.g., FV was selected based on the child's food preferences reported at baseline). Several games were beta-tested, and some were piloted before the final intervention.

Formative evaluations used quantitative (e.g., surveys) and qualitative methods (e.g., focus groups, observation) to assess children's interest in the game's story (or what their preferred story genre was), or which characters were more appealing, but also, play issues (frequency of play, motives, and favorite games). Several followed iterative methodologies during game development, such as a user-centered design.

All these results are systematized in Table A1.

4. Discussion

This study analyzes interventions using serious games to improve children's and adolescents' knowledge and practices of a healthy diet and PA.

The papers reviewed were published in peer-reviewed journals before September 2022 and scrutinized regarding the interventions' characteristics and effectiveness and specific games' characteristics/concrete features that push serious games away from solely cognitive forms of communication.

Our results confirm previous findings, which point to promising results in using serious games for health promotion and obesity prevention in terms of interventions in nutrition. The vast majority of interventions had a positive impact, with changes in knowledge and behavior. Only one game [49] did not significantly impact the tested variables. This is very positive, considering that in some cases the intervention was very brief and the players were only briefly exposed to the game (e.g., in one study, only 30 min–2 h/day, during one week). Therefore, we sought to find out if implementing some interventions over a more extended period of time could have a more significant impact.

In reality, as in other reviews [16], we found that the effects were relatively small. Moreover, there was also a need for long-term follow-up evaluations in most studies that could confirm if the results were sustainable. Our sample is very diverse in its goals, evaluation methods, and tools.

Unfortunately, the interventions targeted at PA were ineffective in the postgame. However, changes in attitudes and intentions were promising, but we were expecting positive changes in PA (besides PA knowledge) because nearly half of the serious games involved motor skills and some cognitive information, although this concurs with previous findings [18]. Some factors that could justify this result is the rather brief duration of the interventions, a higher resistance of less physically active players to the PA messages diffused in interventions [52], or the need to integrate the game intervention in a broader multi-component program [16].

Despite this drawback, we registered the positive influence of in-game PA, and in one study, it led the group to an average speed equaling "moderate to vigorous" aerobic activity levels [43]. This accords with previous research, which points to the effectiveness of active video games in supporting children's PA and energy expenditure [53] (even if not reaching the daily PA recommendations) versus sedentary games more linked to children's health education.

This output encourages the mentioned alternative approach of serious games in nutrition with a performative facet: that could foster sensory education by including natural healthy foods as tangible elements in the game, as opposed to solely cognitive-based games. The hypothesis is that effectiveness can be prompted by including taste/sensory activities in the game, such as having PA in active videogames. In the studies reviewed, real foods were never present in games, following the trend of serious educational games that revolve around cognitive skills [17]. Nutrition communication is always cognitive-based.

The foreseen perspective can be added to the extent of theories applied in serious games for nutrition and PA. In our review, most games included behavior change theories, such as the social cognitive theory or self-determination theory in their design, seeking to extend information to attitudes and behavior change. Moreover, other theories and concepts influenced by psychology were also used—namely, the idea of persuasive gaming or the positive gaming concept; concepts such as enjoyment and experience; or the Situated and Embodied Cognition.

It is interesting to see that, alongside the demand for a more solid research base in design and evaluation [20], the research community is also concerned about exploring different theories in serious games. Embodied learning, for example, could be linked to sensorial education with foods, or self-efficacy [54] in researching and preparing foods. In this trend, there are already two games (Squire Quest! I and II) that prompt players to establish goals to make recipes at home, offering small cooking demonstration videos.

In our attempt to approach children's reality in serious games, we have analyzed the (possible) use of a formative evaluation in the game/intervention design and the (possible) acknowledgment of the children's food environment in the game narrative and concept.

Formative evaluations are crucial, helping to create the game/interventions for the target audience. Moreover, we found that twelve out of the eighteen games were designed following these evaluations using quantitative (e.g., surveys) and qualitative methods. Two also included tailoring mechanisms to suit the game to their players. Only a few games used formative evaluation to access nutritional or PA issues (versus play profiles, story, and character topics). In these examples, preferences, reasons, needs for nutritional information, or parental attitudes towards and support for their child's PA were accessed. In one challenging particular game, recipes presented in a "Virtual Kitchen" were tested before their inclusion to ensure they were child-friendly, tasted good, and looked attractive [55].

Five of the reviewed serious games somehow recognize the children's (occidental) food environment. However, there is a lack of games that expose the truth about the food industry and our social/eating environment. Some online games (not object to evaluation) [56] revolve their narrative around these problems as behavior change issues in the story [18] and as sparks of motivation. In our review, three games acknowledge these limitations and ask players to set solutions for environmental barriers to FV consumption and PA.

Finally, most serious games were targeted to 8–15-year-old children (as reflected in the interventions). This is a suitable age range as kids in this age group are progressively more autonomous in their food choices, making it essential that they are aware of options of what is good for their health and especially that they feel motivated to choose well. Additionally, it would be interesting to see more multiple-component interventions (vs. individual interventions) or simply interventions aimed at parents. As mentioned before, diet changes should be supported by the family and the family environment (and we only found two games that included parents and their offspring).

In our review, all the games were developed in Western countries (nine in the USA), which may indicate the regional prevalence of the obesity epidemic and the easy access to funding or technological means, while also setting the tone for the problems addressed in the games. It would be desirable to find studies in other parts of the world where children's and adolescents' eating habits and leisure time may differ.

Lastly, evaluation methods mostly comprised self-report (or parent-reported) questionnaires and interviews, or some objective measurements, such as the measurement of PA using accelerometers or biometrics—the latter generally not advancing positive results. Some qualitative methodologies could enrich these variables, bringing different indicators of efficacy, for example, through experiments evaluating whether kids positively respond to a food environment change (e.g., in school) in conjunction with a serious game intervention. Food-tasting tests could also be exciting tools to evaluate the game's impact, especially if sensorial education is involved.

This study has some limitations that could interfere with the results. Its primary focus is nutrition, leaving some PA games and exergames out of the analysis. Even so, previous reviews confirm our results. The low number of scientific articles retrieved can indicate that this subject has yet to be fully explored, and more games should be developed with different theoretical perspectives and tested.

5. Conclusions

This review provides an overview of research interventions using serious games as strategies to promote healthy eating and PA in children. Despite some inconsistencies, our findings confirm that most studies in nutrition have been effective in increasing knowledge and/or changing kids' diets to healthier ones. Notwithstanding PA, results seem to be mainly limited to the gameplay. The intrinsic entertainment and motivation of games, coupled with accurate information and a solid theoretical psychology ground, bring some hope for progress in obesity prevention.

All serious games analyzed, approached nutrition through cognition and only two versions of the same game elicited players to prepare recipes at home. A performative facet, using sensorial experiences with foods (seeking transformation in the course of the game), was never present. There is a need for more diversity of games because playing with foods is a good way for kids to get to know and appreciate novel foods, especially healthy ones with bitter tastes.

Although formative evaluation is sometimes used in the game design, only a few examples gathered information about the player's needs and behaviors about the intervention theme. Moreover, although some games acknowledged the children's food environment and food choice pressures, these issues are mostly subtly referred to. From our point of view, serious games should pursue new perspectives other than the mainstream accountability of kids' behaviors for the obesity epidemic. A broader and more ecological perspective is needed.

Finally, as argued by other authors, interventions would benefit from being more research-based, possibly by having more prolonged intervention periods and more long-term evaluation follow-ups. To these claims, we add the benefit of exploring new theoretical grounds for serious games and possibly new evaluation methods to explore all the possibilities of communication in this area of research.

Author Contributions: The authors' responsibilities are as follows: H.S. and N.Z. are responsible for the research project within this review arose. S.R., jointly with E.P. and S.L., established the study design. S.R. and S.L. conducted the search and data collection. S.R., S.L. and S.d.C. drafted the first version manuscript. All authors revised and approved the final manuscript. All authors have read and agreed to the published version of the manuscript.

Funding: The authors would like to acknowledge POCI-FEDER (Programa Operacional para a Competividade e Internacionalização do Fundo Europeu de Desenvolvimento Regional) and FCT (Fundação para a Ciência e a Tecnologia) for funding this Project, under the Grant Agreement No. POCI-01-0145-FEDER-031024. This research was supported by National Funds from FCT—Fundação para a Ciência e Tecnologia through project UIDB/50016/2020.

Institutional Review Board Statement: Not applicable.

Informed Consent Statement: Not applicable.

Data Availability Statement: Not applicable.

Conflicts of Interest: The authors declare no conflict of interest.

Appendix A

Table A1. Characteristics of the included studies.

Reference	Intervention Area	Description of the Intervention				Results	Theory Behind the Game	Performative Aspects			Acknowledgment of the Environment	Formative Evaluation or Tailoring
		Sample/Type of the Study	Duration and Intensity	Assessment Tools	Control			Application Domain	Interactional Elements	Contract with Real Foods		
Vepsäläinen et al., 2022. (Finland) [47] Mole's Veggie Adventures app: a Mobile App to Increase Fruit and Vegetable Acceptance	N	3–6 y n = 221 Experimental	3–10 players; 4 sessions of which includes 6 FV each	Background questionnaire to parents (T0). Acceptability to try the FV presented during the game (questionnaire to parents) (T1)	CG had no play sessions with Mole's Veggie Adventures app	Compared with the CG, the participants in the intervention arm had higher FV acceptance scores at follow-up 3–4 weeks after baseline.	No specific theory.	Cog	Mobile phone	No	No	No
Vlieger at al., 2022 (Australia) [45] Vita Village: improving child nutrition knowledge	N	9–12 y n = 189 Experimental	2 sessions (~20 min)	Nutrition knowledge questionnaire (T0, T1)	CG played mathematics games	Compared to the control group, the intervention group's overall nutrition knowledge was found to increase after playing Vita Village.	No specific theory.	Cog	Tablet	No	No	No
Wengreen et al., 2021 (USA) [44] FIT Game's: Increase Fruit and Vegetable Consumption.	N	5–11 y n = 978 Experimental	32 episodes presented; 3 min each episode looped continuously throughout the lunch time	Daily FV consumption of all the children eating school-prepared lunch was estimated using a waste-based measure: before/after lunch-tray photos were taken and height (T0, T1, T2)—BMI and skin-carotenoid concentrations (T0, T1, T2)	CG had no play session with FIT Game	During the intervention phase, children attending the FIT Game schools consumed significantly more consumption FV compared to the baseline. This increase in at-school consumption was reflected in their skin carotenoid concentrations, which was also significantly different between the IG and CG.	No specific theory.	Cog	Television	Yes (game involves eating FV)	No	No
Frome et al., 2020 (Canada) [46] Foodbot Factory: a Mobile Serious Game to Increasing Nutrition Knowledge in Children	N	8–10 y n = 73 Experimental	10–15 min each day over a five-day period	Nutrition knowledge questionnaire (T0, T1). Nutrition knowledge for each of the four sub-scores measured with the validated Nutrition Attitudes and Knowledge (NAK) Questionnaire. BMI calculated based on parent-reported weight and height (T0)	CG played a control app called "My Salad Shop Bar"	Compared to the control group, children who used Foodbot Factory had significant increases in overall nutrition knowledge, and in Vegetables and Fruits, Protein Foods, and Whole Grain Foods sub-scores. No significant difference in knowledge was observed in the Drinks sub-score	No specific theory.	Cog	Android Tablet	No	No	No
Mack et al., 2020 (Germany) [42] Kids Obesity Prevention program (KOI serious game for children with knowledge-based activities addressing the areas of nutrition, physical activity, and stress coping	N PA	9–12 y n = 82 Experimental	The IG played the game twice, over a 2-week period, with a different selection of game modules (45 min./session).	Knowledge questionnaire (T0, T1, T2). Changes in dietary behavior, Physical activity and Media consumption questionnaires (T0 + T2; child and parents reports) Acceptance of the game and Emotions during game play questionnaires (T1; child self-reports). Analysis of game data (Int) T2= 2 weeks after play	CG received a brochure with basic information about a healthy lifestyle—"How to make food fun" (food pyramid and PA).	Total knowledge increased with the game and remained at the 2-week follow-up. No positive changes were observed in PA.	No specific theory. Game extensively targets the Dietary Energy Density Principle (DED-P).	Cog Mot	Motion control interface (for moving the avatar in the game) + Tablet (choice selection)	No	No	No
Espinosa-Curiel et al., 2020a (Mexico) [57] FoodRateMaster: teaches the characteristics of healthy/unhealthy foods, bearing in mind children's environment.	N PA	8–10 y n = 60 Quasi-experimental	12 game sessions of at least 15 min each, during 6 weeks (45 days)	Food knowledge and Food frequency questionnaires (T0, T1). Parent perception questionnaire (T1)	No control	Increased nutritional knowledge after gameplay. Increased frequency intake of two healthy foods, and decreased intake of 10 unhealthy foods. Positive influence in children's attitudes (parent reported).	Game is grounded on the constructs of Behavioral Theory, Cognitive Theory and Social Cognitive Theory.	Cog Mot	Microsoft Kinect V2 sensor (basic physical movements in avoiding obstacles and for classifying food) + PC	Yes (6 levels that replicate real food establishments (e.g., a food truck, a restaurant, or a grocery store))	No	Interdisciplinary team and iterative methodology (user-centered design).
Espinosa-Curiel et al., 2020b (Mexico) [48] FoodRateMaster:				EGameFlow and GUESS questionnaires (T1)		Enjoyment and user experience satisfaction with the game were positively correlated and significant predictors of learning.						

Table A1. *Cont.*

Reference	Intervention Area	Description of the Intervention				Results	Theory Behind the Game	Performative Aspects			Acknowledgment of the Environment	Formative Evaluation or Tailoring
		Sample/Type of the Study	Duration and Intensity	Assessment Tools	Control			Application Domain	Interactional Elements	Contract with Real Foods		
Holzmann et al., 2019 (Germany) [37] Fit, Food, Fun (FFF): a serious game with European country-specific food items, to increase food knowledge and PA	N PA	12–14 y n = 83 Quasi-experimental	IG played the FFF game individually for 3 consecutive days, 15 min/session.	Dietary behavior, physical activity, and healthy eating attitudes accessed by questionnaire (T0). Nutritional knowledge questionnaire (T0, T1)	CG received a teaching intervention, performed in a classic lecture format (with similar content).	Total knowledge increased in both groups, especially in the CG.	Game of the NUDGE platform. Influenced by the concept of serious gaming, the theory of persuasive gaming, and the concept of positive gaming.	Cog	Tablet	No	No	Pre-game design survey, conducted with 300 adolescents. On preferences, motives, and needs regarding nutritional information and digital gameplay. Usability tests and focus groups.
Baranowski et al., 2019b (USA) [49] Escape from Diab and Nanoswarm: Invasion from Inner Space: 2 video games designed to lower risks of type 2 diabetes and obesity by changing youth diet and physical activity behaviors.	N PA	10–12 y n = 145 (Children in the 85th—99th %ile of BMI) Experimental	Each game had 9 sessions (each episode/session lasting 60 min). Treatment group played Diab and Nano in sequence (total of 2 to 3 months)	BMI assessment; parent self-reported data (T0). Fasting insulin assessment; 32-item Fruits and Vegetables Food Frequency Questionnaire (FV-FFQ); 22- item sweetened beverage FFQ (T0, T1). PA assessed using accelerometer ($\leq$7 days). Gameplay data collected over the Internet (Int) T2 = 2 months after play	CG was a wait list group that received the intervention at the end of the 5-month postbaseline assessment.	No significant differences were detected in any of the tested outcome variables.	Several theories, including Social Cognitive Theory, Self-Determination Theory, Behavioral Inoculation and Transportation Theories and the Elaboration Likelihood Model.	Cog	Computer	No	Yes (barriers to attain diet and physical activity goals were included in "Escape from Diab")	Quantitative and qualitative methods applied to examine child preferences for storyline genres and plot content of nonviolent video games; also, computer access, knowledge, and game-play frequency. Tailoring: goal-settings were selected according to the player's behaviors and preferences reported at the baseline.
Baranowski et al., 2011 (USA) [58] Escape from Diab and Nanoswarm: Invasion from Inner Space		10–12 y n = 145 (Children in the 85th—99th %ile of BMI) Experimental		3 nonconsecutive days of 24 h dietary recalls. 5 consecutive days of physical activity using accelerometers. Self-reported height, weight, waist circumference and triceps skinfold assessments (T0, P1, P2, P3). P1 = immediately after Diab P2 = immediately after Nano P3 = 2 months after intervention.	CG received 2 kits (booklet+ CD), comprising a knowledge-based nutrition game and 8 sessions of web-based online games (related to diet, PA and obesity), with questions after each session.	Significant increase in FV intake, in the IG when compared with the CG, including 5 months later. No positive changes in water intake, physical activity, or body composition.						

Table A1. *Cont.*

Reference	Intervention Area	Description of the Intervention					Theory Behind the Game	Performative Aspects			Acknowledgment of the Environment	Formative Evaluation or Tailoring
		Sample/Type of the Study	Duration and Intensity	Assessment Tools	Control	Results		Application Domain	Interactional Elements	Contract with Real Foods		
Hermans et al., 2018 (Nederlands) [59] Alien Health Game (AHG): videogame designed to teach elementary school children about nutrition and healthy food choices, while engaging in short cardio exercises. (Dutch version)	N PA	10–13 y n = 108 Experimental	30-min long-play sessions, on 2 consecutive days at children's school.	BMI assessment (T0) Nutrition Knowledge questionnaire (T0, T1, T2) Food-taste test (T1, T2) T2 = 2-week after play.	CG played a web-based nutrition game for the same period of time (Super Shopper).	No substantial differences between IG and CG. IG revealed better knowledge only shortly after playing the game (vs. CG). No evidence for behavior change.	"Mixed-reality" platform (AHG uses both digital components as well as tangible, physical components). Theoretically grounded in Situated and Embodied Cognition, including Gestural congruency, and also Behavior Change procedures from Michie inventory.	Cog Mot	SMALLab (mixed-reality educational platform, that uses motion-tracking cameras mounted in a ceiling or on a trussing system, and trackable wands) + interactive whiteboard.	No	No	No
Johnson-Glenberg et al., 2014 [40] (USA) Alien Health Game (AHG)		10–13 y n = 20	50 min of play and play-observing (9 min of actual play/dyad).	Nutrition Knowledge questionnaire (T0, T1)	CG: the same performative food choices at the interactive whiteboard, without a game narrative or cardio exercises.	Total knowledge increased in both groups after intervention, but IG outperformed the CG (especially in the follow-up).						
Johnson-Glenberg et al., 2013 (USA) [60] Alien Health Game (AHG)		Experimental 9–10 y n = 19 Quase-experimental	45 min of play and		No Control	Knowledge regarding food choices increased significantly. Evidence of knowledge transfer of general nutrition principles.						
Thompson et al., 2017 (USA) [55] Squire's Quest! II (SQ2): 10-episode online serious videogame promoting FV intake to preadolescent children, by testing the effect of implementation intentions on FV goal attainment and consumption.	N	9–11 y n = 400 parent/child dyads Experimental Four groups: Action; Coping; Action+ Coping; Control. Action plans state "how" a goal will be achieved. Coping plans identify a potential barrier and corresponding solution.	10-episode, online videogame; each session/episode lasting about 25 min; up to three months to play all 10 episodes.	Telephone interviews with children (T1). Game-play data (INT)	Control condition did not create implementation intentions. Parents were involved through newsletters and a dedicated website.	Overall, mean goal attainment was high (FV consumption goals and recipe goals), with no statistically significant differences between groups. Children were more likely to select the F recipe. Program satisfaction was high.	SQ2 is theoretically grounded in SCT, SDT, Behavioral Inoculation Theory, Maintenance Theory and Elaboration Likelihood Model.	Cog		Yes (brief demonstration videoclips taught players how to make simple FV recipes ('Virtual Kitchen')Players set goals to make a recipe at home)	Yes (children selected barrier-specific solutions to potential obstacles to FV intake)	Extensive formative work conducted to ensure children understood the behavioral procedures and could complete them, and also that the game was appealing (e.g., interviews, alpha testing, beta testing). Recipes tested to ensure they were child-friendly, tasted good, and looked attractive. Pilot study to test procedures (enrollment, data collection, intervention delivery) and as final beta test of the online game.
DeSmet et al., 2017 (USA) [61] Squire's Quest! II (SQ2)				Asking behavior and home FV availability questionnaires, (child-reported and parent-reported, respectively) (T0, T1, T2). T2 = 3 months after play.		Despite increasing (and decreasing, at follow-up), children asking behaviors did not lead to an increase in FV at home or to more FV consumption.						
Cullen et al., 2016 (USA) [62] Squire's Quest! II (SQ2)				24 h dietary recalls conducted via phone (3 unannounced 24 h dietary recalls, FV intake averaged) (T0, T2). T2 = 3 months after play.		Action and coping groups participants reported higher V intake at dinner. Significant increases over time of F intake at breakfast, lunch, and snack (at follow-up).						

Table A1. *Cont.*

Reference	Intervention Area	Description of the Intervention: Sample/Type of the Study	Duration and Intensity	Assessment Tools	Control	Results	Theory Behind the Game	Performative Aspects: Application Domain	Interactional Elements	Contract with Real Foods	Acknowledgment of the Environment	Formative Evaluation or Tailoring
Thompson et al., 2015 (USA) [63] Squire's Quest! II (SQ2)		9–11 y $n = 387$ parent/child dyads Experimental (Four groups)		24 h dietary recalls conducted via phone (3 unannounced 24 h dietary recalls, food and beverage intake averaged) (T0, T1, T2). Demographic data (T0) T2 = 3 months after play.		Children who only created action plans showed increased intake of FVs at follow-up, and favorable changes in energy density and key nutrients. F intake increased over time, regardless individual IG results.						
Sharma et al., 2015 (USA) [51] Quest to Lava Mountain (QTLM): an action-adventure game that requires children to make simulated appropriate food choices and stay physically active to move steadily through the game and succeed.	N PA	9–11 y $n = 94$ Quase-experimental	90 min/week for 6 weeks recommended	Demographic data (T0). Two random 24 h dietary recall interviews. Child self-report surveys to assess Diet and Physical Activity Habits and Related Psychosocial Mediators; anthropometric measures (T0, T1) QTLM usability, exposure to, and progress achieved (INT)	CG were children in three comparison schools (wait list to play QTLM)	Children in IG reported decreased sugar consumption and higher N/PA attitudes pre- to post intervention. No significant effects on PA.	Social Cognitive Theory and the Theory of Reasoned Action	Cog	Computer	No	No	No
Marchetti et al., 2015 (Italy) [64] Gustavo in Gnam's Planet: a game to improve knowledge on healthy foods and increase their consumption.	N	14–18 y $n = 83$ Qusai-experimental	30 min–2 h/day, during one week.	Healthy food knowledge questionnaire, Food frequency questionnaire, and Interest questionnaire (T0, T1)	No control	Knowledge on healthy diet improved with the game. Increased consumption of different healthy foods and lower consumption of sugary snacks post-play.	Theoretically grounded in the Transtheoretical Model of Change, the SCT, the SDT, and the Elaboration Likelihood Model.	Cog	Computer	No	No	No
Saksono et al., 2015 (USA) [39] Spaceship Launch (SL): game with Fitbit activity trackers, to increase parent and child PA.	PA	3–8 y $n = 14$ (and 15 caregivers) Quase-experimental	≥once a week total of 3 weeks	Demographics, PA intention and parental PA modeling and support (T0). PA intention survey. Experience with the game and impact in intentions and modeling behavior (semi-structured interviews with parents) (T1).	No control	Children and parents reported an increase in the intention to be physically more active.	Informed by SCT, SDT, and concepts of Parental PA modeling (as predictor of children's PA) and collaborative games in family	Mot	Fitbit activity trackers + Web app (home devices and large interactive display in gym sessions).	No	No	Formative and post-gameplay studies, to guide the game design. Focus groups with parents to probe parental attitudes towards, and support for, their child's PA.
Majumdar et al., 2013 (USA) [50] Creature-101: online game to promote energy balance-related behaviors (EBRBs)	N PA	11–13 y $n = 590$ Quasi-experimental	7 sessions, 30 min each, for 1 month	Frequency and amount of the targeted behaviors (Eat-Move instrument) and demographic data (T0, T1)	CG played 8 minigames (Whyville). matching standard science/health curriculums of NYC. Nutrition games excluded and networking activities deactivated.	Decrease in the consumption of SB and PS. No significant positive effects in FV and water intake, PA, or screen time.	Based on SCT and SDT. Behavioral change procedures based on Michie inventory. Embedded in a social networking structure (Elgg).	Cog	PC (game experience mostly through a MMO virtual world (Tween)	No	No	Focus groups and in-class observations to obtain feed-back about game structure and if it met behavior change objectives (link of the game to real-life behaviors). Beta-testing.

Table A1. *Cont.*

Reference	Intervention Area	Description of the Intervention				Results	Theory Behind the Game	Performative Aspects			Acknowledgment of the Environment	Formative Evaluation or Tailoring
		Sample/Type of the Study	Duration and Intensity	Assessment Tools	Control			Application Domain	Interactional Elements	Contract with Real Foods		
Macvean et al., 2012 (UK) [43] iFitQuest: Location-aware mobile exergame, played on the iPhone, by using Google Maps. The game is made up of a number of "mini-games", each designed to target a different type of fitness.	PA	12–15 y $n = 25$ Experimental	3 h session, with 30 min of play (15-min/mini game)	Background questionnaire (T0). Exertion and enjoyment of exercise with the game assessed through questionnaire; interview of expert PA teacher (that observed sessions) (T1). In-game log-files and rating collected during play (INT)	No control	IG achieved levels of speed representing "moderate to vigorous" activity, while playing iFitQuest.	No specific theory. Being physically demanding, iFitQuest grounds itself in published exergames design requirements to maintain motivation and enjoyment.	Mot	iPhone (exercise of game-players in real world physical movements are used to control the virtual character).	No	No	Preliminary school-based field study to guide the game development
Amaro et al., 2006 (Italy) [4] Kalèdo: a board-game to teach nutrition knowledge and to influence dietary behavior, regarding Mediterranean diet.	N PA	11–14 y $n = 241$ Experimental	2 to 4 players; 24 play sessions (15–30-min-long play sessions, once a week)	Nutrition knowledge, dietary intake, and physical activity questionnaires (T0, T1). BMI measurement (T0)	CG had no play sessions with Kalèdo.	Significant increase in nutrition knowledge and in weekly vegetable intake (vs. CG).	Unspecified. Combined purpose of promoting/discouraging specific dietary behaviors.	Cog	Board Game (cards, paws, play pieces, dice, "kaleido-scopes")	No	No	No
Cullen et al., 2005 (USA) [65] Squire's Quest! I: a 10-session interactive game to enable children to increase FJV intake, through activities promoting increasing asking behaviors and increasing skills in FJV preparation through virtual recipes.	N	8–12 y $n = 1578$ Experimental	25 min/session, in a total of 10 sessions/episodes, for 5 weeks.	4 days of dietary intake assessment using FIRSSt, (T0, T1).	GC without intervention	IG increased the consumption of fruit and 100% juice at snacks and the consumption of regular vegetables at lunch.	Based on social cognitive theory, the game used multiple exposure and fun in educational activities to increase preferences for and FJV consumption.	Cog	Computer	Yes (game involves students preparing FJV recipes in a virtual kitchen, and then setting goals to make recipes at home).	Yes (game involves a problem-solving routine to help players think of practices to increase the likelihood of eating more FJV).	Focus group discussions with fourth-grade children to assess interest in the story line and to identify child-desired characters' characteristics. Tailoring: FJV were selected based on the child's food preferences reported at baseline.
Baranowski et al., 2003 (USA) [66] Squire's Quest! I						IG increased their FJV consumption by 1.0 servings more than the CG.						

CG—Control Group; Cog—Cognitive skills; FJV—Fruit, 100% fruit Juice and non-fried Vegetables; FV—Fruit and vegetable GUESS—Game User Experience Satisfaction Scale; IG—Intervention Group; INT—During Intervention; MMO—Massively Multiplayer Online game; Mot—Motor skills; N—Nutrition; NA—Not Applicable; NYC—New York City; PA—Physical activity; PC—Personal computer; PS—Packaged Snacks; SB—Sweetened Beverages; SCT—Social Cognitive Theory; SDT—Self-Determination Theory; T0—Intervention baseline; T1—Immediately post-game; T2—a few months post-game; V—Vegetable.

References

1. Morales Camacho, W.J.; Molina Díaz, J.M.; Plata Ortiz, S.; Plata Ortiz, J.E.; Morales Camacho, M.A.; Calderón, B.P. Childhood obesity: Aetiology, comorbidities, and treatment. *Diabetes Metab. Res. Rev.* **2019**, *35*, e3203. [CrossRef]
2. Anderson, K.L. A Review of the Prevention and Medical Management of Childhood Obesity. *Child Adolesc. Psychiatr. Clin. N. Am.* **2018**, *27*, 63–76. [CrossRef] [PubMed]
3. Yoo, H.; Suneja, U. *Pediatric Obesity Nutritional Guidelines*; StatPearls Publishing: Tampa, FL, USA, 2021.
4. Brown, T.; Moore, T.H.; Hooper, L.; Gao, Y.; Zayegh, A.; Ijaz, S.; Elwenspoek, M.; Foxen, S.C.; Magee, L.; O'Malley, C.; et al. Interventions for preventing obesity in children. *Cochrane Database Syst. Rev.* **2019**, *7*, CD001871. [CrossRef] [PubMed]
5. Sanyaolu, A.; Okorie, C.; Qi, X.; Locke, J.; Rehman, S. Childhood and Adolescent Obesity in the United States: A Public Health Concern. *Glob. Pediatr. Health* **2019**, *6*, 2333794X19891305. [CrossRef] [PubMed]
6. Weihrauch-Blüher, S.; Schwarz, P.; Klusmann, J.H. Childhood obesity: Increased risk for cardiometabolic disease and cancer in adulthood. *Metab. Clin. Exp.* **2019**, *92*, 147–152. [CrossRef] [PubMed]
7. Lanigan, J. Prevention of overweight and obesity in early life. *Proc. Nutr. Soc.* **2018**, *77*, 247–256. [CrossRef]
8. Huang, J.Y.; Qi, S.J. Childhood obesity and food intake. *World J. Pediatr. WJP* **2015**, *11*, 101–107. [CrossRef]
9. Rosiek, A.; Maciejewska, N.F.; Leksowski, K.; Rosiek-Kryszewska, A.; Leksowski, Ł. Effect of Television on Obesity and Excess of Weight and Consequences of Health. *Int. J. Environ. Res. Public Health* **2015**, *12*, 9408–9426. [CrossRef]
10. Romanelli, R.; Cecchi, N.; Carbone, M.G.; Dinardo, M.; Gaudino, G.; Del Giudice, E.M.; Umano, G.R. Pediatric obesity: Prevention is better than care. *Ital. J. Pediatr.* **2020**, *46*, 103. [CrossRef]
11. Stenseng, F.; Hygen, B.W.; Wichstrøm, L. Time spent gaming and psychiatric symptoms in childhood: Cross-sectional associations and longitudinal effects. *Eur. Child Adolesc. Psychiatry* **2020**, *29*, 839–847. [CrossRef]
12. ESA. 2021 Sales, Demographic, and Usage Data: Essential Facts about the Video Game Industry. Entertainment Software Association. Available online: http://www.theesa.com/wp-content/uploads/2021/08/2021-Essential-Facts-About-the-Video-Game-Industry-1.pdf (accessed on 17 September 2021).
13. Thompson, D. Designing serious video games for health behavior change: Current status and future directions. *J. Diabetes Sci. Technol.* **2012**, *6*, 807–811. [CrossRef]
14. Rego, P.; Moreira, P.M.; Reis, L.P. Serious games for rehabilitation: A survey and a classification towards a taxonomy. In Proceedings of the 5th Iberian Conference on Information Systems and Technologies, Santiago de Compostela, Spain, 16–19 June 2010; pp. 1–6.
15. Kato, P.M.; Cole, S.W.; Bradlyn, A.S.; Pollock, B.H. A video game improves behavioral outcomes in adolescents and young adults with cancer: A randomized trial. *Pediatrics* **2008**, *122*, e305–e317. [CrossRef] [PubMed]
16. DeSmet, A.; Van Ryckeghem, D.; Compernolle, S.; Baranowski, T.; Thompson, D.; Crombez, G.; Poels, K.; Van Lippevelde, W.; Bastiaensens, S.; Van Cleemput, K.; et al. A meta-analysis of serious digital games for healthy lifestyle promotion. *Prev. Med.* **2014**, *69*, 95–107. [CrossRef] [PubMed]
17. Wattanasoontorn, V.; Boada, I.; García, R.; Sbert, M. Serious games for health. *Entertain. Comput.* **2013**, *4*, 231–247. [CrossRef]
18. Baranowski, T.; Buday, R.; Thompson, D.I.; Baranowski, J. Playing for real: Video games and stories for health-related behavior change. *Am. J. Prev. Med.* **2008**, *34*, 74–82. [CrossRef]
19. Mack, I.; Bayer, C.; Schäffeler, N.; Reiband, N.; Brölz, E.; Zurstiege, G.; Fernandez-Aranda, F.; Gawrilow, C.; Zipfel, S. Chances and Limitations of Video Games in the Fight against Childhood Obesity-A Systematic Review. *Eur. Eat. Disord. Rev. J. Eat. Disord. Assoc.* **2017**, *25*, 237–267. [CrossRef]
20. Baranowski, T.; Ryan, C.; Hoyos-Cespedes, A.; Lu, A.S. Nutrition education and dietary behavior change games: A scoping review. *Games Health J.* **2019**, *8*, 153–176. [CrossRef]
21. Chow, C.Y.; Riantiningtyas, R.R.; Kanstrup, M.B.; Papavasileiou, M.; Liem, G.D.; Olsen, A. Can games change children's eating behaviour? A review of gamification and serious games. *Food Qual. Prefer.* **2020**, *80*, 103823. [CrossRef]
22. Guy, S.; Ratzki-Leewing, A.; Gwadry-Sridhar, F. Moving beyond the stigma: Systematic review of video games and their potential to combat obesity. *Int. J. Hypertens.* **2011**, *2011*, 179124. [CrossRef]
23. Blüher, M. Obesity: Global epidemiology and pathogenesis. *Nat. Rev. Endocrinol.* **2019**, *15*, 288–298. [CrossRef]
24. Kadomura, A.; Tsukada, K.; Siio, I. EducaTableware: Sound Emitting Tableware for Encouraging Dietary Education. *J. Inf. Process.* **2014**, *22*, 325–333. [CrossRef]
25. Mustonen, S.; Tuorila, H. Sensory education decreases food neophobia score and encourages trying unfamiliar foods in 8–12-year-old children. *Food Qual. Prefer.* **2010**, *21*, 353–360. [CrossRef]
26. Dovey, T.M.; Staples, P.A.; Gibson, E.L.; Halford, J.C. Food neophobia and 'picky/fussy' eating in children: A review. *Appetite* **2008**, *50*, 181–193. [CrossRef]
27. Moher, D.; Liberati, A.; Tetzlaff, J.; Altman, D.G. Preferred reporting items for systematic reviews and meta-analyses: The PRISMA statement. *BMJ* **2009**, *339*, b2535. [CrossRef]
28. Bandura, A. *Social Foundations of Thought and Action: A Social Cognitive Theory*; Prentice-Hall, Inc.: Hoboken, NJ, USA, 1986.
29. Ryan, R.M.; Deci, E.L. Self-determination theory and the facilitation of intrinsic motivation, social development, and well-being. *Am. Psychol.* **2000**, *55*, 68–78. [CrossRef] [PubMed]
30. Petty, R.E.; Cacioppo, J.T. (Eds.) *Communication and Persuasion: Central and Peripheral Routes to Attitude Change*; Springer: New York, NY, USA, 1986.

31. Prochaska, J.O.; DiClemente, C.C. Stages and processes of self-change of smoking: Toward an integrative model of change. *J. Consult. Clin. Psychol.* **1983**, *51*, 390–395. [CrossRef]
32. McGuire, W.J. Resistance to persuasion conferred by active and passive prior refutation of the same and alternative counterarguments. *J. Abnorm. Soc. Psychol.* **1961**, *63*, 326–332. [CrossRef]
33. Rothman, A.J. Toward a theory-based analysis of behavioral maintenance. *Health Psychol.* **2000**, *19*, 64–69. [CrossRef]
34. Fishbein, M. A theory of reasoned action: Some applications and implications. *Neb. Symp. Motiv.* **1980**, *27*, 65–116.
35. Green, M.C.; Brock, T.C. The role of transportation in the persuasiveness of public narratives. *J. Personal. Soc. Psychol.* **2000**, *79*, 701–721. [CrossRef] [PubMed]
36. Michie, S.; Johnston, M.; Francis, J.; Hardeman, W.; Eccles, M. From Theory to Intervention: Mapping Theoretically Derived Behavioural Determinants to Behaviour Change Techniques. *Appl. Psychol.* **2008**, *57*, 660–680. [CrossRef]
37. Holzmann, S.L.; Schäfer, H.; Groh, G.; Plecher, D.A.; Klinker, G.; Schauberger, G.; Hauner, H.; Holzapfel, C. Short-Term Effects of the Serious Game "Fit, Food, Fun" on Nutritional Knowledge: A Pilot Study among Children and Adolescents. *Nutrients* **2019**, *11*, 2031. [CrossRef] [PubMed]
38. Schäfer, H.; Plecher, D.A.; Holzmann, S.L.; Groh, G.; Klinker, G.; Holzapfel, C.; Hauner, H. NUDGE-NUtritional, Digital Games in Enable. In *Positive Gaming: Workshop on Gamification and Games for Wellbeing, at CHI PLAY '17*; University of Waterloo Library: Waterloo, ON, Canada, 2017; pp. 15–18.
39. Saksono, H.; Ranade, A.; Kamarthi, G.; Castaneda-Sceppa, C.; Hoffman, J.A.; Wirth, C.; Parker, A.G. Spaceship Launch: Designing a Collaborative Exergame for Families. In Proceedings of the 18th ACM Conference on Computer Supported Cooperative Work & Social Computing (CSCW '15), Vancouver, BC, Canada, 14–18 March 2015; Association for Computing Machinery: New York, NY, USA, 2015; pp. 1776–1787. [CrossRef]
40. Johnson-Glenberg, M.C.; Savio-Ramos, C.; Henry, H. "Alien Health": A Nutrition Instruction Exergame Using the Kinect Sensor. *Games Health J.* **2014**, *3*, 241–251. [CrossRef] [PubMed]
41. Amaro, S.; Viggiano, A.; Di Costanzo, A.; Madeo, I.; Viggiano, A.; Baccari, M.E.; Marchitelli, E.; Raia, M.; Viggiano, E.; Deepak, S.; et al. Kalèdo, a new educational board-game, gives nutritional rudiments and encourages healthy eating in children: A pilot cluster randomized trial. *Eur. J. Pediatr.* **2006**, *165*, 630–635. [CrossRef]
42. Mack, I.; Reiband, N.; Etges, C.; Eichhorn, S.; Schaeffeler, N.; Zurstiege, G.; Gawrilow, C.; Weimer, K.; Peeraully, R.; Teufel, M.; et al. The Kids Obesity Prevention Program: Cluster Randomized Controlled Trial to Evaluate a Serious Game for the Prevention and Treatment of Childhood Obesity. *J. Med. Internet Res.* **2020**, *22*, e15725. [CrossRef]
43. Macvean, A.; Robertson, J. FitQuest: A school based study of a mobile location-aware exergame for adolescents. In Proceedings of the 14th International Conference on Human-Computer Interaction with Mobile Devices and Services (MobileHCI'12), San Francisco, CA, USA, 21–25 September 2012; Association for Computing Machinery: New York, NY, USA, 2012; pp. 359–368. [CrossRef]
44. Wengreen, H.J.; Joyner, D.; Kimball, S.S.; Schwartz, S.; Madden, G.J. A Randomized Controlled Trial Evaluating the FIT Game's Efficacy in Increasing Fruit and Vegetable Consumption. *Nutrients* **2021**, *13*, 2646. [CrossRef] [PubMed]
45. de Vlieger, N.M.; Sainsbury, L.; Smith, S.P.; Riley, N.; Miller, A.; Collins, C.E.; Bucher, T. Feasibility and Acceptability of 'VitaVillage': A Serious Game for Nutrition Education. *Nutrients* **2021**, *14*, 189. [CrossRef]
46. Froome, H.M.; Townson, C.; Rhodes, S.; Franco-Arellano, B.; LeSage, A.; Savaglio, R.; Brown, J.M.; Hughes, J.; Kapralos, B.; Arcand, J. The Effectiveness of the Foodbot Factory Mobile Serious Game on Increasing Nutrition Knowledge in Children. *Nutrients* **2020**, *12*, 3413. [CrossRef]
47. Vepsäläinen, H.; Skaffari, E.; Wojtkowska, K.; Barlińska, J.; Kinnunen, S.; Makkonen, R.; Heikkilä, M.; Lehtovirta, M.; Ray, C.; Suhonen, E.; et al. A Mobile App to Increase Fruit and Vegetable Acceptance Among Finnish and Polish Preschoolers: Randomized Trial. *JMIR Mhealth Uhealth* **2022**, *10*, e30352. [CrossRef]
48. Espinosa-Curiel, I.E.; Pozas-Bogarin, E.E.; Martínez-Miranda JPérez-Espinosa, H. Relationship Between Children's Enjoyment, User Experience Satisfaction, and Learning in a Serious Video Game for Nutrition Education: Empirical Pilot Study. *JMIR Serious Games* **2020**, *8*, e21813. [CrossRef]
49. Baranowski, T.; Baranowski, J.; Chen, T.A.; Buday, R.; Beltran, A.; Dadabhoy, H.; Ryan, C.; Lu, A.S. Videogames That Encourage Healthy Behavior Did Not Alter Fasting Insulin or Other Diabetes Risks in Children: Randomized Clinical Trial. *Games Health J.* **2019**, *8*, 257–264. [CrossRef]
50. Majumdar, D.; Koch, P.A.; Lee, H.; Contento, I.R.; Islas-Ramos, A.D.; Fu, D. "Creature-101": A Serious Game to Promote Energy Balance-Related Behaviors Among Middle School Adolescents. *Games Health J.* **2013**, *2*, 280–290. [CrossRef]
51. Sharma, S.V.; Shegog, R.; Chow, J.; Finley, C.; Pomeroy, M.; Smith, C.; Hoelscher, D.M. Effects of the Quest to Lava Mountain Computer Game on Dietary and Physical Activity Behaviors of Elementary School Children: A Pilot Group-Randomized Controlled Trial. *J. Acad. Nutr. Diet.* **2015**, *115*, 1260–1271. [CrossRef]
52. Greszczuk, C. Making Messages Work. The Health Foundation, 21 April 2020. Available online: https://www.health.org.uk/thinking-differently-about-health/making-messages-work (accessed on 17 September 2021).
53. Parisod, H.; Pakarinen, A.; Kauhanen, L.; Aromaa, M.; Leppänen, V.; Liukkonen, T.N.; Smed, J.; Salanterä, S. Promoting Children's Health with Digital Games: A Review of Reviews. *Games Health J.* **2014**, *3*, 145–156. [CrossRef]
54. Bandura, A. Self-efficacy: Toward a unifying theory of behavioral change. *Psychol. Rev.* **1977**, *84*, 191–215. [CrossRef]

55. Thompson, D. Incorporating Behavioral Techniques into a Serious Videogame for Children. *Games Health J.* **2017**, *6*, 75–86. [CrossRef] [PubMed]
56. FatWorld: A Game about the Politics of Nutrition. Persuasive Games. Available online: http://persuasivegames.com/game/fatworld (accessed on 17 July 2021).
57. Espinosa-Curiel, I.E.; Pozas-Bogarin, E.E.; Lozano-Salas, J.L.; Martínez-Miranda, J.; Delgado-Pérez, E.E.; Estrada-Zamarron, L.S. Nutritional Education and Promotion of Healthy Eating Behaviors Among Mexican Children Through Video Games: Design and Pilot Test of FoodRateMaster. *JMIR Serious Games* **2020**, *8*, e16431. [CrossRef]
58. Baranowski, T.; Baranowski, J.; Thompson, D.; Buday, R.; Jago, R.; Griffith, M.J.; Islam, N.; Nguyen, N.; Watson, K.B. Video game play, child diet, and physical activity behavior change a randomized clinical trial. *Am. J. Prev. Med.* **2011**, *40*, 33–38. [CrossRef]
59. Hermans, R.; van den Broek, N.; Nederkoorn, C.; Otten, R.; Ruiter, E.; Johnson-Glenberg, M.C. Feed the Alien! The Effects of a Nutrition Instruction Game on Children's Nutritional Knowledge and Food Intake. *Games Health J.* **2018**, *7*, 164–174. [CrossRef] [PubMed]
60. Johnson-Glenberg, M.C.; Hekler, E.B. "Alien Health Game": An Embodied Exergame to Instruct in Nutrition and MyPlate. *Games Health J.* **2013**, *2*, 354–361. [CrossRef]
61. DeSmet, A.; Liu, Y.; De Bourdeaudhuij, I.; Baranowski, T.; Thompson, D. The effectiveness of asking behaviors among 9–11 year-old children in increasing home availability and children's intake of fruit and vegetables: Results from the Squire's Quest II self-regulation game intervention. *Int. J. Behav. Nutr. Phys. Act.* **2017**, *14*, 51. [CrossRef] [PubMed]
62. Cullen, K.W.; Liu, Y.; Thompson, D.I. Meal-Specific Dietary Changes from Squires Quest! II: A Serious Video Game Intervention. *J. Nutr. Educ. Behav.* **2016**, *48*, 326–330.e1. [CrossRef]
63. Thompson, D.; Bhatt, R.; Vazquez, I.; Cullen, K.W.; Baranowski, J.; Baranowski, T.; Liu, Y. Creating action plans in a serious video game increases and maintains child fruit-vegetable intake: A randomized controlled trial. *Int. J. Behav. Nutr. Phys. Act.* **2015**, *12*, 39. [CrossRef]
64. Marchetti, D.; Fraticelli, F.; Polcini, F.; Lato, R.; Pintaudi, B.; Nicolucci, A.; Fulcheri, M.; Mohn, A.; Chiarelli, F.; Di Vieste, G.; et al. Preventing Adolescents' Diabesity: Design, Development, and First Evaluation of "Gustavo in Gnam's Planet". *Games Health J.* **2015**, *4*, 344–351. [CrossRef] [PubMed]
65. Cullen, K.W.; Watson, K.; Baranowski, T.; Baranowski, J.H.; Zakeri, I. Squire's Quest: Intervention changes occurred at lunch and snack meals. *Appetite* **2005**, *45*, 148–151. [CrossRef] [PubMed]
66. Baranowski, T.; Baranowski, J.; Cullen, K.W.; Marsh, T.; Islam, N.; Zakeri, I.; Honess-Morreale, L.; deMoor, C. Squire's Quest! Dietary outcome evaluation of a multimedia game. *Am. J. Prev. Med.* **2003**, *24*, 52–61. [CrossRef]

nutrients

MDPI

Systematic Review

Differential Gene Expression of Subcutaneous Adipose Tissue among Lean, Obese, and after RYGB (Different Timepoints): Systematic Review and Analysis

Elena Marisol Cruz-García [1], María E. Frigolet [1], Samuel Canizales-Quinteros [2] and Ruth Gutiérrez-Aguilar [1,3,*]

[1] Laboratorio de Investigación en Enfermedades Metabólicas: Obesidad y Diabetes, Hospital Infantil de México "Federico Gómez", Mexico City 06720, Mexico
[2] Unidad de Genómica de Poblaciones Aplicada a la Salud, Facultad de Química, UNAM/Instituto Nacional de Medicina Genómica (INMEGEN), Mexico City 14610, Mexico
[3] División de Investigación, Facultad de Medicina, Universidad Nacional Autónoma de México (UNAM), Mexico City 04510, Mexico
* Correspondence: ruthgutz@unam.mx; Tel.: +52-5552289917 (ext. 4509)

Abstract: The main roles of adipose tissue include triglycerides storage and adipokine secretion, which regulate energy balance and inflammation status. In obesity, adipocyte dysfunction leads to proinflammatory cytokine production and insulin resistance. Bariatric surgery is the most effective treatment for obesity, the gold-standard technique being Roux-en-Y gastric bypass (RYGB). Since metabolic improvements after RYGB are clear, a better understanding of adipose tissue molecular modifications could be derived from this study. Thus, the aim of this systematic review was to find differentially expressed genes in subcutaneous adipose tissue of lean, obese and post-RYGB (distinct timepoints). To address this objective, publications from 2015–2022 reporting gene expression (candidate genes or transcriptomic approach) of subcutaneous adipose tissue from lean and obese individuals before and after RGYB were searched in PubMed, Elsevier, and Springer Link. Excluded publications were reviews, studies analyzing serum, other types of tissues, or bariatric procedures. A risk-of-bias summary was created for each paper using Robvis, to finally include 17 studies. Differentially expressed genes in post-RYGB vs. obese and lean vs. obese were obtained and the intersection among these groups was used for analysis and gene classification by metabolic pathway. Results showed that the lean state as well as the post-RYGB is similar in terms of increased expression of insulin-sensitizing molecules, inducing lipogenesis over lipolysis and downregulating leukocyte activation, cytokine production and other factors that promote inflammation. Thus, massive weight loss and metabolic improvements after RYGB are accompanied by gene expression modifications reverting the "adipocyte dysfunction" phenomenon observed in obesity conditions.

Keywords: obesity; subcutaneous adipose tissue; RYGB; gene expression; gene candidate; transcriptome

1. Introduction

Obesity is defined as abnormal or excessive fat accumulation that presents a risk to health [1]. The obesity rates have increased dramatically in the past decades, with a global prevalence of overweight/obesity of ~30% [2]. It is associated with increased risk of diabetes, hypertension, cardiovascular disease, certain types of cancer, and osteoarthritis, among other abnormalities [3].

The main role of adipose tissue (AT) is the storage of triglycerides when circulating fuels are available, namely lipogenesis. An important molecule involved in adipose lipogenesis is fatty acid synthase (FASN) [4]. On the other hand, lipolysis occurs when energy is limited, and the release of fatty acids from AT triglycerides is fundamental to maintaining peripheral organ function [5]. Additional to triglycerides, cholesterol metabolism and transport in adipocytes, a process mediated by apoprotein E (APOE), is modified during obesity due to an increase in intracellular free cholesterol concentrations causing adipocyte enlargement [6,7]. Thus, AT promotes energy homeostasis partly through the regulation of the lipogenesis and lipolysis processes.

However, it is now well known that AT is not only an energy reservoir, but it also actively participates as an endocrine organ producing peptides or "adipokines" as adiponectin (ADIPOQ), which regulates glucose and fatty acid metabolism, and exerts anti-inflammatory effects in target organs [8,9]. Apart from metabolic and endocrine actions, many other functions of AT, such as angiogenesis, adipogenesis, extracellular matrix dissolution and reformation, steroid metabolism, immune response, and hemostasis have been described [10].

These functions are changed during AT expansion [11], when adipogenesis, defined as preadipocyte differentiation into mature adipocytes, is upregulated [12]. A key factor involved in adipogenesis is peroxisome proliferator activating receptor gamma (PPARγ), which mediates physiological AT growth through an increased cell number or hyperplasia which is accompanied by angiogenesis, regulated adipokine production, a low number of immune cells, and balanced lipolysis and lipogenesis [13–16].

In contrast to physiological AT expansion, fat accumulation due to chronic energy intake leads to obesity. In these conditions, AT growth is mainly associated with increased cell size or hypertrophy and with lower expression of adipogenic factors as PPARγ [17]. Obese adipose depots are characterized by extracellular matrix remodeling to allow adequate tissue expansion, in addition to increased lipolysis, lower secretion of ADIPOQ, and immune cells infiltration (mainly, accumulation of macrophages) [14,18–20]. In these conditions, the innate and adaptive immune system is activated by mobilizing several type of leukocytes (lymphocytes, neutrophils, eosinophils, etc.) and local macrophages [21]. In fact, a "healthy" AT contains around 10–15% of macrophages, but under obesity conditions they increase up to 50% [22]. Polarization and activation of AT proinflammatory macrophages contributes greatly to the chronic low-grade inflammation observed in obesity conditions [23]. The M1 macrophages' pro-inflammatory responses initiate via the toll-like receptors (TLRs), leading to the signaling pathways mediated by chemokines and cytokines, as tumor necrosis factor (TNF) and interleukins 1 (IL-1) and 6 (IL-6), among other inflammatory mediators. The interleukin signaling provokes the activation of further leukocytes involved in the immune response. One feature of dysfunction is proinflammatory cytokine production from adipocytes or infiltrated macrophages [24]. Signaling of such factors in target cells leads to impaired insulin signaling, diabetes, and metabolic syndrome establishment [25,26].

It has been shown that AT metabolism is greatly modified after massive weight loss induced by bariatric surgery [27]. Bariatric surgery is the most effective treatment for obesity and for sustained weight loss over time [28]. The bariatric gold-standard technique is the Roux en Y gastric bypass (RYGB), and it involves the construction of a gastric pouch and the bypass of the duodenum, reducing gastric volume and nutrient absorption [29]. RYGB yields an estimated weight loss of 73% and remission of diabetes and hypertension in 95 and 81% of cases, respectively [30]. AT biopsies from obese and post-RYGB individuals have been used to evaluate candidate gene expression or transcriptome analysis. These reports have demonstrated gene expression modifications after RYGB in subcutaneous adipose tissue (SAT) with focus on adipocyte volume, lipid metabolism and inflammation [31,32].

Significant weight loss is achieved as early as 4 weeks and 3 months after RYGB; in addition, the loss is maintained at 2–5 years. At these early timepoints (4 weeks and 3 months) diabetes remission indicators such as the HOMA index, oral glucose tolerance tests, and glycated hemoglobin (HbA1c) are significantly lower [33,34]. Another metabolic improvement after RYGB related to adipocyte function is adiponectin concentration, which is attained at one week to 3 months after RYGB [35]. After 2 years, serum adiponectin, adipose lipolysis and fat cell size are still lower than before the surgery, however, at 5 years post-surgery, no further changes in circulating adiponectin were found compared to before surgery, while increased lipolysis was suggested [36].

Some authors have focused on short-term and others on long-term effects of RYGB due to the difficulty and cost of sampling SAT after the surgery. Therefore, this review includes several studies to achieve the comparisons between lean, obese, and different timepoints after surgery. If SAT gene expression in RYGB subjects resembles SAT in lean subjects, then we could confirm that adipocyte functionality is ameliorated after surgery, reverting the "adiposopathy" process observed during obesity.

Thus, the aim of this systematic review was to find differentially expressed genes in the SAT of lean, obese, and post-RYGB individuals at different timepoints.

2. Materials and Methods

2.1. Protocol and Data

This systematic review and analysis was performed according to the Preferred Reporting Items for Systematic Reviews and Meta-Analyses (PRISMA) guidelines [37]. Complete data as raw values from the microarrays, reported and calculated gene expression, gene expression fold change, among others, can be found in Supplementary Materials.

2.2. Information Sources and Search Strategy

Original publications reporting gene expression of SAT before and after RGYB were searched in the electronic bibliographic databases PubMed, Elsevier, and Springer Link using the terms "bariatric surgery" and "AT transcriptome", "AT RYGB microarrays", "before and after RYGB microarrays", "RYGB bariatric surgery RNAseq", "RYGB SAT transcriptome", and "bariatric surgery SAT expression or microarrays". Data from publications between 2015 and 2022 were included. This search was finalized in July 2022. The detailed search approach is described in Figure 1.

2.3. Eligibility Criteria

The main criteria for this review were gene expression studies carried out in SAT from lean individuals and obese patients before and after RYGB at different timepoints. The inclusion criteria included studies analyzing mRNA expression of either candidate genes or transcriptomic analysis of SAT from obese patients who underwent RYGB, adults older than 18 years. Studies required gene expression comparison between: (1) obese vs. post-RYGB at different time points, or (2) lean vs. obese. All studies included in our review manifest having obtained the biopsy from the periumbilical regions close to the openings of the trocars during the surgery either by needle aspiration or tissue extraction. When post-bariatric surgery samples were taken the same region (periumbilical) was used for tissue extraction. Thus, the region that was reported to be utilized for gene expression is characterized as a homogenous sample (regarding cell type composition) among individuals. Moreover, we included all the papers meeting the including criteria, regardless of the ethnicity of the patients (Table S1).

The exclusion criteria were: review papers, studies analyzing serum or another type of AT, other types of bariatric procedures (gastric band, sleeve gastrectomy, RGYB combined with another bariatric surgery, etc.), metabolic or proteomic analysis, DNA methylation pattern or transcriptomic regulation via miRNAs or lnRNAs.

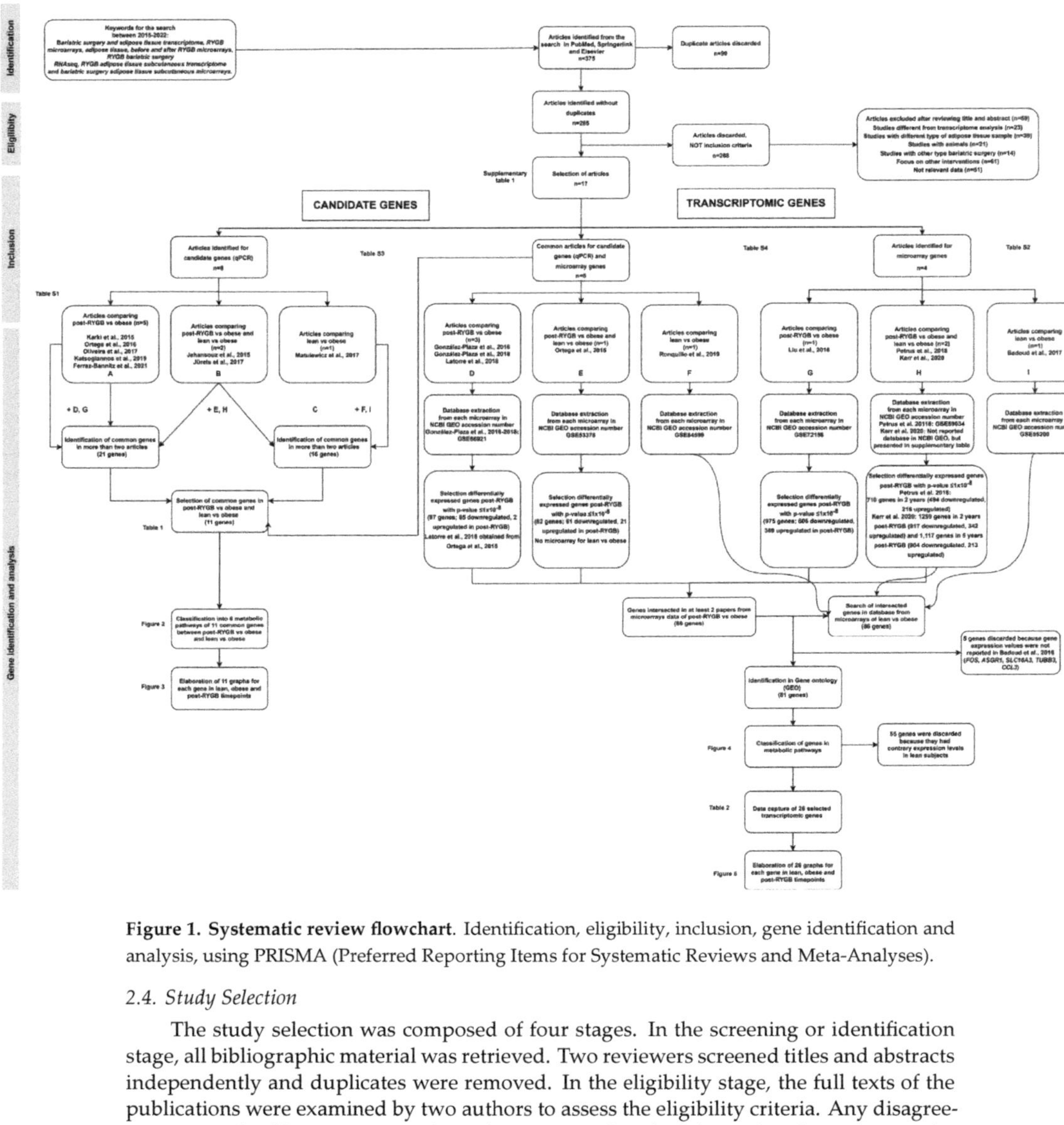

Figure 1. Systematic review flowchart. Identification, eligibility, inclusion, gene identification and analysis, using PRISMA (Preferred Reporting Items for Systematic Reviews and Meta-Analyses).

2.4. Study Selection

The study selection was composed of four stages. In the screening or identification stage, all bibliographic material was retrieved. Two reviewers screened titles and abstracts independently and duplicates were removed. In the eligibility stage, the full texts of the publications were examined by two authors to assess the eligibility criteria. Any disagreement was solved by consensus. The inclusion stage classified the studies depending on the approach: candidate genes or transcriptomic genes. In the gene identification and analysis stage, we selected the genes and extracted raw data. In addition, analysis of data to compare gene expression between post-RYGB vs. obese and lean vs. obese was performed (Figure 1).

2.5. Data Collection and Risk of Bias Assessment

A predesigned extraction sheet was used for relevant information such as: authors, publication year, participants characteristics (number of patients, gender, mean age, and recruitment hospital), mean body mass index (BMI before and after surgery), mean BMI loss, type of bariatric surgery, timepoints post-RYGB, gene expression method used (qPCR or microarray), and change fold gene expression between lean vs. obese and obese vs. post-bariatric surgery (different sample collection time points) (Table S1). A risk-of-bias summary was created for each paper that was included in this systematic review, analyzing each criteria using the risk of bias visualization tool from Robvis (Figure S1) [38].

2.6. Synthesis Methods and Effect Measures

Once the papers meeting the inclusion criteria were selected, and papers matching the exclusion criteria were discarded, the papers were divided in two different approaches: (a) candidate genes (genes with known functions implicated in AT metabolism), or (b) transcriptomic genes (genes obtained from microarrays, but not necessarily with known functions). Raw data for the candidate genes was obtained directly from the figures or tables from each paper. Concerning the transcriptomic genes, microarray data was obtained using the NCBI GEO accession number (GSE66921, GSE53378, GSE84599, GSE72158, and GSE55200) or the raw data contained in the supplementary materials. Genes with a p-value under $p \leq 1 \times 10^{-8}$ were considered for the next stage restricting our analysis to the most significant and differentially expressed genes between groups in each microarray analysis (File S1).

Each study presented the gene expression levels relative to either lean, obese or post-bariatric expression and sometimes only raw data was available. Therefore, to be able to compare between different studies, we needed to calculate the fold change expression relative to obese samples values. For this purpose, lean or post-bariatric values were divided by the obese values and 1 was subtracted. The resulting value was named "calculated fold change" = ((lean or post-RYGB)/obese) − 1). The interpretation of these data was: (a) for values higher than 0, the expression of that gene is upregulated in lean and post-bariatric subjects compared to obese subjects; (b) values lower than 0 mean that the expression of that gene is downregulated in lean and post-bariatric subjects compared to obese subjects (Tables S1–S3).

Once we obtained the calculated fold change, a comparison of the gene expression among all the papers of post-RYGB vs. obese and lean vs. obese was performed. Then, only the genes that were differentially expressed between groups, in at least two different papers, were selected. Only the intersected genes between post-bariatric vs. obese and lean vs. obese were selected for the next stage.

A list of genes was created and catalogued in different metabolic pathways. For candidate genes, the gene function and pathway are already known (Figure 2). However, for the transcriptomic genes, the pathway classification was performed using several bioinformatics tools: Gene Ontology (http://geneontology.org/), Reactome (https://reactome.org/PathwayBrowser/, accessed on 14 September 2022), and Topp Gene (https://toppgene.cchmc.org/), (Figure 4).

Finally, graphs were created comparing gene expression fold change among lean, obese and post-RYGB SAT samples at different time points, using Prism V8 (Figures 3 and 5).

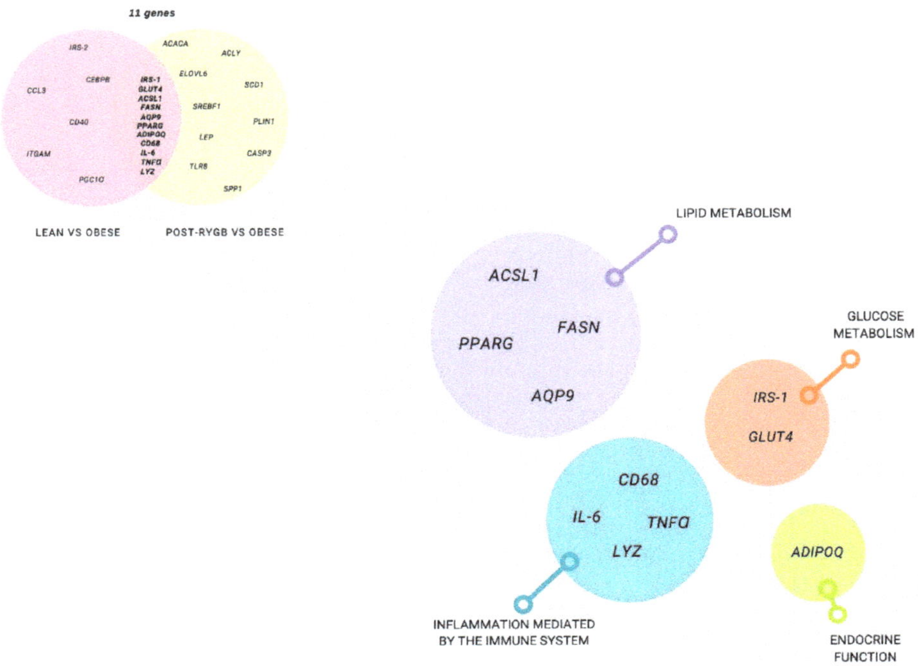

Figure 2. Subcutaneous adipose tissue differentially expressed genes using a candidate gene approach. Genes that were studied at least in two papers in post-RYGB vs. obese (yellow) and lean vs. obese (pink) are represented. Gene classification by function: glucose metabolism (orange), lipid metabolism (purple), endocrine function (green), and inflammation (blue).

3. Results

Our initial search identified 375 publications using PubMed, Springerlink, and Elsevier; however, 90 papers were duplicated, and were discarded. The 285 non-duplicated articles were read in detail and 268 were discarded, because inclusion criteria were not met, as shown in Figure 1. Therefore, 17 publications were eligible and included in this systematic review and analysis.

As mentioned above, the main objective of this review is to compare gene expression of SAT before and after RYGB bariatric surgery (different timepoints), as well as with lean samples. Therefore, we selected the publications based on studies comparing post-RYGB vs. obese, as well as lean vs. obese. Then, we divided the publications depending on the methodological approach: (1) candidate genes (qPCR) or (2) transcriptomic genes (microarrays).

Ten studies were selected for the candidate gene approach, based on known gene functions in AT metabolism and those genes were analyzed by qPCR. Five studies compared post-RYGB vs. obese samples, two studies compared post-RYGB and lean vs. obese samples, and only one study compared lean vs. obese samples. Moreover, four studies used both approaches (qPCR and microarray), three studies compared post-RYGB vs. obese, one study compared post-RYGB and lean vs. obese samples, and one study compared or lean vs. obese sample. On the other hand, for the transcriptomic gene approach, one study for each comparison was found: post-RYGB vs. obese, post-RYGB, and lean vs. obese samples.

In the next sections, we will describe these studies and identify the genes that were differentially expressed in SAT between post-RYGB vs. obese and lean vs. obese in at least two studies and from different recruitment countries. A summarized description of each article is presented below, highlighting only the differentially expressed genes for each comparison, i.e., post-RYGB vs. obese or lean vs. obese in at least two studies.

3.1. Candidate Gene Approach

In this section, we describe studies that reported candidate genes, because of their known function in AT metabolism. In the papers where microarrays were performed, we took into consideration the candidate genes selection presented by each author.

3.1.1. SAT Candidate Gene Differential Gene Expression between Post-RYGB vs. Obese

Karki et al., 2015 analyzed gene expression by qPCR of SAT samples from 19 obese subjects ($\geq$18 years), with an initial BMI of 42 $\pm$ 5 kg/m^2 and a final BMI of ~10 kg/m^2 after 8 $\pm$ 5 months post-RYGB. It is important to notice that the samples were not taken at the same time, which is a reason why this information should be considered cautiously. The expression levels were measured by qPCR. The selected candidate genes are implicated in lipolysis and triglyceride metabolism and their expression was increased after RYGB and inversely correlated with lipids and glucose markers [39] (Table S1). From the studied genes, only perilipin 1 (*PLIN1*) was selected for the next stage using our inclusion criteria.

Ortega et al., 2016 analyzed the expression of 17 candidate genes associated with adipocytes differentiation, de novo lipogenesis, fatty-acid transport, glycerol recycling, glucose uptake, insulin sensitivity, adipokines, and inflammation. The samples were obtained from 17 obese individuals with RYGB surgery (initial BMI 45 $\pm$ 3 kg/m^2, age 46 $\pm$ 10 years) during the RYGB surgery (90–120 min). At this timepoint, there is no effect on BMI. Therefore, we excluded these data for the following analysis (Table S1) [40].

Oliveira et al., 2017 analyzed SAT samples from 13 obese patients (~33 $\pm$ 9 years) with an initial BMI of ~45 $\pm$ 6 kg/m^2 and reducing about ~10 kg/m^2 before and after 6 months post-RYGB. They analyzed *UCP2* and *PLIN1* expression by qPCR, reporting that *UCP2* is overexpressed after RYGB. In addition, *UCP2* and *PLIN1* expression influenced the resting metabolic rate in obese individuals, suggesting that they could be used as predictors for percentage of weight loss after RYGB (Table S1) [41]. However, only *PLIN1* was selected for the next stage of our review.

Katsogiannos et al., 2019 analyzed samples for obese individuals before and after 1 and 6 months post-RYGB. SAT samples were obtained from 13 obese individuals with an initial BMI of 37 $\pm$ 4 kg/m^2, aged 55 $\pm$ 9 years. The BMI reduced ~4 kg/m^2 after 1 month and ~8 kg/m^2 after 6 months post-surgery, respectively. Genes implicated in glucose metabolism (*SLC2A4* (solute carrier family 2 member4)/*GLUT4, IRS-1,* etc.), adipogenesis, lipid metabolism (ADIPOQ, among others), and cellular proliferation were analyzed by qPCR. They reported that 1 month after RYGB, leptin (*LEP*) was downregulated and *ADIPOQ* (among others) was overexpressed, and even more after 6 months. At 6 months, *PPARG, FAS, GLUT4,* and *IRS1* were overexpressed (Table S1) [34]. All these genes were selected for the next stage of our review.

Ferraz-Bannitz et al., 2021 reported SAT differential expression in 13 obese subjects (BMI 42 $\pm$ 4 kg/m^2) aged 38 $\pm$ 8 years, before and 3 and 6 months post-surgery, reducing ~6 kg/m^2 and ~9 kg/m^2, respectively. The authors analyzed 24 candidate genes involved in inflammation, lipid transport, adipogenesis, aminoacid metabolism, glucose homeostasis and oxidative stress by qPCR. The genes that were differentially expressed, were selected for the next stage of our review were: *ADIPOQ* and *PGC1α* were overexpressed and *PPARG, TNFα* (at 6 months), and *IL-6* (at 3 months) were downregulated. Therefore, these authors concluded that bariatric surgery can acutely modulate inflammation and ER-stress (Table S1) [31].

González-Plaza et al., 2016 analyzed samples from eight obese individuals (52 $\pm$ 7 kg/m^2, ~41 $\pm$ 11 years) who, after 2 years, lost ~18 kg/m^2 (final BMI ~34 $\pm$ 9 kg/m^2).

They performed a microarray analysis on more than 62,000 transcripts before and after bariatric surgery. They reported that 172 genes were overexpressed and were implicated in lipids synthesis, Krebs cycle, glucolysis, glucogenolysis, and glucogenesis. Moreover, 731 genes were downregulated and were implicated in the immune system and inflammation. However, the authors validated only 8 candidate genes by qPCR in 20 obese individuals (BMI~56 ± 7 kg/m^2, ~46 ± 10 years) after two years of RYGB with a loss of ~17 kg/m^2. These authors concluded that RYGB improves the expression of genes involved in lipid metabolism and in inflammation in SAT, because *IRS-1*, *ACACA*, and *FASN* were overexpressed and *IL-6* and *TNFα* were downregulated (Table S1) [42]. All these genes were included in the next stage of our review.

González-Plaza et al., 2018 used the data published previously by the same first author in 2016. Then, they subdivided the samples in two groups based on insulin resistance: four low insulin resistant obese individuals (49.5 ± 5.2 kg/m^2, 39.0 ± 13.1 years, losing ~17.6 kg/m^2 after 2 years) and four high insulin resistant obese individuals (52.2 ± 6.8 kg/m^2, 43.2 ± 10.7 years and losing ~15.6 kg/m^2 after 2 years). For the low resistant group, 227 overexpressed and 619 downregulated genes were reported. For the high resistant group, 153 genes were overexpressed, and 865 genes downregulated. The intersection of these two groups showed that genes implicated in lipids biosynthesis were overexpressed; on the other hand, genes implicated in chemotaxis, immune response, and signaling transduction were downregulated. Specifically, for the low insulin resistant group the overexpressed genes were associated with carbohydrate metabolism, and for the high insulin resistant group the overexpressed genes were implicated in immune response, inflammation, phosphatidil-3-kinase protein, cellular proliferation and differentiation, cytokines interaction, and cancer. The authors concluded that insulin resistance state modifies gene expression after RYGB. Then, only eight genes were validated by qPCR using 20 obese subjects before and after 2 years post-surgery, divided in low insulin resistant (45 ± 13 years, with a BMI loss of ~18 kg/m^2) and high insulin resistant (47 ± 9 years, with a BMI loss of ~17 kg/m^2). However, for the validated genes, *IRS-1* was overexpressed and *TNFα* was downregulated post-RYGB in both low and high insulin resistance (Table S1) [43].

Latorre et al., 2018 analyzed the microarray data previously reported by Ortega et al., 2015 (described in the next section), selecting only 14 candidate genes implicated in inflammation, glucose transport and toll-like receptors, and validated by qPCR. They reported that *IRS1*, *GLUT4*, *ADIPOQ* were overexpressed and *IL6*, *TNFα*, *LEP*, and *TLR8* were downregulated 2 years post-RYGB (Table S1), among other genes [44].

Liu et al., 2016 performed a microarray with 47,231 transcripts from SAT samples of 42 obese individuals (~47 ± 6 kg/m^2, ~43 ± 11 years), comparing before and 12 months post-RYGB (final BMI 33 ± 5 kg/m^2, losing ~15 kg/m^2). After one year, 4236 genes were overexpressed, and 2989 genes were downregulated in post-RYGB. The authors validated the expression of 64 genes involved in the extracellular matrix, collagen accumulation, synthesis and degradation. However, 10 genes were overexpressed and 41 downregulated after 1 year of RYGB (Table S1). These results suggest that increased collagen degradation and decreased cross-linking are modulated after RYGB, mediating extracellular matrix adaptation after fat mass loss [45]. However, none of these candidate genes were considered for the next stage of our review.

3.1.2. SAT Candidate Gene Differential Gene Expression between Post-RYGB or Lean vs. Obese

Jahansouz et al., 2015 analyzed an acute effect comparing gene expression before and one week after bariatric surgery. They analyzed SAT samples from eight obese individuals (initial BMI ~40 ± 2 kg/m^2, ~50 ± 3 years) with a loss of ~1 kg/m^2 after one week. Moreover, they analyzed lean SAT samples (BMI ~24 ± 1 kg/m^2, 45 ± 6 years). Genes implicated in mitochondrial biogenesis, oxidative stress, and protein carbonylation were analyzed by qPCR (Table S1). The authors concluded that RYGB increases mitochondrial biogenesis gene expression (like *PGC1α*) in SAT [46], gene that was included for the next stage of our review.

Jürets et al., 2017 reported differential gene expression of SAT samples from lean individuals and obese individuals before and one year after RYGB. The samples were obtained from 20 lean individuals (~25 ± 3 kg/m^2 de 43 ± 9 years) and from 26 obese individuals (~46 ± 6 kg/m^2 and ~42 ± 12 years), and after one year of surgery the loss was ~15 kg/m^2. Expression of 20 candidate genes implicated in inflammation, growth factors, metabolic markers, cellular surface, lipolysis, and apoptosis were analyzed by qPCR (Table S1). *TNFα* and *CASP3* were overexpressed and *IL6, PPARG, ADIPOQ, CD68, PLIN1*, and *GLUT4* were downregulated one year post-RYGB compared to obese individuals [47], and these genes were included in the next stage of our review.

Ortega et al. (2015) performed a microarray with 13,885 transcripts using SAT samples from 16 obese individuals before and after 2 years post-RYGB (BMI ~43 ± 5 kg/m^2, 48 ± 10 years, losing ~14 kg/m^2) were analyzed. The results demonstrated the overexpression of 2432 genes implicated in lipids metabolism, energy production, Krebs cycle, oxidative phosphorylation, and mithocondrial disfunction after 2 years of RYGB. Moreover, 2586 genes were downregulated, implicated in lipid metabolism, cell-cell interaction and signaling, and carbohydrate metabolism. They validated 29 genes by qPCR, demonstrating overexpression of *FASN, ACLY, ACACA, ACSL1, GLUT4, IRS1*, among others, and downregulation of *LYZ, TNFα, AQP9*, and *IL-6* after 2 years of RYGB. In addition, samples from 26 lean individuals (BMI 24.15 ± 2.3 kg/m^2, 45 ± 5 years) were also analyzed and compared against obese samples. We realized that most of the genes validated by qPCR presented the same expression in lean as in post-RYGB, except for *ACACA*. However, *TNFα* and *IL-6* were upregulated in controls vs. obese (Table S1) [48]. Therefore, all the genes described here were included for the next stage of our review.

Petrus et al., 2018 analyzed SAT samples from 16 obese subjects (BMI 41 ± 1 kg/m^2, 46 ± 2 years) before and after 2 years of RYGB (losing ~16 kg/m^2), as well as 16 lean individuals (~25 ± 1 kg/m^2, 48 ± 2 years). Gene expression using a microarray containing more than 28,000 transcripts was performed. The authors focused on associated genes with adipocyte number change in obesity and post-RYGB, obtaining 79 genes. The upregulated genes were growth factors (*TGFB3, CXCL2, FGF7, OGN*, and *PDGFD*) and extracellular matrix organization; on the other hand, the downregulated genes were involved in cell growth and proliferation [49] (Table S1). However, none of these 5 genes were considered for the next stage of our review.

Kerr et al., 2020 analyzed SAT samples from 50 obese subjects (BMI 43 ± 5 kg/m^2, 43 ± 9 years) before and after 2 and 5 years post-RYGB (losing ~14 y 11 kg/m^2, respectively), as well as 28 lean individuals (27 ± 5 kg/m^2, 44 ± 9 years). At 2 and 5 years post-surgery, only 49 and 38 samples were obtained, and analyzed gene expression using a microarray containing more than 19,000 transcripts. After 2 years of-RYGB, 2420 genes were overexpressed and were involved in processes of protein translation, metabolism and adipocyte differentiation. Moreover, 3576 genes were downregulated and involved in immune and inflammatory responses. In addition, after 5 years of RYGB, 1653 were overexpressed, involved in lipid metabolism, adipocyte differentiation and function, and 3930 genes were downregulated and involved in immune response and cytokines production. For the comparison among lean, obese, and post-bariatric samples, they reported 5583 genes were differentially expressed. However, they were focused in only 60 inflammatory genes. They found that *CD68, ITGAM, LYZ*, and *TLR8* expression was higher in the obese compared to lean and post-surgery (2 and 5 years) among other genes (Table S1). In addition, *AQP9* was downregulated, but FASN was upregulated post-RYGB. The authors concluded that, inflammatory gene expression continuously improved after RYGB, despite body weight loss [32]. These genes were considered for the next stage of our study.

3.1.3. SAT Candidate Gene Differential Gene Expression between Lean vs. Obese

After selecting the candidate genes that were differentially expressed between post-RYGB and obese, we wanted to compare their expression between lean and obese. We found one article using qPCR and two with microarray methodology.

Using qPCR, Matulewicz et al., 2017 evaluated genes related to adipogenesis, extracellular matrix remodeling, and inflammation. The samples were obtained from 19 obese individuals (BMI ~33 $\pm$ 3 kg/m^2 aged ~26 $\pm$ 5 years), 83 lean individuals (BMI ~22 $\pm$ 2 kg/m^2, aged ~23 $\pm$ 2 years). They reported that adipogenic and insulin signaling genes (CEBPB, PPARG, ADIPOQ, IRS-1, IRS-2, GLUT4, among others) were downregulated in obesity. Moreover, *ADIPOQ, IRS-1, IRS-2,* and *GLUT4* were associated with insulin sensitivity independently of BMI. On the other hand, pro-inflammatory and immune cell marker genes (*CD68, ITGAM,* among others) were upregulated in obese compared to lean individuals (Table S1) [50]. All these genes were considered for the next stage of this review.

Ronquillo et al., 2019 performed a microarray (over 18,000 genes) of SAT samples from eight obese individuals (BMI ~33.03 + $-$3.15 kg/m^2, ~41 + $-$8.59 years) compared to eight lean individuals (BMI ~24 + $-$1.34 kg/m^2, ~36 + $-$9.3 years). Then, validation by qPCR in 37 obese and 35 lean subjects was performed. They showed that 12 genes were overexpressed in the obese, which were implicated in glycolysis, gluconeogenesis, inflammation, insulin, and leptin signaling, lipids and carbohydrate metabolism, and oxidative stress. On the other hand, genes related to endorine function, β-oxidation, lipids synthesis, insulin and leptin signaling were downregulated (Table S1) [51]. However, for this review we only considered *PPARG, ACSL1,* and *IRS2* for the next stage.

In a transcriptomic microarray analysis (more than 10,000 transcripts), Badoud et al., 2017 studied SAT samples from eleven obese subjects (35 $\pm$ 1.2 kg/m^2, 46 $\pm$ 1.5 years) and nine lean subjects (BMI 22.1 $\pm$ 0.5 kg/m^2, ~50 $\pm$ 3 years). They found 353 differentially expressed genes (130 overexpressed and 91 downregulated) in the obese samples. The overexpressed genes were implicated in cytokine receptor interaction and signaling pathways. On the other hand, the downregulated genes are implicated in lipolysis and AMPc signaling [52]. None of the candidate genes studied in this paper were selected for the next stage of our review. However, the database of the gene expression was used to look for the candidate genes in the next stage.

3.1.4. Analysis of SAT Candidate Gene Expression in Lean, Obese and Post-RYGB (Different Timepoints)

As described above, we analyzed 11 articles where differential gene expression between obese vs. post-RYGB (different timepoints) was reported. We found 21 candidate genes that were common in at least two papers. We classified them upon their function in different metabolic pathways: glucose metabolism (*IRS-1* and *GLUT4*), lipogenesis (*ACSL1, ACACA, ACLY, AQP9, ELOVL6, FASN, SCD1,* and *SREBF1*), lipolysis (*PLIN1*), adipogenesis (*PPARG*), endocrine function (*ADIPOQ* and *LEP*), and inflammation (*CASP3, CD68, IL-6, TLF8, TNFα, SPP1,* and *LYZ*).

Then, five papers were analyzed for SAT differential gene expression between lean vs. obese samples. We obtained 16 genes that were common in at least two papers between lean and obese. We classified them according to their function in glucose metabolism (*GLUT4, IRS-1,* and *IRS-2*), lipogenesis (*ACSL1, FASN*), lipolysis (*AQP9*), adipogenesis (*PPARG* and *CEBPB*), endocrine function (*ADIPOQ*), and inflammation (*CCL3, CD40, CD68, IL-6, ITGAM, TNFα,* and *LYZ*).

We then intersected all of these genes, analyzing the ones that were common between obese vs. post-RYGB and obese vs. lean, finding 11 genes *IRS-1, GLUT4, ACSL1, FASN, AQP9, PPARG, ADIPO, CD68, IL-6, TNFα,* and *LYZ*), shown in Table 1 and Figure 2.

Table 1. Summary of candidate genes differentially expressed in subcutaneous adipose tissue among lean, obese and post-RGYB.

Pathways	Gene Abbreviation	Gene Name
Glucose metabolism	*IRS-1*	Insulin Receptor Substrate 1
	GLUT4	Solute Carrier Family 2 Member 4
Lipids metabolism	*ACSL1*	Acyl-CoA Synthetase Long Chain Family Member 1
	FASN	Fatty Acid Synthase
	AQP9	Aquaporin 9
	PPARG	Peroxisome Proliferator Activated Receptor Gamma
Endocrine function	*ADIPOQ*	Adiponectin
Inflammation	*CD68*	Antigen CD68
	IL-6	Interleukin 6
	TNFα	Tumor Necrosis Factor
	LYZ	Lysozyme

Then, we were interested in comparing and analyzing their expression among different studies and the time after RYGB (Table S2). We observed that genes involved in glucose and lipid metabolism (*IRS-1, GLUT4, ACSL1,* and *FASN*) were overexpressed in lean compared to obese subjects. In addition, some of those genes were already overexpressed at 6 months, but all were upregulated at 2 and 5 years after RYGB, consistent in different studies (Figure 3, panels 1–4). For *AQP9,* we observed that in lean and in post-RYGB subjects (2 and 5 years) (Figure 3, panel 5), expression levels were downregulated compared to obese. For *PPARG,* we found that it was overexpressed in lean compared to obese subjects; however, after RYGB there is not a clear trend (Figure 3, panel 6).

For *ADIPOQ,* we observed that the gene expression is barely increased in lean subjects compared to obese ones. Then, in the earlier timepoints (3, 6 months after RYGB) its expression increases from 3–12 fold. However, in 2 and 5 years its expression is reduced to similar levels of lean subjects (Figure 3, panel 7).

For *LYZ,* gene expression was downregulated in lean subjects, increasing for obese ones, but downregulated or reverted after 2 and 5 years post-RYGB (Figure 3, panel 11). Moreover, *CD68* is similar to *LYZ,* but it seems to be downregulated from 12 months after RYGB (Figure 3, panel 8). In addition, two inflammatory gene expressions, *IL-6* and *TNFα,* were inconsistent in lean subjects. However, it is clear that after 3 months post-RYGB their expression is extremely reduced in post-surgery compared to obese subjects (Figure 3, panels 9,10).

These results suggest that RYGB reverts the gene expression of *IRS-1, GLUT4, ACSL1, FASN,* and *ADIPOQ* compared to obese subjects, having an overexpression as compared to lean subjects. On the other hand, *AQP9, LYZ, CD68, IL-6,* and *TNFα* are downregulated in lean, overexpressed in obese, and post-RYGB they are again downregulated, showing that RYGB reverts their expression (Figure 3).

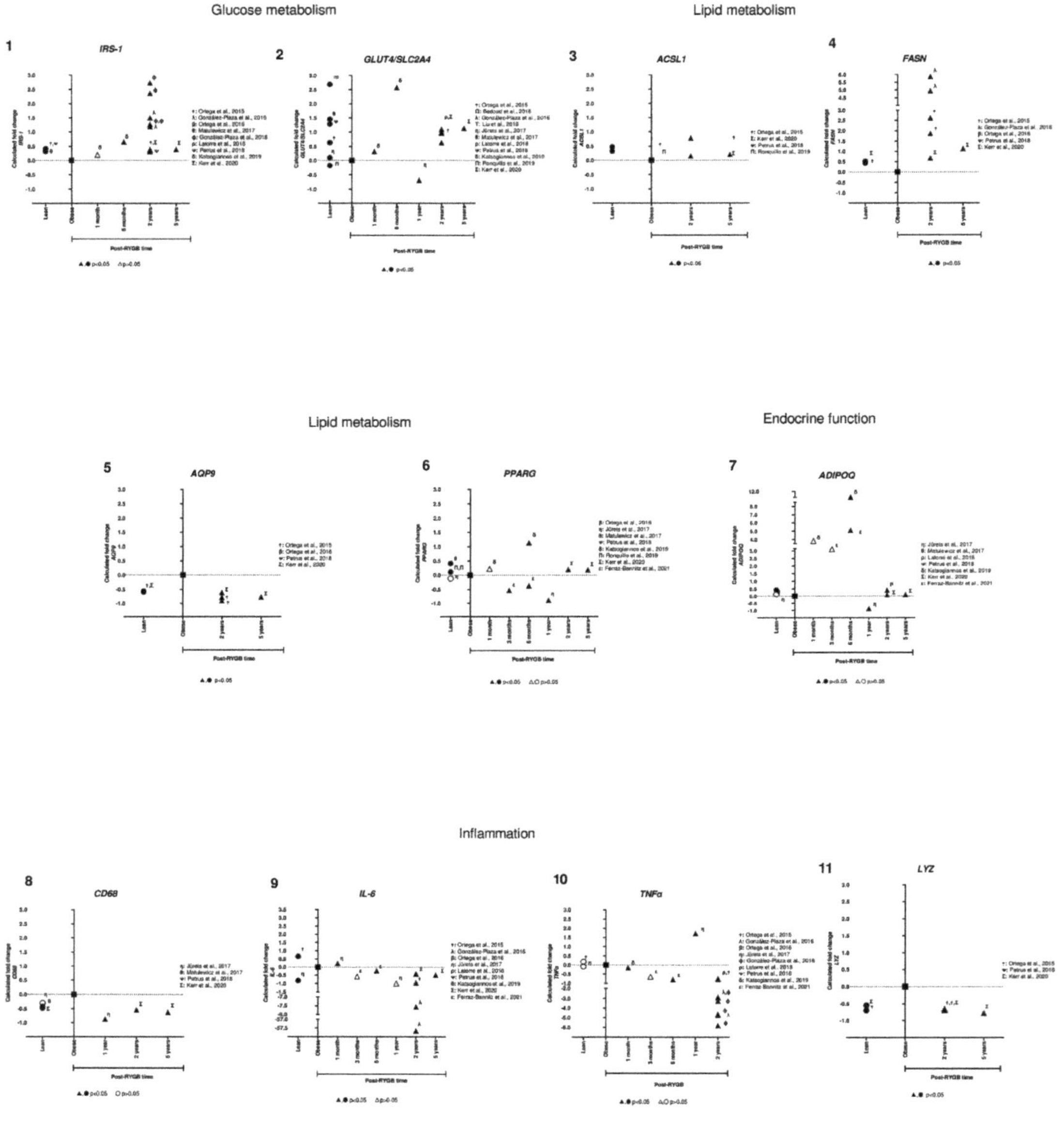

Figure 3. Subcutaneous adipose tissue candidate gene expression among lean, obese, and post-RYGB (different timepoints). Comparison of expression levels of each gene among different studies, identified by the Calculated fold change was significant (p-value < 0.05, ▲, •) or not (p-value > 0.05, △, ○). (α: [38]; ☨: [47]; Ω: [51]; λ: [41]; T: [44]; γ: [40]; η: [46]; θ: [49]; ϕ: [42]; ρ: [43]; Ψ: [48]; δ: [34]; Π: [50]; Σ: [32]; ε: [31]).

3.2. Transcriptomic Gene Approach

In this section, we describe studies that reported SAT gene differential expression obtained by microarrays. As mentioned above, the authors chose the candidate genes based on their known function and implication in AT metabolism. In fact, for some of the microarray papers, the authors focused their discussion on a particular pathway, leading to a limitation of the analysis of the microarray data.

To avoid this limitation, in this section, we obtained the raw data from the microarray of the studies described above. We previously described six papers showing differential gene expression between obese vs. post-RGYB (different timepoints) and two papers comparing obese vs. lean subjects, using a transcriptomic approach (Figure 1). However, from the obese vs. post-RGYB papers, two were discarded from this section (Latorre et al., 2018 and Gonzalez-Plaza et al., 2018), because they used microarray data already published by Ortega et al., 2015 and Gonzalez-Plaza et al., 2016.

For this section, we selected all the genes that had a differential expression with a p-value $\leq 1 \times 10^{-8}$.

3.2.1. SAT Differential Gene Expression between Post-RYGB vs. Obese from Microarrays

From the microarray reported by Gonzalez-Plaza et al., 2016, we obtained 2 genes upregulated and 85 downregulated in samples from 2 years post-RYGB compared to obese [42]. Ortega et al., 2015 analyzed samples of obese vs. 2 years post-RYGB. The raw data that we extracted from this microarray showed 21 genes overexpressed and 61 downregulated in post-RYGB [48]. In addition, Liu et al., 2016 studied samples of 1 year post-surgery vs. obesity and we obtained a 369 upregulated and 606 downregulated in post-surgery [45].

3.2.2. SAT Differential Gene Expression between Post-RYGB or Lean vs. Obese from Microarrays

From the microarray reported by Petrus et al., 2018, we obtained 710 genes for 2 years post-RYGB (216 upregulated and 494 downregulated in post-RYGB) [49]. From another database from Kerr et al., 2020, we obtained 1259 genes for 2 years post-RYGB (342 upregulated and 917 downregulated in post-RYGB) and for 5 years post-RYGB, we extracted 1117 genes (213 upregulated and 904 downregulated in post-RYGB) [32].

We then intersected all these genes obtained from microarrays and selected those that were reported in at least 2 papers. We obtained 86 genes differentially expressed in SAT samples between post-RYGB vs. obese.

3.2.3. SAT Differential Gene Expression between Lean vs. Obese from Microarrays

Once we had these 86 genes, we searched them in the raw data from microarrays comparing lean vs. obese published [32,51,52]. We discarded 5 genes, because their expression values were not available [52].

For the 81 genes left, we performed a Gene Ontology analysis (GEO), classifying these genes in different metabolic pathways: lipid and aminoacid metabolism, glycerol transport, acetyl-COA and acyl-COA metabolic process, cell surface, signaling transduction, apoptosis signaling. In addition, most of the genes were classified on inflammation and immune system pathways such as: anti-inflammatory response, innate immune system, inflammation mediated by chemokine and cytokine signaling, interleukins signaling, leukocyte activation and involve in immune response, regulation of leukocyte differentiation, antigen processing cross presentation, neutrophil degranulation, phagocytic cells, and regulation of cytokine production (Figure 4).

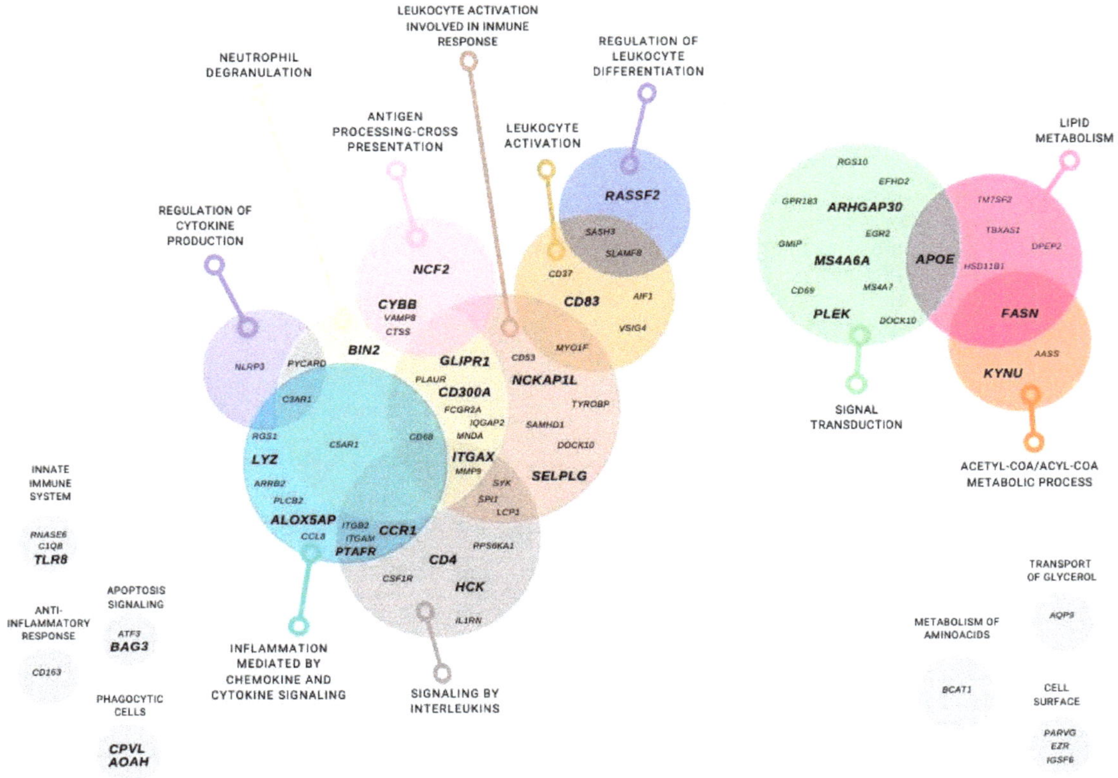

Figure 4. Subcutaneous adipose tissue differentially expressed genes using a transcriptomic gene approach. Genes that were differentially expressed in at least two microarrays in post-RYGB vs. obese and were found in lean vs. obese are represented. Gene classification by function: lipid and aminoacid metabolism, glycerol transport, acetyl-COA and acyl-COA metabolic process, cell surface, signaling transduction, apoptosis signaling. In addition, inflammation and immune system pathways such as: anti-inflammatory response, innate immune system, inflammation mediated by chemokine and cytokine signaling, interleukins signaling, leukocyte activation and involve in immune response, regulation of leukocyte differentiation, antigen processing cross presentation, neutrophil degranulation, phagocytic cells, and regulation of cytokine production.

After the genes were classified into different pathways, we then analyzed the expression data of lean vs. obese. We discarded 55 genes, because they showed contrary expression levels in lean subjects within different studies.

We ended with 26 genes that are summarized in Table 2. Fold change expression among lean, obese, and post-RYGB (different timepoints) is presented on Table S3. Then, the expression levels of each gene were plotted, representing lean, obese and post-RYGB different timepoints.

Table 2. Summary of transcriptomic genes differentially expressed in subcutaneous adipose tissue among lean, obese and post-RGYB.

Pathways	Gene Abbreviation	Gene Name
Lipids metabolism	*FASN*	Fatty Acid Synthase
	APOE	Apolipoprotein E
Innate immune system	*TLR8*	Toll like receptor 8
Inflammation mediated by chemokine and cytokine signaling pathway	*ALOX5AP*	Arachidonate 5-lipoxygenase activating protein
	PTAFR	Platelet activating factor receptor
	CCR1	Chemokine, cc motif, receptor 1
	LYZ	Lysozyme
Signaling by interleukins	*ITGAX*	Integrin Subunit Alpha X
	HCK	HCK proto-oncogene, Src family tyrosine kinase
	CD4	Antigen CD4
Leukocyte activation	*CD83*	Antigen CD83
Leukocyte activation involved in immune response	*NCKAP1L*	NCK Associated Protein 1 Like
	SELPLG	Selectin P ligand
Regulation of leukocyte differentiation	*RASSF2*	Ras association domain family member 2
Antigen processing-cross presentation	*NCF2*	Neutrophil cytosolic factor 2
	CYBB	Cytochrome b (−245), beta subunit
Neutrophil degranulation	*BIN2*	Bridging Integrator 2
	CD300A	CD300a molecule
	GLIPR1	Glioma pathogenesis-related protein 1
Phagocytic cells	*CPVL*	Carboxypeptidase Vitellogenic Like
	AOAH	Acyloxyacyl hydrolase
Apoptosis signaling pathway	*BAG3*	BAG cochaperone 3
Signaling transduction	*ARHGAP30*	Rho GTPase activating protein 30
	MS4A6A	Membrane-spanning 4-domains, subfamily A, member 6A
	PLEK	Pleckstrin
Acetyl-CoA/Acyl-CoA metabolic process	*KYNU*	Kynureninase

We identified only two genes implicated in lipid metabolism (*FASN* and *APOE*) that were overexpressed in lean compared to obese, and after RYGB the expression was reverted to even higher expression levels (Figure 5, panels 1,2). Interestingly, the rest of the genes showed lower expression in lean, increased in obese, and were downregulated after RYGB involved in: innate immune system (*TLR8*, Figure 5, panel 3), inflammation mediated by chemokine and cytokine signaling pathway (*ALOX5AP, PTAFR, CCR1, LYZ,* Figure 5, panels 4–7), signaling by interleukins (*ITGAX, HCK, CD4,* Figure 5, panels 8–10), leukocyte activation involved in immune response (*CD83, NCKAP1L, SELPLG,* Figure 5, panels 11–13), phagocytic cells (*CPVL, AOAH,* Figure 5, panels 20, 21), regulation of leukocyte differentiation (*RASSF2,* Figure 5, panel 14), neutrophil degranulation (*BIN2, GLIPR1, CD300A,* Figure 5, panels 17–19), antigen processing-cross presentation (*CYBB, NCF2,* Figure 5, panels 15,16), acetyl-CoA/Acyl-CoA metabolic process (*KYNU,* Figure 5, panel 26), signaling transduction (*ARHGAP30, MS4A6A, PLEK,* Figure 5, panel 23–25), and apoptosis signaling (BAG3, Figure 5, panel 22).

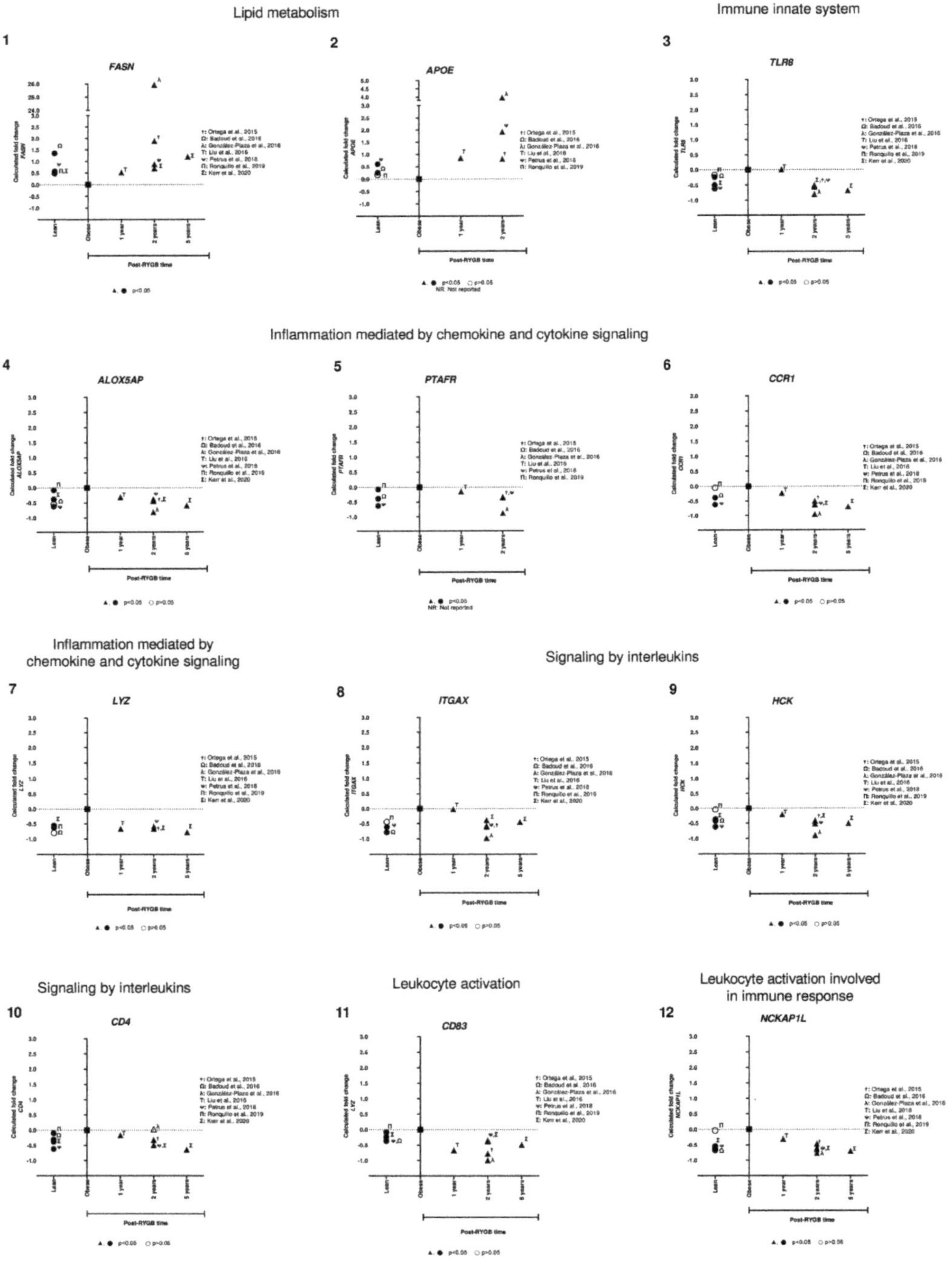

Figure 5. *Cont.*

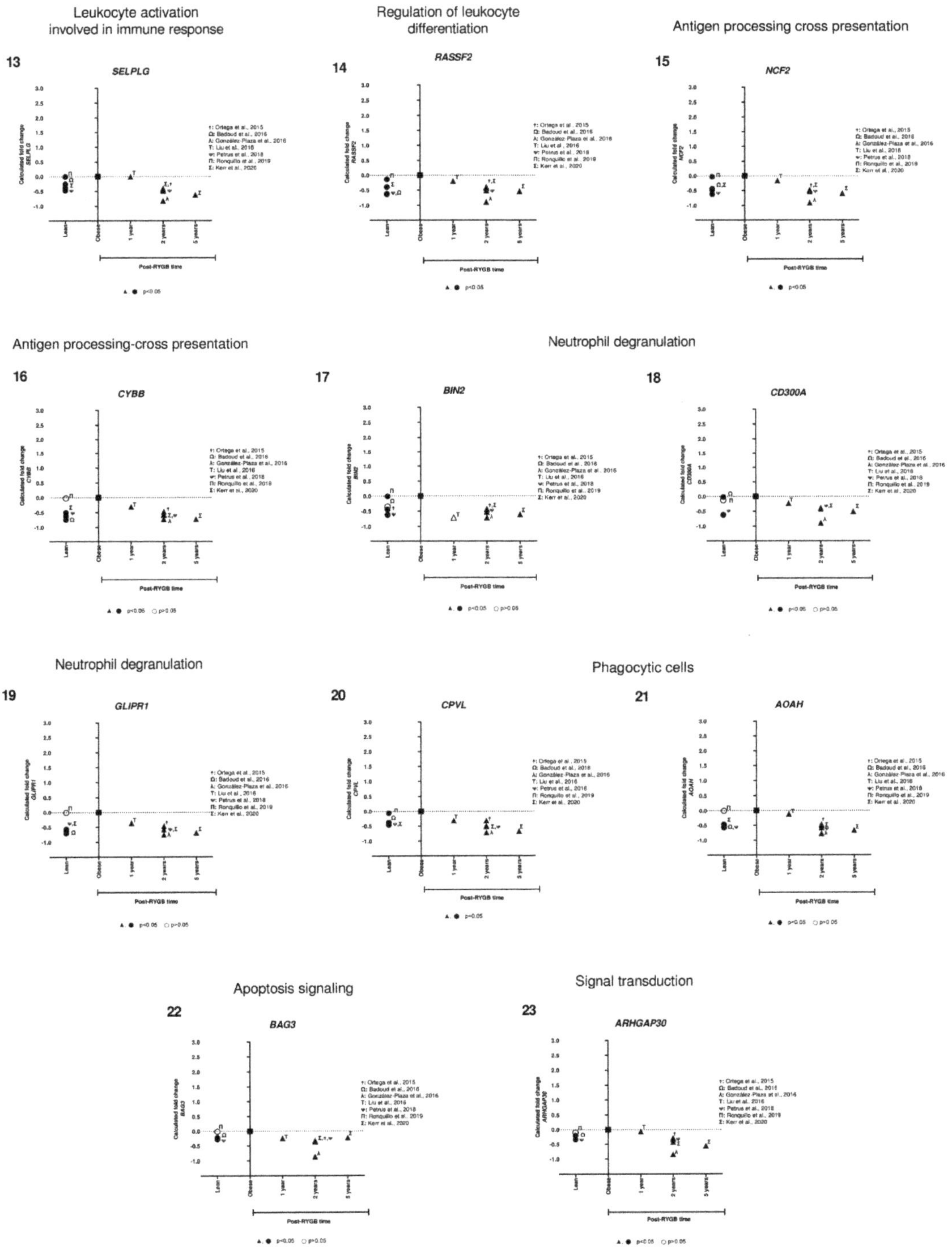

Figure 5. *Cont.*

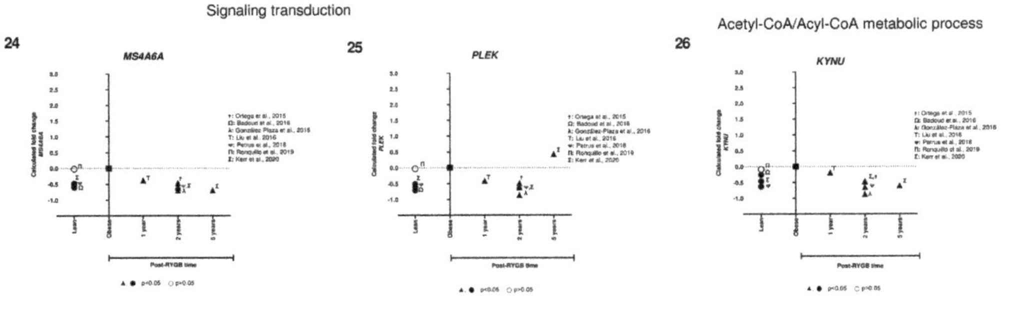

Figure 5. Subcutaneous adipose tissue transcriptomic gene expression among lean, obese, and post-RYGB (different timepoints). Comparison of expression levels of each gene among different studies, identified by the author (ϯ: [47]; Ω: [51]; λ: [41]; T: [44]; Ψ: [48]; Π: [50]; Σ: [32]). Calculated fold change was significant (p-value < 0.05, ▲, •) or not (p-value > 0.05, △, ○).

In general, we observed that expression levels of all these genes were lower in lean compared to obese samples. However, one-year post-RYGB, downregulation of all these genes was similar to lean expression level. Moreover, after 2 years post-RYGB, the expression of these genes reduced even more compared to obese and 1-year post-RYGB (Figure 5).

4. Discussion

To our knowledge, this is the first systematic review that compares SAT expression levels between lean and obese (before and after RYGB different timepoints).

In the past decades, bariatric surgery has become an effective intervention to lose weight and revert type 2 diabetes or dyslipidemias. A recent meta-analysis showed that RGYB was one of the most effective bariatric procedures, improving metabolic parameters, such as insulin sensitivity and serum lipids [53]. However, the underlying mechanisms promoting such metabolic changes are unknown, as well as the impact that it exerts over different organs that regulate metabolism, such as AT. In addition, several authors have demonstrated that important adipocyte function features are modified after RYGB, i.e., decreased adipocyte volume [49] (along with decreased lipolysis, immune response and inflammation.

Therefore, the aim of this systematic review was to collect data from SAT gene expression among lean, obese and post-RYGB to start dissecting the pathways and genes influencing obesity establishment and massive weight loss after bariatric surgery.

4.1. Candidate Gene Approach

From gene candidate approach, we show that metabolic pathways associated with obesity development and weight loss after bariatric surgery include glucose and lipid metabolism, adipogenesis, endocrine function, and inflammation.

Regarding glucose metabolism, glucose uptake in target cells requires insulin binding to its receptor causing downstream activation of signaling molecules as insulin receptor substrate-1 (IRS-1). After IRS1 activation, GLUT4 can be translocated to the membrane to promote glucose internalization. IRS-1 and GLUT4 expression in AT is typically decreased in obesity and associated with insulin resistance [34,42–44,48,54–56]. Our findings are consistent with this observation since the expression of *IRS-1* and *GLUT4* is lower in obese individuals. After RYGB, both *IRS-1* and *GLUT4* expression was increased at 6 months, 2, and 5 years. Thus, while insulin signaling molecules expression are decreased in obesity, RYGB increases such expression. After six months, 2, and 5 years insulin sensitivity is augmented and diabetes remission occurs [28,57].

Apart from glucose metabolism, lipid metabolism is also modified after bariatric surgery. ACSL1 (acyl-CoA synthetase long chain family member 1) induces lipid transport and accumulation in adipocytes [58]. These effects are associated with increased insulin sensitivity, since lipid storage in AT prevents lipid accumulation in non-adipose organs. Also, FASN (fatty acid synthase) is a molecular complex that allows fatty acid synthesis from acetyl-CoA [59]. Normally, lipogenesis in AT during obesity is decreased due to chronic energy excess. We found that the expression of both genes was decreased in obese in comparison with lean subjects, and reverted 2 and 5 years after RYGB, suggesting that adipose lipogenesis concurs with metabolic improvements driven by the surgery. On the other hand, lipolysis, which is the hydrolysis of triglycerides to fatty acids and glycerol has been found increased in AT of obese subjects leading to higher circulating levels of free fatty acids. Aquaporins are glycerol and water transporters in AT and liver. Evidence shows that aquaporin 9 (AQP9) could be implicated in adipose lipolysis during obesity conditions [60,61] because lean subjects have decreased *AQP9* expression in contrast to obese patients. After 2 and 5 years of *RYGB, AQP9* expression is decreased. Thus, the expression of key molecules involved in lipid metabolism is significantly modified after bariatric surgery, with downregulation of lipolysis and upregulation of lipogenesis, which is similar to metabolism in fat depots of lean subjects.

The transcription factor PPARγ is also implied in lipid metabolism promoting the expression of lipogenic enzymes; however, its main role is to regulate adipogenesis [62]. Since obesity requires adequate energy storage, the recruitment of new adipocytes represents a metabolic advantage. Nevertheless, as chronic energy consumption becomes excessive, the expression of PPARγ and consequent adipogenesis is decreased. These observations are here reflected, since lean subjects have increased PPARγ expression [47,50]. In post-RYGB patients, expression of *PPAR*γ after 3–12 months is either down or upregulated, however, 2–5 years after RYGB, this expression appears to be increased. Thus, long-term overexpression of *PPAR*γ is consistent with the decreased cell size phenomenon observed after RYGB [27].

One target gene of PPARγ is *ADIPOQ*, which is the most abundant adipokine in circulation. ADIPOQ generates anti-inflammatory effects and is decreased in serum of obese subjects. In fact, hypoadiponectinemia appears to play an important role in obesity-linked insulin resistance [63]. Here we show that *ADIPOQ* expression in AT of lean was lightly increased compared to obese individuals. Also, *ADIPOQ* was 4–8 times overexpressed after 3–6 months of undergoing RYGB. Nevertheless, 2–5 years after RYGB, *ADIPOQ* expression is decreased in comparison with earlier timepoints, but still higher than in obese patients. Finally, short and long-term overexpression of *ADIPOQ* after RYGB could partly explain improved insulin sensitivity and anti-inflammatory processes.

Chronic low-grade inflammation is a feature of obesity, with many related events occurring in AT [64]. The expression of inflammatory markers as CD68, IL-6, TNFα and lysozyme is increased during obesity and associated with insulin resistance [65–70]. On the other hand, the lower expression of such factors is related with improved adipocyte function [66,71,72]. We found that the expression of these markers was upregulated in obese individuals and downregulated in post-RYGB patients, especially after 2–5 years. In the short term (before 1 year after RYGB), mixed results regarding up-or downregulation of inflammatory markers was observed. These results suggest that RYGB reduces AT inflammation.

Interestingly, another systematic review analyzed SAT gene expression after lifestyle interventions (diet, exercise, etc.). They observed that *LEP* was downregulated and *ADIPOQ* was upregulated after lifestyle interventions [73]. In our study, LEP was not in the intersected genes, but we observed that *ADIPOQ* was also increased after RYGB. Moreover, for *TNF-α* and *IL-6* expression after lifestyle interventions had contradictory effects [73]. However, our findings showed that for lean subjects the expression was contradictory, but after RYGB both genes were clearly downregulated. This means that weight loss, independent of metabolic modifications driven by the surgery, could regulate gene expression of adipokines, proinflammatory cytokines, among others.

In summary, gene candidate studies show that post-RYGB AT expression reflects a "healthy metabolism" while augmenting insulin-sensitizing molecules, inducing lipogenesis over lipolysis, and downregulating inflammation. Such healthy metabolism is reflected by modification of several genes implicated in these pathways which are reverted few months after RYGB and maintained up to 5 years.

4.2. *Transcriptomic Gene Approach*

As mentioned above, the candidate gene approach is limited to the knowledge of the gene's function. However, a transcriptomic approach could lead to the discovery of new pathways or genes involved in the AT functionality.

Our results from the transcriptomic approach showed several pathways involved in lipid metabolism (*FASN, APOE*), innate immune system (*TLR8*), inflammation mediated by chemokine and cytokine signaling pathway (*LYZ, CCR1, ALOX5AP, PTAFR*), signaling by interleukins (*ITGAX, CD4, HCK*), leukocyte activation involved in immune response (*CD83, NCKAP1L, SELPLG*), among others.

We compared the genes from candidate and transcriptomic approach. We identified *CD68* and *AQP9* as candidate genes, but during the transcriptomic analysis, these two genes were part of the 81 differentially expressed genes discarded due to their contradictory expression levels in lean vs. obese subjects. However, *FASN* and *LYZ* were common in both approaches, suggesting an important implication of both genes in AT metabolism in lean and post-RYGB compared to obesity. Moreover, *FASN* is involved in lipogenesis and is downregulated in obese SAT compared to lean and post-RYGB, as explained before. Another gene implicated in lipid metabolism is *APOE*, which controls lipoprotein metabolism. *APOE* is expressed and secreted by adipocytes [74]. *APOE* KO mice present smaller adipocytes and downregulation of lipogenic genes, as well as hypercholesterolemia and atherosclerotic lesions [75,76]. Our results showed higher expression of *APOE* in lean compared to obese and it was upregulated at 1 and 2 years post-RYGB. It has been reported that adipocyte volume is reduced post-RYGB [49]. The exact role of *APOE* in AT and this inverse correlation between expression level and size of the adipocyte has not yet been explained, therefore, it would be important to explore the role of *APOE* in SAT during weight gain and loss

Besides these two genes involved in lipid metabolism, most of the genes that we obtained in our analysis were related to different phases of the innate or adaptative immune response and inflammation. Obesity is characterized by a low-grade chronic inflammation and the mechanism by which the immune response leads to AT hypertrophy remains to be fully elucidated. In addition, little is known of the mechanism by which AT diminishes its size after bariatric surgery. Our transcriptomic results showed common immune response pathways between the expandability and reduction of the AT by comparing lean, obese and post-RYGB are explained below.

First, the initiation of the innate immune response starts with the Toll-like receptors (TLR), which are responsible for the recognition of pathogens or molecular patterns of cellular stress; then, a signaling cascade recruits and activates leukocytes and macrophages [77]. In particular, our results showed that *TLR8* expression was higher in obese SAT compared to lean, as previously reported [78]. *TLR8* has been positively correlated with levels of *IL-6*, *TNFα*, and *CD68* [78]. Interestingly, after bariatric surgery, all these markers were downregulated as well as *TLR8* expression. This suggests that during obesity, *TLR8* must be present to initiate the activation of the immune system, responsible for AT expansion. On the contrary, upon AT size reduction, TLR8 is downregulated at 2 and 5 years post-RYGB, reducing inflammation and AT remodeling.

After the initiation of the immune response, then the secretion of cytokines such as chemokines and interleukins will lead to the mobilization of the leukocytes and macrophages, also known as chemiotaxis, to the site of inflammation. *ALOX5AP* (arachidonate 5-lipoxygenase activating protein) is involved in the synthesis of leukotrienes from arachidonic acid as part of a proinflammatory system. This protein acts together with

ALOX5 to oxygenate and dehydrate fatty acids by sequential reactions, to finally obtain leukotriene B4, which is a chemiotactic molecule. Pharmacological inhibition of ALOX5AP provoked decreased macrophage infiltration, reduced TNF-α, IL6, and free fatty acid concentrations, resulting in a beneficial response [79]. Our results showed that *ALOX5AP* was upregulated in obesity compared to lean and post-RYGB, suggesting that its downregulation, starting at 1-year and maintained up to 5-years post-RYGB, could be responsible for a better AT functionality. Similar expression results were obtained for *PTAFR* (platelet activating factor receptor), which is another chemotactic mediator, involved in angiogenesis and inflammation, but their specific function in AT is still unknown.

Afterwards, the chemokines bind to their specific receptors, for example, CCR1 (chemokine receptor 1). *CCR1* is highly expressed in AT derived stromal cells, participating in the multipotency of these cells and inflammation/migration mediated by chemokine signaling pathway [80]. *CCR1* is highly expressed in obese fat tissue [81], consistent with our results. Moreover, *CCR1* downregulation at 1 and 2 years post-RGYB suggests that macrophage migration would be reduced, as well as inflammation.

A gene that modulates chemokines as well as chemokines receptors is *LYZ*. *LYZ* codes for the lysozyme, generating a proper innate immune system response [82]. *LYZ* was one of the genes that we obtained by the candidate and transcriptomic approach. Our results showed that, *LYZ* was overexpressed in obese AT compared to lean. After 1 year and up to 5 years post-RYGB, its expression was reverted to similar levels of lean AT. *LYZ* function in AT has recently been dissected, demonstrating upregulation in diet-induced obese mice, and being positively correlated with *IL-6* and *TNF-α* (pro-inflammatory cytokines), and *ITGAX* and *CCR2* (macrophage markers). Consistently, when *LYZ* was knockdowned in those animals, increased adipogenesis, decreased inflammation, and improvement of AT functions were observed [72]. This is congruent with our results, where we demonstrated that after RYGB, *LYZ* was downregulated (after 1-year and maintained up to 5-years post-RYGB), as well as *IL-6*, *TNF-α*, and *ITGAX*, indicating that *LYZ* is important for the adequate AT functionality.

ITGAX (integrin subunit alpha X) is a member of the integrin family. It is important for chemotaxis and monocyte adhesion, as well as a macrophage marker. During inflammatory responses, *ITGAX* mediates cell-cell interaction. In endothelial cells, *ITGAX* stimulates proliferation, migration and tumor angiogenesis [83]. Our results showed that *ITGAX* expression levels were lower in lean, overexpressed in obese, and downregulated at 2 and 5 years post-RYGB, showing that bariatric surgery reverts its expression. However, its exact function in AT is not yet understood. Another macrophage marker is *HCK* (hemopoietic cell kinase), a member of the Src family of tyrosine kinases. It is expressed in myeloid cells and highly expressed in macrophages. It has been implicated in the signaling of cell surface receptors, regulation of the innate immune response, release of inflammatory molecules, phagocytosis, mobilization of secretory lysosomes, and activation of the NRLP3 (NLR family pyrin domain containing 3) inflammasome [84]. *HCK* is important for macrophage activation and the TNF-α secretion, involved in diabetes progression [85]. Our results showed that *HCK* was downregulated in lean, increased in obese, and reverted to lean levels, after 1 year and maintained up to 5-years post-RYGB. Therefore, this suggests that the macrophage marker, *HCK*, is downregulated in lean and post-RYGB, because of reduced macrophage number.

In addition, adaptive immune response is also regulated during AT expansion and reduction (lean to obese and post-RYGB). One of the genes implicated in this adaptive immune response is *CD4* (CD4 antigen), which encodes a glycoprotein that serves as a surface marker of T-cell and dendritic cells. The CD4+ T-cell surface glycoprotein has been considered another crosstalk molecule between AT and immune system. CD4+ T-cells could secrete pro-inflammatory cytokines, such as interferon (IFN)-γ and IL-17 that will stimulate M1 macrophages, leading to the secretion of IL-6 and TNF-α. On the other hand, CD4+ T-cells could also secrete anti-inflammatory factors (IL-4 or IL-10). Nevertheless, the exact implication of CD4 in AT inflammation is yet to be determined [86]. High *CD4* expression has been associated with higher BMI and obesity-related diseases [87], similar to what we observed in our results between obese vs. lean comparison. Interestingly, this gene was downregulated 1 year after RYGB, and diminished even more at 2 and 5 years post-RYGB. It is plausible that the number of T-cells and dendritic cells decrease after bariatric surgery, as well as their marker *CD4*, but more research is needed to understand its implication in AT functionality.

Another maturation dendritic cell marker and B-cell marker is *CD83* antigen (activated B lymphocytes, immunoglobulin superfamily) [88]. Our results demonstrated that *CD83* is downregulated in lean and post-RYGB (starting at 1-year and maintained up to 5-years) compared to obesity. However, its function in AT is yet to be discovered.

Our results showed several genes implicated in other pathways as: leukocyte activation involved in immune response (*NCKAP1L, SELPLG*), regulation of leukocyte differentiation (*RASSF2*), antigen processing-cross presentation (*CYBB, NCF2*), neutrophil degranulation (*BIN2, GLIPR1, CD300A*), phagocytic cells (*CPVL, AOAH*), apoptosis signaling (*BAG3*), signaling transduction (*ARHGAP30, MS4A6A, PLEK*), acetyl-CoA/Acyl-CoA metabolic process (*KYNU*). Most of these genes were downregulated in lean, overexpressed in obese, and reverted its expression after 1-year post-RYGB and continuing to reduce its expression at 2 and 5-years after surgery. However, their implication in AT expandability, as well as their specific function in AT is still unknown. Therefore, this opens the horizon of possibilities to explore new pathways and genes and better understand the mechanism how the AT is modulated during the establishment of obesity and during weight loss.

Recently, two studies performed a similar analysis to what we presented in this review. The study performed by Liu et al., 2020, used two database: (1) Hoggard et al., 2012 (obese vs. vertical banded gastroplasty, comparing SAT vs. omental VAT) and (2) Petrus et al., 2018, as previously reported [49,89]. The authors reported similar GO enrichment pathways to our results, such as toll-like receptor signaling pathway, chemokine and cytokine signaling pathway, leukocyte migration and chemotaxis, among others. Moreover, they further analyzed genes methylation and miRNA interaction [90]. The common genes between our study and Liu's are: *AQP9*, *TLR8* and *HCK*.

The second study performed by Chen et al., 2022, used the database from Hoggard et al., 2012, Ortega et al., 2015, Liu et al., 2016, and Petrus et al., 2018, also obtaining similar results to ours. They showed that the enriched pathways were mainly related to inflammatory response, secretion, defense response, toll-like receptor binding, arachidonic acid binding, neutrophil degranulation and neutrophil activation involved in immune response, among others. In addition, they focused their search on the immunomodulation and immune cell infiltration [91]. The common genes between our analysis and Chen′s were: *AQP9*, *LYZ*, and *APOE*. Even though we found common genes with these two studies, we have to highlight the differences: in our study, we did not consider Hoggard et al., 2022 database, because it did not meet our inclusion criteria. These two papers only compared obese vs. post-bariatric surgery; however, our analysis compared lean vs. obese vs. post-RYGB. Therefore, our results highlight SAT differential expression pathways during gaining or losing weight at different timepoints post-RYGB.

In summary, genes involved in lipid metabolism are highly expressed in SAT from lean, reduced in obese, and upregulated after RYGB (1-year and increased even more after 2-years). In addition, genes involved in several phases of the innate and adaptive immune response are downregulated in lean subjects, elevated in obese and reduced post-RYGB (1-year and further downregulated at 2 and 5-years after surgery).

4.3. Strength and Limitation of the Study

The strength of this systematic review was the comparison between two different approaches (candidate and transcriptomic), obtaining a few genes in common. From the transcriptomic approach, we obtained new genes that need be studied to understand their implication in AT functionality. Moreover, the comparisons performed between lean vs.

obese and obese vs. post-RYGB highlight the shared pathways and genes of AT plasticity required for weight gain or loss. In addition, showing the gene expression through different timepoints leads to the understanding of processes that happen as acute response, due to body weight loss, or chronic response as the result of sustained weight. Nevertheless, our systematic review has some limitations that must be acknowledge: (1) the candidate approach only identified genes with known functions; (2) each paper reported different sampling timepoints of post-RYGB; therefore, we calculated the fold change from raw databases to compare expression values among studies. Moreover, we could not have the expression of all the genes at all the timepoints reported in several papers; (3) we could not perform meta-analysis, because of the heterogeneity of the samples (individuals number, age, BMI, etc.) and distinct sampling timepoints; (4) several papers did not report the ethnicity of the patients from whom the samples were taken; (5) diet and nutritional data from the patients before sampling is not here described because information was not available, but all the samples were taken under fasting conditions. However, we perform the risk of bias for each paper included in this review and we observed that each one is of high scientific quality, concluding that the results that we present in this manuscript are reliable.

In this systematic review, we summarized the differential gene expression in SAT by comparing lean, obese and post-RYGB. However, we noticed that most of the studies were performed using samples of 1, 2 or 5-years after RYGB. In the future, it would be interesting to perform more studies using samples of previous timepoints, as 1, 3, 6, or 9 months post-RYGB, to understand the acute response on gene expression after this surgery.

5. Conclusions

This review summarizes the gene expression patterns in SAT of lean, obese and post-RYGB patients. We conclude obesity leads to adipose tissue dysfunction by promoting impaired adipogenesis and adipokine secretion, increased lipolysis over lipogenesis, insulin resistance, immune response, and inflammation. However, RYGB reverts these effects switching the "unhealthy" features of AT metabolism into a functional version of this organ. These effects are reflected by reverting gene expression post-RYGB, starting 1 year and maintaining such expression up to 5-years after the surgery.

Supplementary Materials: The following supporting information can be downloaded at: https://www.mdpi.com/article/10.3390/nu14224925/s1, Figure S1. Risk of bias graph; Table S1. Characteristics of all the studies included in this systematic review; File S1. Raw expression levels of the genes extracted from different microarrays post-RYGB vs. obese and lean vs. obese; Table S2. Summary of the genes with differential expression in subcutaneous adipose tissue using a candidate gene approach; Table S3. Summary of the genes that are differential expression subcutaneous adipose tissue using a transcriptomic gene approach.

Author Contributions: Data acquisition, E.M.C.-G.; data analysis, E.M.C.-G. and R.G.-A.; data interpretation, M.E.F. and R.G.-A.; writing, M.E.F. and R.G.-A.; review and editing, E.M.C.-G., M.E.F., S.C.-Q. and R.G.-A.; conceptualization and funding acquisition: R.G.-A. All authors have read and agreed to the published version of the manuscript.

Funding: This work was funded by Programa de Apoyo a Proyectos de Investigación e Innovación Tecnológica (PAPIIT grant number IA203919)/Dirección General de Asuntos del Personal Académico (DGAPA)/Universidad Nacional Autónoma de México (UNAM); División de Investigación de la Facultad de Medicina, UNAM; Hospital Infantil de México Federico Gómez (grant number HIM/2018/028 SSA. 1494); and partially supported by CONACyT-FOSSIS 289699.

Institutional Review Board Statement: Not applicable.

Informed Consent Statement: Not applicable.

Data Availability Statement: Complete data as raw values from the microarrays, reported and calculated gene expression, gene expression fold change, among others, can be found in Supplementary Materials.

Conflicts of Interest: The authors declare no conflict of interest. The funders had no role in the design of the study; in the collection, analyses, or interpretation of data; in the writing of the manuscript; or in the decision to publish the results.

References

1. OMS Obesidad y Sobrepeso. Available online: https://www.who.int/es/news-room/fact-sheets/detail/obesity-and-overweight (accessed on 16 January 2022).
2. Health Effects of Overweight and Obesity in 195 Countries over 25 Years. *N. Engl. J. Med.* **2017**, *377*, 13–27. [CrossRef] [PubMed]
3. Von Schnurbein, J.; Manzoor, J.; Brandt, S.; Denzer, F.; Kohlsdorf, K.; Fischer-Posovszky, P.; Weißenberger, M.; Frank-Podlech, S.; Mahmood, S.; Wabitsch, M. Leptin Is Not Essential for Obesity-Associated Hypertension. *Obes. Facts* **2019**, *12*, 460–475. [CrossRef] [PubMed]
4. Song, Z.; Xiaoli, A.M.; Yang, F. Regulation and metabolic significance of De Novo lipogenesis in adipose tissues. *Nutrients* **2018**, *10*, 1383. [CrossRef] [PubMed]
5. Birsoy, K.; Festuccia, W.T.; Laplante, M. A comparative perspective on lipid storage in animals. *J. Cell Sci.* **2013**, *126*, 1541–1552. [CrossRef] [PubMed]
6. Yu, B.L.; Zhao, S.P.; Hu, J.R. Cholesterol imbalance in adipocytes: A possible mechanism of adipocytes dysfunction in obesity. *Obes. Rev.* **2010**, *11*, 560–567. [CrossRef]
7. Basu, S.K.; Ho, Y.K.; Brown, M.S.; Bilheimer, D.W.; Anderson, R.G.; Goldstein, J.L. Biochemical and genetic studies of the apoprotein E secreted by mouse macrophages and human monocytes. *J. Biol. Chem.* **1982**, *257*, 9788–9795. [CrossRef]
8. Yamauchi, T.; Kamon, J.; Minokoshi, Y.; Ito, Y.; Waki, H.; Uchida, S.; Yamashita, S.; Noda, M.; Kita, S.; Ueki, K.; et al. Adiponectin stimulates glucose utilization and fatty-acid oxidation by activating AMP-activated protein kinase. *Nat. Med.* **2002**, *8*, 1288–1295. [CrossRef]
9. Takemura, Y.; Ouchi, N.; Shibata, R.; Aprahamian, T.; Kirber, M.T.; Summer, R.S.; Kihara, S.; Walsh, K. Adiponectin modulates inflammatory reactions via calreticulin receptor-dependent clearance of early apoptotic bodies. *J. Clin. Investig.* **2007**, *117*, 375–386. [CrossRef]
10. Bays, H.E.; González-Campoy, J.M.; Bray, G.A.; Kitabchi, A.E.; Bergman, D.A.; Schorr, A.B.; Rodbard, H.W.; Henry, R.R. Pathogenic potential of adipose tissue and metabolic consequences of adipocyte hypertrophy and increased visceral adiposity. *Expert Rev. Cardiovasc. Ther.* **2008**, *6*, 343–368. [CrossRef]
11. Orsso, C.E.; Colin-Ramirez, E.; Field, C.J.; Madsen, K.L.; Prado, C.M.; Haqq, A.M. Adipose Tissue Development and Expansion from the Womb to Adolescence: An Overview. *Nutrients* **2020**, *12*, 2735. [CrossRef]
12. Hausman, G.J.; Hausman, D.B. Search for the preadipocyte progenitor cell. *J. Clin. Investig.* **2006**, *116*, 3103–3106. [CrossRef] [PubMed]
13. Herold, J.; Kalucka, J. Angiogenesis in Adipose Tissue: The Interplay Between Adipose and Endothelial Cells. *Front. Physiol.* **2021**, *11*, 624903. [CrossRef] [PubMed]
14. Klöting, N.; Fasshauer, M.; Dietrich, A.; Kovacs, P.; Schön, M.R.; Kern, M.; Stumvoll, M.; Blüher, M. Insulin-sensitive obesity. *Am. J. Physiol.-Endocrinol. Metab.* **2010**, *299*, E506–E515. [CrossRef] [PubMed]
15. O'Connell, J.; Lynch, L.; Cawood, T.J.; Kwasnik, A.; Nolan, N.; Geoghegan, J.; McCormick, A.; O'Farrelly, C.; O'Shea, D. The relationship of omental and subcutaneous adipocyte size to metabolic disease in severe obesity. *PLoS ONE* **2010**, *5*, e9997. [CrossRef]
16. Primeau, V.; Coderre, L.; Karelis, A.D.; Brochu, M.; Lavoie, M.E.; Messier, V.; Sladek, R.; Rabasa-Lhoret, R. Characterizing the profile of obese patients who are metabolically healthy. *Int. J. Obes.* **2011**, *35*, 971–981. [CrossRef]
17. Vishvanath, L.; Gupta, R.K. Contribution of adipogenesis to healthy adipose tissue expansion in obesity. *J. Clin. Investig.* **2019**, *129*, 4022–4031. [CrossRef]
18. Gustafson, B.; Hedjazifar, S.; Gogg, S.; Hammarstedt, A.; Smith, U. Insulin resistance and impaired adipogenesis. *Trends Endocrinol. Metab.* **2015**, *26*, 193–200. [CrossRef]
19. Lee, M.J.; Wu, Y.; Fried, S.K. Adipose tissue remodeling in pathophysiology of obesity. *Curr. Opin. Clin. Nutr. Metab. Care* **2010**, *13*, 371–376. [CrossRef]
20. Sun, K.; Kusminski, C.M.; Scherer, P.E. Adipose tissue remodeling and obesity. *J. Clin. Investig.* **2011**, *121*, 2094–2101. [CrossRef]
21. Ferrante, A.W. The immune cells in adipose tissue. *Diabetes Obes. Metab.* **2013**, *15*, 34–38. [CrossRef]
22. Weisberg, S.P.; McCann, D.; Desai, M.; Rosenbaum, M.; Leibel, R.L.; Ferrante, A.W.J. Obesity is associated with macrophage accumulation in adipose tissue. *J. Clin. Investig.* **2003**, *112*, 1796–1808. [CrossRef] [PubMed]
23. Castoldi, A.; De Souza, C.N.; Saraiva Câmara, N.O.; Moraes-Vieira, P.M. The macrophage switch in obesity development. *Front. Immunol.* **2016**, *6*, 637. [CrossRef] [PubMed]
24. Unamuno, X.; Gómez-Ambrosi, J.; Rodríguez, A.; Becerril, S.; Frühbeck, G.; Catalán, V. Adipokine dysregulation and adipose tissue inflammation in human obesity. *Eur. J. Clin. Investig.* **2018**, *48*, e12997. [CrossRef] [PubMed]
25. Danforth, E.J. Failure of adipocyte differentiation causes type II diabetes mellitus? *Nat. Genet.* **2000**, *26*, 13. [CrossRef]
26. Vidal-Puig, A. Adipose tissue expandability, lipotoxicity and the metabolic syndrome. *Endocrinol. Nutr.* **2013**, *60*, 39–43. [CrossRef]

27. Frikke-Schmidt, H.; O'Rourke, R.W.; Lumeng, C.N.; Sandoval, D.A.; Seeley, R.J. Does bariatric surgery improve adipose tissue function? *Obes. Rev.* **2016**, *17*, 795–809. [CrossRef]
28. Baheeg, M.; Tag El-Din, M.; Labib, M.F.; Elgohary, S.A.; Hasan, A. Long-term durability of weight loss after bariatric surgery; a retrospective study. *Int. J. Surg. Open* **2021**, *28*, 37–40. [CrossRef]
29. Arterburn, D.E.; Courcoulas, A.P. Bariatric surgery for obesity and metabolic conditions in adults. *BMJ* **2014**, *349*, g3961. [CrossRef]
30. Chang, S.H.; Stoll, C.R.T.; Song, J.; Varela, J.E.; Eagon, C.J.; Colditz, G.A. The effectiveness and risks of bariatric surgery an updated systematic review and meta-analysis, 2003–2012. *JAMA Surg.* **2014**, *149*, 275–287. [CrossRef]
31. Ferraz-Bannitz, R.; Welendorf, C.R.; Coelho, P.O.; Salgado, W.; Nonino, C.B.; Beraldo, R.A.; Foss-Freitas, M.C. Bariatric surgery can acutely modulate ER-stress and inflammation on subcutaneous adipose tissue in non-diabetic patients with obesity. *Diabetol. Metab. Syndr.* **2021**, *13*, 1–11. [CrossRef]
32. Kerr, A.G.; Andersson, D.P.; Rydén, M.; Arner, P.; Dahlman, I. Long-term changes in adipose tissue gene expression following bariatric surgery. *J. Intern. Med.* **2020**, *288*, 219–233. [CrossRef] [PubMed]
33. Ji, G.; Li, W.; Li, P.; Tang, H.; Yu, Z.; Sun, X.; Li, R.; Zhu, L.; Zhu, S. Effect of Roux-en-Y Gastric Bypass for Patients with Type 2 Diabetes Mellitus and a BMI < 32.5 kg/m^2: A 6-Year Study in Chinese Patients. *Obes. Surg.* **2020**, *30*, 2631–2636. [CrossRef] [PubMed]
34. Katsogiannos, P.; Kamble, P.G.; Boersma, G.J.; Karlsson, F.A.; Lundkvist, P.; Sundbom, M.; Pereira, M.J.; Eriksson, J.W. Early Changes in Adipose Tissue Morphology, Gene Expression, and Metabolism After RYGB in Patients With Obesity and T2D. *J. Clin. Endocrinol. Metab.* **2019**, *104*, 2601–2613. [CrossRef] [PubMed]
35. Seridi, L.; Leo, G.C.; Lynis Dohm, G.; Pories, W.J.; Lenhard, J. Time course metabolome of Roux-en-Y gastric bypass confirms correlation between leptin, body weight and the microbiome. *PLoS ONE* **2018**, *13*, e0198156. [CrossRef]
36. Hoffstedt, J.; Andersson, D.P.; Hogling, D.E.; Theorell, J.; Näslund, E.; Thorell, A.; Ehrlund, A.; Rydén, M.; Arner, P. Long-term protective changes in adipose tissue after gastric bypass. *Diabetes Care* **2017**, *40*, 77–84. [CrossRef] [PubMed]
37. Page, M.J.; McKenzie, J.E.; Bossuyt, P.M.; Boutron, I.; Hoffmann, T.C.; Mulrow, C.D.; Shamseer, L.; Tetzlaff, J.M.; Akl, E.A.; Brennan, S.E.; et al. The PRISMA 2020 statement: An updated guideline for reporting systematic reviews. *BMJ* **2021**, *372*, 1–9. [CrossRef]
38. McGuinness, L.A.; Higgins, J.P.T. Risk-of-bias VISualization (robvis):An R package and Shiny web app for visualizingrisk-of-bias assessments. *Res. Synth. Methods* **2021**, *12*, 55–61. [CrossRef]
39. Karki, S.; Farb, M.G.; Myers, S.; Apovian, C.; Hess, D.T.; Gokce, N.; Sverdlov, A.L. Effect of Bariatric Weight Loss on the Adipose Lipolytic Transcriptome in Obese Humans. *Mediat. Inflamm.* **2015**, *2015*, 1–7. [CrossRef]
40. Ortega, F.J.; Vilallonga, R.; Xifra, G.; Sabater, M.; Ricart, W.; Fernández-Real, J.M. Bariatric surgery acutely changes the expression of inflammatory and lipogenic genes in obese adipose tissue. *Surg. Obes. Relat. Dis.* **2016**, *12*, 357–362. [CrossRef]
41. de Oliveira, B.A.P.; de Souza Pinhel, M.A.; Nicoletti, C.F.; de Oliveira, C.C.; Quinhoneiro, D.C.G.; Noronha, N.Y.; Fassini, P.G.; da Silva Júnior, W.A.; Junior, W.S.; Nonino, C.B. UCP2 and PLIN1 Expression Affects the Resting Metabolic Rate and Weight Loss on Obese Patients. *Obes. Surg.* **2017**, *27*, 343–348. [CrossRef]
42. González-Plaza, J.J.; Gutiérrez-Repiso, C.; García-Serrano, S.; Rodriguez-Pacheco, F.; Garrido-Sánchez, L.; Santiago-Fernández, C.; García-Arnés, J.; Moreno-Ruiz, F.J.; Rodríguez-Cañete, A.; García-Fuentes, E. Effect of Roux-en-Y gastric bypass-induced weight loss on the transcriptomic profiling of subcutaneous adipose tissue. *Surg. Obes. Relat. Dis.* **2016**, *12*, 257–263. [CrossRef] [PubMed]
43. González-Plaza, J.J.; Santiago-Fernández, C.; Gutiérrez-Repiso, C.; García-Serrano, S.; Rodriguez-Pacheco, F.; Ho-Plagaro, A.; Garrido-Sánchez, L.; Moreno-Ruiz, F.J.; Rodríguez-Cañete, A.; García-Fuentes, E. The changes in the transcriptomic profiling of subcutaneous adipose tissue after bariatric surgery depend on the insulin resistance state. *Surg. Obes. Relat. Dis.* **2018**, *14*, 1182–1191. [CrossRef] [PubMed]
44. Latorre, J.; Moreno-Navarrete, J.M.; Sabater, M.; Buxo, M.; Rodriguez-Hermosa, J.I.; Girones, J.; Fort, J.M.; Vilallonga, R.; Ricart, W.; Simo, R.; et al. Decreased TLR3 in Hyperplastic Adipose Tissue, Blood and Inflamed Adipocytes is Related to Metabolic Inflammation. *Cell. Physiol. Biochem.* **2018**, *51*, 1051–1068. [CrossRef] [PubMed]
45. Liu, Y.; Aron-Wisnewsky, J.; Marcelin, G.; Genser, L.; Le Naour, G.; Torcivia, A.; Bauvois, B.; Bouchet, S.; Pelloux, V.; Sasso, M.; et al. Accumulation and Changes in Composition of Collagens in Subcutaneous Adipose Tissue After Bariatric Surgery. *J. Clin. Endocrinol. Metab.* **2016**, *101*, 293–304. [CrossRef] [PubMed]
46. Jahansouz, C.; Serrot, F.J.; Frohnert, B.I.; Foncea, R.E.; Dorman, R.B.; Slusarek, B.; Leslie, D.B.; Bernlohr, D.A.; Ikramuddin, S. Roux-en-Y Gastric Bypass Acutely Decreases Protein Carbonylation and Increases Expression of Mitochondrial Biogenesis Genes in Subcutaneous Adipose Tissue. *Obes. Surg.* **2015**, *25*, 2376–2385. [CrossRef]
47. Jürets, A.; Itariu, B.K.; Keindl, M.; Prager, G.; Langer, F.; Grablowitz, V.; Zeyda, M.; Stulnig, T.M. Upregulated TNF Expression 1 Year After Bariatric Surgery Reflects a Cachexia-Like State in Subcutaneous Adipose Tissue. *Obes. Surg.* **2017**, *27*, 1514–1523. [CrossRef]
48. Ortega, F.J.; Mercader, J.M.; Moreno-Navarrete, J.M.; Nonell, L.; Puigdecanet, E.; Rodriquez-Hermosa, J.I.; Rovira, O.; Xifra, G.; Guerra, E.; Moreno, M.; et al. Surgery-Induced Weight Loss Is Associated With the Downregulation of Genes Targeted by MicroRNAs in Adipose Tissue. *J. Clin. Endocrinol. Metab.* **2015**, *100*, E1467–E1476. [CrossRef]

49. Petrus, P.; Mejhert, N.; Corrales, P.; Lecoutre, S.; Li, Q.; Maldonado, E.; Kulyté, A.; Lopez, Y.; Campbell, M.; Acosta, J.R.; et al. Transforming Growth Factor-β3 Regulates Adipocyte Number in Subcutaneous White Adipose Tissue. *Cell Rep.* **2018**, *25*, 551–560. [CrossRef]
50. Matulewicz, N.; Stefanowicz, M.; Nikołajuk, A.; Karczewska-Kupczewska, M. Markers of Adipogenesis, but Not Inflammation, in Adipose Tissue Are Independently Related to Insulin Sensitivity. *J. Clin. Endocrinol. Metab.* **2017**, *102*, 3040–3049. [CrossRef]
51. Ronquillo, M.; Mellnyk, A.; Cárdenas-Rodríguez, N.; Martínez, E.; Comoto, D.; Carmona-Aparicio, L.; Herrera, N.; Lara, E.; Pereyra, A.; Floriano-Sánchez, E. Different gene expression profiles in subcutaneous & visceral adipose tissues from Mexican patients with obesity. *Indian J. Med. Res.* **2019**, *149*, 616–626. [CrossRef]
52. Badoud, F.; Brewer, D.; Charchoglyan, A.; Cuthbertson, D.J.; Mutch, D.M. Multi-omics Integrative Investigation of Fatty Acid Metabolism in Obese and Lean Subcutaneous Tissue. *Omi. A J. Integr. Biol.* **2017**, *21*, 371–379. [CrossRef] [PubMed]
53. Liu, D.F.; Ma, Z.Y.; Zhang, C.S.; Lin, Q.; Li, M.W.; Su, K.Z.; Dong, J. The effects of bariatric surgery on dyslipidemia and insulin resistance in overweight patients with or without type 2 diabetes: A systematic review and network meta-analysis. *Surg. Obes. Relat. Dis.* **2021**, *17*, 1655–1672. [CrossRef] [PubMed]
54. Eissing, L.; Scherer, T.; Tödter, K.; Knippschild, U.; Greve, J.W.; Buurman, W.A.; Pinnschmidt, H.O.; Rensen, S.S.; Wolf, A.M.; Bartelt, A.; et al. De novo lipogenesis in human fat and liver is linked to ChREBP-β and metabolic health. *Nat. Commun.* **2013**, *4*, 1–11. [CrossRef] [PubMed]
55. Kraus, D.; Yang, Q.; Kong, D.; Banks, A.S.; Zhang, L.; Rodgers, J.T.; Pirinen, E.; Pulinilkunnil, T.C.; Gong, F.; Wang, Y.C.; et al. Nicotinamide N-methyltransferase knockdown protects against diet-induced obesity. *Nature* **2014**, *508*, 258–262. [CrossRef] [PubMed]
56. Poletto, A.C.; David-Silva, A.; de Yamamoto, A.P.M.; Machado, U.F.; Furuya, D.T. Reduced Slc2a4/GLUT4 expression in subcutaneous adipose tissue of monosodium glutamate obese mice is recovered after atorvastatin treatment. *Diabetol. Metab. Syndr.* **2015**, *7*, 1–6. [CrossRef] [PubMed]
57. Yan, Y.; Sha, Y.; Yao, G.; Wang, S.; Kong, F.; Liu, H.; Zhang, G.; Zhang, H.; Hu, C.; Zhang, X. Roux-en-Y Gastric Bypass Versus Medical Treatment for Type 2 Diabetes Mellitus in Obese Patients: A Systematic Review and Meta-Analysis of Randomized Controlled Trials. *Medicine* **2016**, *95*, e3462. [CrossRef] [PubMed]
58. Zhan, T.; Poppelreuther, M.; Ehehalt, R.; Füllekrug, J. Overexpressed FATP1, ACSVL4/FATP4 and ACSL1 Increase the Cellular Fatty Acid Uptake of 3T3-L1 Adipocytes but Are Localized on Intracellular Membranes. *PLoS ONE* **2012**, *7*, e45087. [CrossRef]
59. Long, K.R.; Ma, J.D.; Chen, L.; Wang, P.J.; He, D.F.; Li, M.Z.; Li, X.W. Promoter and first exon methylation regulate porcine FASN gene expression. *Genet. Mol. Res.* **2015**, *14*, 8443–8450. [CrossRef]
60. Méndez-Giménez, L.; Becerril, S.; Moncada, R.; Valentí, V.; Fernández, S.; Ramírez, B.; Catalán, V.; Gómez-Ambrosi, J.; Soveral, G.; Malagón, M.M.; et al. Gastric Plication Improves Glycemia Partly by Restoring the Altered Expression of Aquaglyceroporins in Adipose Tissue and the Liver in Obese Rats. *Obes. Surg.* **2017**, *27*, 1763–1774. [CrossRef]
61. Rodríguez, A.; Gena, P.; Méndez-Giménez, L.; Rosito, A.; Valentí, V.; Rotellar, F.; Sola, I.; Moncada, R.; Silva, C.; Svelto, M.; et al. Reduced hepatic aquaporin-9 and glycerol permeability are related to insulin resistance in non-alcoholic fatty liver disease. *Int. J. Obes.* **2014**, *38*, 1213–1220. [CrossRef]
62. Medina-Gomez, G.; Gray, S.L.; Yetukuri, L.; Shimomura, K.; Virtue, S.; Campbell, M.; Curtis, R.K.; Jimenez-Linan, M.; Blount, M.; Yeo, G.S.H.; et al. PPAR gamma 2 prevents lipotoxicity by controlling adipose tissue expandability and peripheral lipid metabolism. *PLoS Genet.* **2007**, *3*, 0634–0647. [CrossRef] [PubMed]
63. Kadowaki, T.; Yamauchi, T.; Kubota, N.; Hara, K.; Ueki, K. Adiponectin and adiponectin receptors in obesity-linked insulin resistance. *Novartis Found. Symp.* **2007**, *286*, 164–203. [CrossRef] [PubMed]
64. Kawai, T.; Autieri, M.V.; Scalia, R. Adipose tissue inflammation and metabolic dysfunction in obesity. *Am. J. Physiol. Cell Physiol.* **2021**, *320*, C375–C391. [CrossRef]
65. Guebre-Egziabher, F.; Debard, C.; Drai, J.; Denis, L.; Pesenti, S.; Bienvenu, J.; Vidal, H.; Laville, M.; Fouque, D. Differential dose effect of fish oil on inflammation and adipose tissue gene expression in chronic kidney disease patients. *Nutrition* **2013**, *29*, 730–736. [CrossRef] [PubMed]
66. Moreno-Navarrete, J.M.; Latorre, J.; Lluch, A.; Ortega, F.J.; Comas, F.; Arnoriaga-Rodríguez, M.; Ricart, W.; Fernández-Real, J.M. Lysozyme is a component of the innate immune system linked to obesity associated-chronic low-grade inflammation and altered glucose tolerance. *Clin. Nutr.* **2021**, *40*, 1420–1429. [CrossRef] [PubMed]
67. Braune, J.; Weyer, U.; Hobusch, C.; Mauer, J.; Brüning, J.C.; Bechmann, I.; Gericke, M. IL-6 Regulates M2 Polarization and Local Proliferation of Adipose Tissue Macrophages in Obesity. *J. Immunol.* **2017**, *198*, 2927–2934. [CrossRef] [PubMed]
68. Challier, J.C.; Basu, S.; Bintein, T.; Minium, J.; Hotmire, K.; Catalano, P.M.; Hauguel-de Mouzon, S. Obesity in Pregnancy Stimulates Macrophage Accumulation and Inflammation in the Placenta. *Placenta* **2008**, *29*, 274–281. [CrossRef]
69. Hotamisligil, G.S.; Shargill, N.S.; Spiegelman, B.M. Adipose expression of tumor necrosis factor-α: Direct role in obesity-linked insulin resistance. *Science* **1993**, *259*, 87–91. [CrossRef]
70. Tzanavari, T.; Giannogonas, P.; Karalis, K.P. TNF-α and obesity. *Curr. Dir. Autoimmun.* **2010**, *11*, 145–156. [CrossRef]
71. Di Gregorio, G.B.; Hensley, L.; Lu, T.; Ranganathan, G.; Kern, P.A. Lipid and carbohydrate metabolism in mice with a targeted mutation in the IL-6 gene: Absence of development of age-related obesity. *Am. J. Physiol. Endocrinol. Metab.* **2004**, *287*, E182–E187. [CrossRef]

72. Latorre, J.; Lluch, A.; Ortega, F.J.; Gavaldà-Navarro, A.; Comas, F.; Morón-Ros, S.; Rodríguez, A.; Becerril, S.; Villarroya, F.; Frühbeck, G.; et al. Adipose tissue knockdown of lysozyme reduces local inflammation and improves adipogenesis in high-fat diet-fed mice. *Pharmacol. Res.* **2021**, *166*, 105486. [CrossRef] [PubMed]
73. Campbell, K.L.; Landells, C.E.; Fan, J.; Brenner, D.R. A Systematic Review of the Effect of Lifestyle Interventions on Adipose Tissue Gene Expression: Implications for Carcinogenesis. *Obesity* **2017**, *25*, S40–S51. [CrossRef] [PubMed]
74. Zechner, R.; Moser, R.; Newman, T.C.; Fried, S.K.; Breslow, J.L. Apolipoprotein E gene expression in mouse 3T3-L1 adipocytes and human adipose tissue and its regulation by differentiation and lipid content. *J. Biol. Chem.* **1991**, *266*, 10583–10588. [CrossRef]
75. Ewart, M.A.; Kennedy, S.; MacMillan, D.; Raja, A.L.N.; Watt, I.M.; Currie, S. Altered vascular smooth muscle function in the ApoE knockout mouse during the progression of atherosclerosis. *Atherosclerosis* **2014**, *234*, 154–161. [CrossRef] [PubMed]
76. Lasrich, D.; Bartelt, A.; Grewal, T.; Heeren, J. Apolipoprotein E promotes lipid accumulation and differentiation in human adipocytes. *Exp. Cell Res.* **2015**, *337*, 94–102. [CrossRef] [PubMed]
77. Kim, S.J.; Choi, Y.; Choi, Y.H.; Park, T. Obesity activates toll-like receptor-mediated proinflammatory signaling cascades in the adipose tissue of mice. *J. Nutr. Biochem.* **2012**, *23*, 113–122. [CrossRef] [PubMed]
78. Ahmad, R.; Kochumon, S.; Thomas, R.; Atizado, V.; Sindhu, S. Increased adipose tissue expression of TLR8 in obese individuals with or without type-2 diabetes: Significance in metabolic inflammation. *J. Inflamm.* **2016**, *13*, 1–15. [CrossRef]
79. Horrillo, R.; González-Périz, A.; Martínez-Clemente, M.; López-Parra, M.; Ferré, N.; Titos, E.; Morán-Salvador, E.; Deulofeu, R.; Arroyo, V.; Clària, J. 5-Lipoxygenase Activating Protein Signals Adipose Tissue Inflammation and Lipid Dysfunction in Experimental Obesity. *J. Immunol.* **2010**, *184*, 3978–3987. [CrossRef]
80. Kauts, M.L.; Pihelgas, S.; Orro, K.; Neuman, T.; Piirsoo, A. CCL5/CCR1 axis regulates multipotency of human adipose tissue derived stromal cells. *Stem Cell Res.* **2013**, *10*, 166–178. [CrossRef]
81. Sindhu, S.; Kochumon, S.; Thomas, R.; Bennakhi, A.; Al-Mulla, F.; Ahmad, R. Enhanced Adipose Expression of Interferon Regulatory Factor (IRF)-5 Associates with the Signatures of Metabolic Inflammation in Diabetic Obese Patients. *Cells* **2020**, *9*, 730. [CrossRef]
82. Ganz, T. The role of antimicrobial peptides in innate immunity. *Integr. Comp. Biol.* **2003**, *43*, 300–304. [CrossRef] [PubMed]
83. Wang, J.; Yang, L.; Liang, F.; Chen, Y.; Yang, G. Integrin alpha x stimulates cancer angiogenesis through PI3K/Akt signaling–mediated VEGFR2/VEGF-A overexpression in blood vessel endothelial cells. *J. Cell. Biochem.* **2019**, *120*, 1807–1818. [CrossRef] [PubMed]
84. Kong, X.; Liao, Y.; Zhou, L.; Zhang, Y.; Cheng, J.; Yuan, Z.; Wang, S. Hematopoietic Cell Kinase (HCK) Is Essential for NLRP3 Inflammasome Activation and Lipopolysaccharide-Induced Inflammatory Response In Vivo. *Front. Pharmacol.* **2020**, *11*, 581011. [CrossRef] [PubMed]
85. Choi, K.S.; Jun, H.S.; Kim, H.N.; Park, H.J.; Eom, Y.W.; Noh, H.L.; Kwon, H.; Kim, H.M.; Yoon, J.W. Role of Hck in the Pathogenesis of Encephalomyocarditis Virus-Induced Diabetes in Mice. *J. Virol.* **2001**, *75*, 1949–1957. [CrossRef] [PubMed]
86. Zhao, Y.; Lin, L.; Li, J.; Xiao, Z.; Chen, B.; Wan, L.; Li, M.; Wu, X.; Hin Cho, C.; Shen, J. CD4+ T cells in obesity and obesity-associated diseases. *Cell Immunol.* **2018**, *332*, 1–6. [CrossRef]
87. Pecht, T.; Gutman-Tirosh, A.; Bashan, N.; Rudich, A. Peripheral blood leucocyte subclasses as potential biomarkers of adipose tissue inflammation and obesity subphenotypes in humans. *Obes. Rev.* **2014**, *15*, 322–337. [CrossRef]
88. Peckert-Maier, K.; Royzman, D.; Langguth, P.; Marosan, A.; Strack, A.; Sadeghi Shermeh, A.; Steinkasserer, A.; Zinser, E.; Wild, A.B. Tilting the Balance: Therapeutic Prospects of CD83 as a Checkpoint Molecule Controlling Resolution of Inflammation. *Int. J. Mol. Sci.* **2022**, *23*, 732. [CrossRef]
89. Hoggard, N.; Cruickshank, M.; Moar, K.M.; Bashir, S.; Mayer, C.D. Using gene expression to predict differences in the secretome of human omental vs. subcutaneous adipose tissue. *Obesity* **2012**, *20*, 1158–1167. [CrossRef]
90. Liu, Y.; Jin, J.; Chen, Y.; Chen, C.; Chen, Z.; Xu, L. Integrative analyses of biomarkers and pathways for adipose tissue after bariatric surgery. *Adipocyte* **2020**, *9*, 384–400. [CrossRef]
91. Chen, S.; Jiang, Y.; Qi, X.; Song, P.; Tang, L.; Liu, H. Bioinformatics analysis to obtain critical genes regulated in subcutaneous adipose tissue after bariatric surgery. *Adipocyte* **2022**, *11*, 550–561. [CrossRef]

MDPI AG
Grosspeteranlage 5
4052 Basel
Switzerland
Tel.: +41 61 683 77 34

Nutrients Editorial Office
E-mail: nutrients@mdpi.com
www.mdpi.com/journal/nutrients

www.ingramcontent.com/pod-product-compliance
Lightning Source LLC
LaVergne TN
LVHW070445061126
851858LV00011B/167